Modern Applications of 3D/4D Ultrasound Imaging in Radiotherapy

IPEM–IOP Series in Physics and Engineering in Medicine and Biology

About the Series

Series in Physics and Engineering in Medicine and Biology will allow IPEM to enhance its mission to 'advance physics and engineering applied to medicine and biology for the public good.'

Focusing on key areas including, but not limited to:

- clinical engineering
- diagnostic radiology
- informatics and computing
- magnetic resonance imaging
- nuclear medicine
- physiological measurement
- radiation protection
- radiotherapy
- rehabilitation engineering
- ultrasound and non-ionising radiation.

A number of IPEM–IOP titles are published as part of the EUTEMPE Network Series for Medical Physics Experts.

Modern Applications of 3D/4D Ultrasound Imaging in Radiotherapy

Edited by
Emma Harris
The Joint Department of Physics, Institute of Cancer Research and The Royal Marsden NHS Foundation Trust, London, UK

Davide Fontanarosa
School of Clinical Sciences, Queensland University of Technology, Gardens Point Campus, 2 George St, Brisbane, QLD 4000, Australia
Institute of Health & Biomedical Innovation, Queensland University of Technology, Brisbane, QLD 4000, Australia

Saskia Camps
External Beam Ablation Medical Devices (EBAMed) SA, Geneva, Switzerland

Frank Verhaegen
Department of Radiation Oncology (MAASTRO), GROW School for Oncology and Developmental Biology, Maastricht, Netherlands

IOP Publishing, Bristol, UK

Multimedia content is available for this book from http://iopscience.iop.org/book/978-0-7503-2552-3.

ISBN 978-0-7503-2552-3 (ebook)
ISBN 978-0-7503-2550-9 (print)
ISBN 978-0-7503-2553-0 (myPrint)
ISBN 978-0-7503-2551-6 (mobi)

DOI 10.1088/978-0-7503-2552-3

Version: 20210101

IOP ebooks

British Library Cataloguing-in-Publication Data: A catalogue record for this book is available from the British Library.

Published by IOP Publishing, wholly owned by The Institute of Physics, London

IOP Publishing, Temple Circus, Temple Way, Bristol, BS1 6HG, UK

US Office: IOP Publishing, Inc., 190 North Independence Mall West, Suite 601, Philadelphia, PA 19106, USA

This book is dedicated to all those who have contributed to the field of ultrasound imaging applied to radiation therapy.

Contents

Preface

Ultrasound imaging in medicine has been in use for more than 50 years and it is still today one of the most commonly employed medical imaging technologies. Compared to other forms of imaging such as x-ray computed tomography or magnetic resonance imaging, it is much cheaper and more portable. In 21st century radiotherapy image-guided irradiation has played a major role. While most image guidance of radiotherapy has been developed based on x-ray cone beam computed tomography, ultrasound imaging has also been investigated. Today the latter is not a widely used technology, but this is likely to change soon due to rise of automation and artificial intelligence for detecting features in images. A distinct advantage of ultrasound imaging is the real-time aspect of images which is ideal for detecting misdirection of radiation beams with respect to moving organs. As more and more imaging is performed as part of a multi-fraction irradiation regime, ultrasound imaging may offer other advantages such as zero radiation dose (compared to x-rays), the non-interference with treatment beams (compared to strong magnetic fields) and the applicability to the majority of treatment platforms.

The idea for this book about 3D/4D ultrasound imaging specifically for radiotherapy, where quantitative imaging is important for irradiation guidance and treatment adaptation, arose from the need for students and practitioners in image guided radiotherapy to understand better the past and future developments of this field. Robotics, artificial intelligence, miniaturisation, novel imaging sensors etc, are all moving fast and will lead to a whole new generation of ultrasound technology. We brought together many experts in the field to work on this book, and from the outset, our aim was to provide ample animated and interactive material to accompany the text. The book describes existing and developing ultrasound technology, imaging in absolute spatial coordinates registered with treatment equipment, the role of ultrasound imaging in treatment planning, its use for quantifying and mitigating organ motion, and the very novel evolution of automation and robotics. We also dedicated a chapter to ionoacoustics, the exotic and exciting application where radiation beams lead to small acoustic shock waves which can be exploited to verify radiation therapy.

We hope the book will lead to a better appreciation of the potential role of ultrasound imaging in radiotherapy, the technique really has a lot to offer and should be considered against other technologies, which all have their advantages and disadvantages. With the rising use of ion beams for radiotherapy, where image guidance still mostly has to be developed, perhaps ultrasound imaging may find a new application. We hope this book may contribute to this.

Emma Harris

Davide Fontanarosa

Sakia Camps

Frank Verhaegen

Editor biographies

Emma Harris

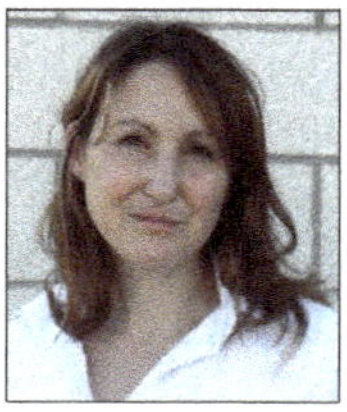

Dr Emma Harris is a Reader of Imaging and Radiation Physics at the Institute of Cancer Research in London, UK. Her research focuses on the application of radiation physics, ultrasound physics engineering and image processing to improve radiotherapy. She has spent more than a decade leading experimental studies of image guided radiotherapy and has devised and conducted a number of clinical studies investigating the use of ultrasound for image guidance of radiotherapy of cervical cancer, prostate cancer and paediatric cancers.

Davide Fontanarosa

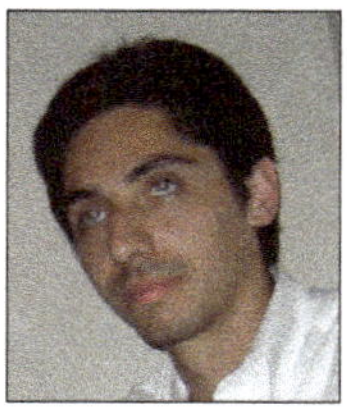

Dr Davide Fontanarosa is a physicist with a solid background in ultrasound imaging and medical physics. He worked in one of the top institutions for radiation therapy (MAASTRO Clinic, in the Netherlands) and in one of the largest industrial research laboratories in the world, Philips Research, as Senior Scientist. Then he moved to Queensland University of Technology (Brisbane, Australia) where he is currently working as Associate Professor and doing research in several fields related to advanced quantitative ultrasound imaging techniques and radiation therapy.

Saskia Camps

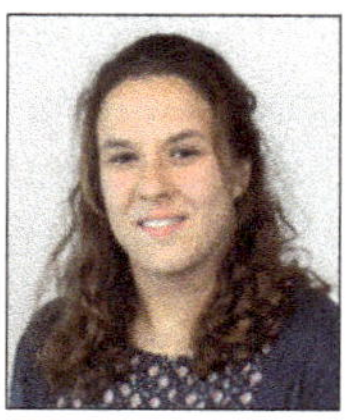

Dr Saskia Camps is a Biomedical R&D engineer at the Swiss startup EBAMed. EBAMed develops and commercialises innovative solutions which allow for non-invasive treatment of cardiac arrhythmias using proton beams. Before joining EBAMed, Saskia earned her PhD at the Eindhoven University of Technology in a collaboration with the Maastro Clinic (Maastricht, the Netherlands) and Philips Research (Eindhoven, the Netherlands). The focus of her PhD work was on automation of ultrasound image acquisition and interpretation for dose guidance in prostate cancer radiotherapy workflows.

Frank Verhaegen

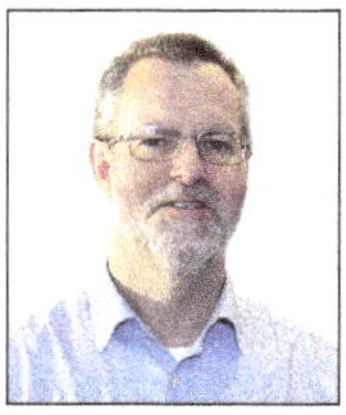

Frank Verhaegen is a professor at the University of Maastricht (Netherlands) and head of the physics research division of Maastro Clinic, a radiotherapy facility with photon, electron and proton beams. Before that, he was an associate professor at McGill University (Montreal, Canada). He is specialised in image guidance and dose calculations for radiotherapy. Both at Maastricht and Montreal he performed several research projects with medical companies developing novel 3D/4D ultrasound imaging devices for radiotherapy. He is the co-author of several studies and review papers in this field.

List of contributors

Maria Antico
School of Mechanical, Medical & Process Engineering, Science and Engineering Faculty, Queensland University of Technology, Brisbane, QLD 4000, Australia
Institute of Health & Biomedical Innovation, Queensland University of Technology, Brisbane, QLD

Walter Assmann
Ludwig-Maximilians-Universität München, Faculty of Physics, Department of Medical Physics, Munich, Germany

Saskia Camps
External Beam Ablation Medical Devices (EBAMed) SA, Geneva, Switzerland

Christopher Edwards
School of Clinical Sciences, Queensland University of Technology, Gardens Point campus, 2 George St, Brisbane, QLD 4000, Australia
Institute of Health & Biomedical Innovation, Queensland University of Technology, Brisbane, QLD
Mater Research Institute, University of Queensland, Level 3, Aubigny Place, Raymond Terrace, South Brisbane, QLD, 4101, Australia

Floris Ernst
Institute for Robotics and Cognitive Systems, University of Lübeck, Lübeck, Germany

Davide Fontanarosa
School of Clinical Sciences, Queensland University of Technology, Gardens Point campus, 2 George St, Brisbane, QLD 4000, Australia
Institute of Health & Biomedical Innovation, Queensland University of Technology, Brisbane, QLD

Alexander Grimwood
Wellcome/EPSRC Centre for Surgical and Interventional Sciences,
Department of Medical Physics and Biomedical Engineering, University College London, London, UK

Emma Harris
The Joint Department of Physics, Institute of Cancer Research and The Royal Marsden NHS Foundation Trust, London, UK

Svenja Ipsen
Institute for Robotics and Cognitive Systems, University of Lübeck, Lübeck, Germany

Sarah Mason
MRC Unit for Lifelong Health and Ageing at UCL, Department of Population Science & Experimental Medicine, UCL Institute of Cardiovascular Science, University College London, London, UK

Katia Parodi
Ludwig-Maximilians-Universität München, Faculty of Physics, Department of Medical Physics, Munich, Germany

Alexander Schlaefer
Institute of Medical Technology and Intelligent Systems, Hamburg University of Technology, Hamburg, Germany

Frank Verhaegen
Department of Radiation Oncology (MAASTRO), GROW School for Oncology and Developmental Biology, Maastricht, Netherlands

Glossary

2D	two-dimensional
3D	three-dimensional
4D	four-dimensional
AAPM	American Association of Physicists in Medicine
ABC	active breathing control
ADC	analogue-to-digital convertor
AGS	assisted gyne segmentation
AI	artificial intelligence
AP	anterior posterior
APBI	accelerated partial breast irradiation
ART	adaptive radiotherapy
BAT	B-mode acquisition and targeting
CBCT	cone beam computed tomography
CEUS	contrast enhanced ultrasound
CMUT	capacitive micromachined ultrasound transducer
CNN	convolutional neural network
CNR	contrast-to-noise ratio
CT	computed tomography
CTV	clinical tumour volume
DDC	discrete dynamic contouring
DGRT	dose-guided radiotherapy
DIR	deformable image registration
DOF	degrees of freedom
DP	defined phantom
DSC	Dice similarity coefficient
EM	electromagnetic
EPI	electronic portal imaging
EBRT	external beam radiotherapy
EA	extended aperture
FM	fiducial marker
FOV	field of view
GPS	global positioning system
GTV	gross tumour volume
FPS	frames per second
HE	hand-eye
IGRT	image-guided radiation therapy
IMRT	intensity modulated radiotherapy
IR	infrared
KIM	kilovoltage intrafraction monitoring
kV	kilovolt
LED	light emitting diode
linac	linear accelerator
LR	left right or lateral resolution
MLC	multi-leaf collimator
MPR	multi-planar reformatting
MR	magnetic resonance
MRI	magnetic resonance imaging

MRS	magnetic resonance spectroscopy
NCC	normalised cross correlation
MV	megavolt
OAR	organ at risk
PET	positron emission tomography
POTD	plan of the day
PRV	positioning reference volume
PTV	planning target volume
PVDF	polyvinylidine difluoride
PZT	lead zirconate titanate
QA	quality assurance
RC	respiratory correlated
RF	radio-frequency or random forest
RMS	root mean square
RMSE	root mean square error
ROI	region of interest
RT	radiotherapy
RTT	radiation therapy technologist
SBRT	stereotactic body radiation therapy
SD	standard deviation
SI	superior inferior
SIM	simulation
SOS	speed of sound
SNR	signal-to-noise ratio
SSD	sum of squared distances
SVD	support vector machine
TAUS	transabdominal ultrasound
TGC	time gain compensation
THI	tissue harmonic imaging
TOF	time of flight
TPS	treatment planning system
TPUS	transperineal ultrasound
TRUS	transrectal ultrasound
US	ultrasound
USgRT	ultrasound-guided radiotherapy
VGA	variable gain amplifier
VMAT	volumetric modulated arc therapy

IOP Publishing

Chapter 1

Introduction

Davide Fontanarosa and Emma Harris

1.1 Image guided and adaptive radiotherapy

Cancer is one of the leading causes of death worldwide, with an estimated 9.6 million deaths in 2018 [1]. Currently, there are three main treatment options available for cancer: surgery, drug-based therapy, and radiation therapy. Radiation therapy uses ionising radiation to deliver a treatment dose to the tumour while sparing, as much as possible, the surrounding normal tissue. Different types of cancer require different treatments, which can involve the use of one or more of these modalities combined in order to maximise treatment effectiveness.

There are three different types of radiation therapy: external beam radiotherapy (EBRT), brachytherapy and internal radionuclide therapy. This book will focus on EBRT, which uses high energy beams of photons, electrons or hadrons delivered by an accelerator. The radiotherapy workflow is represented in figure 1.1, it comprises a simulation stage where a digital model of the patient is generated, a planning stage in which treatment is planned, a delivery stage and an assessment stage.

The simulation stage begins one or two weeks prior to treatment commencement, when a computed tomography (CT) scan (although recently magnetic resonance imaging (MRI) is also considered [2]) of the patient is acquired. To create a useful model of the patient for planning the relevant regions of interest (ROI), the target tissues and neighbouring organs at risk (OAR) are delineated. The target tissues may be the tumour only, an entire organ containing a tumour or an extended volume of tissue encompassing involved (cancerous) lymph nodes. Once these structures have been contoured they are expanded with a margin to take all the possible sources of uncertainty into account, namely: setup errors, organ motion, organ volume change and organ shape change.

At the planning stage, these structures are used to prescribe the treatment dose to the target. The dose is selected from within the therapeutic window, in order to

doi:10.1088/978-0-7503-2552-3ch1

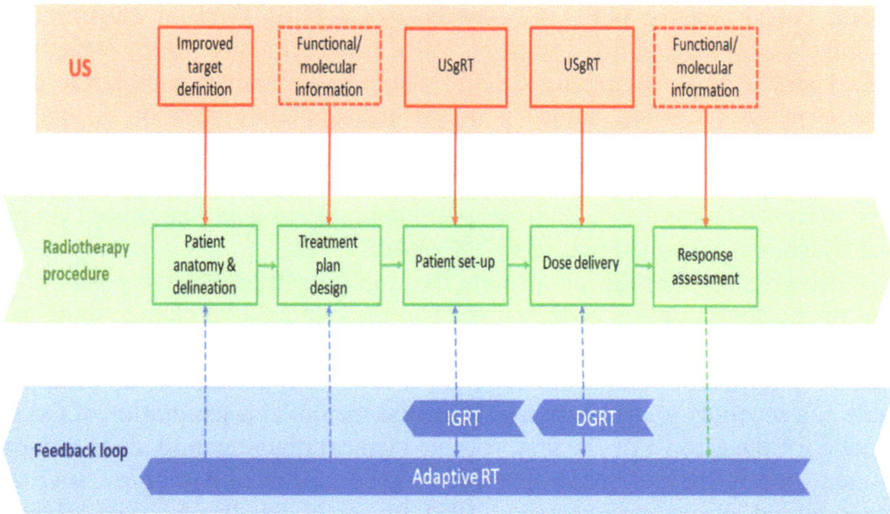

Figure 1.1. Typical radiotherapy workflow (middle) with the input that can be provided by ultrasound (US) (top) and the possible adpative radiotherapy (ART) feedback loops (bottom). The arrows indicate the temporal direction. The dashed components in the top row are the ones not yet clinically available in ultrasound-guided radiotherapy. Adapted from [15]. Copyright IOP Publishing. Reproduced with permission. All rights reserved.

maximise the biological treatment efficacy on the tumour while at the same time minimising toxicity to OAR. To deliver EBRT, the gantry, which is used to deliver the radiation, rotates around the patient while the radiation beam is shaped by collimators and/or beam modifiers. A treatment planning system (TPS) is used to calculate all the accelerator related settings (beam angles, collimator apertures, irradiation times, etc) necessary to deliver the optimal dose distribution to the patient resulting in a patient specific treatment plan. Traditional forward planning employs several beams which are geometrically shaped around the target and delivered from different angles. Contemporary intensity modulated radiotherapy (IMRT) plans are automatically inversely optimised using the prescribed treatment dose, OAR dose constraints and the delineated ROIs. IMRT is also delivered from several different beam angles, however, at each angle a number of multi-leaf collimator shaped fields or segments are superimposed to make up a beam. If these segments are delivered from a continuous distribution of angles, instead of discretised, the treatment type is called arc therapy or rotational therapy.

Conventionally, the treatment is usually delivered to the patient in multiple treatment fractions, so it is essential that the conditions in which the plan was prepared are accurately reproduced before each fraction. Accurate patient setup before treatment reduces (interfraction) positioning errors and allows minimisation of margins around the structures and helps to keep toxicity in the OARs low. For this purpose, imaging systems are used to verify the position of the patient prior to treatment. If the patient is not correctly positioned their position can be adjusted accordingly. Imaging modalities that are the most clinically established are film [3], electronic portal imaging (EPI) [4], cone beam CT (CBCT) [5] or 2D stereoscopic kilovoltage x-ray imaging [6]. Typically, at the treatment stage, bony structures are identified and used as surrogates for the whole tissue distribution in the patient. If these structures are not aligned with the corresponding position at simulation stage, a correction in the patient's setup is applied. This strategy is not very effective when relative changes between the soft tissues (including the target and the OARs) and the bony structures occur. So other positioning technologies have been proposed, among which are implanted markers [7, 8] or MRI [9].

It is also possible that during a single fraction (intrafraction) the position of the patient or the configuration of their tissues in the treated area change significantly. When intrafraction motion occurs, firstly it is essential to have a way to detect the change with respect to the treatment plan preparation conditions as promptly as possible and secondly to take action to minimise the possible irradiation of OARs by correcting for the error. For the first, specific medical imaging modalities to monitor the patient during the treatment have been introduced in radiotherapy, such as for example global positioning system (GPS) for body localisation [8], kilovoltage intrafraction monitoring (KIM) [10] or optical surface guidance [11]. The second is typically achieved using gating or tracking of the beam [12].

Radiotherapy that includes the use of the technologies described above to measure (and correct for) inter- and intrafraction motion is referred to as image-guided radiotherapy (IGRT)[13]. More recently, a new and rapidly developing branch of radiotherapy called adaptive radiotherapy (ART) [14] has been introduced. ART focuses on strategies to modify the radiation delivery plan to match the changed conditions of the patient. This process can happen at different timescales: offline, if the plan is adapted between treatment fractions; online if it is adapted immediately prior to a treatment fraction; in real time if it is adapted during treatment delivery. Different levels of complexity have been proposed for the different ART strategies. The simplest approach considers several possible anatomical changes at the planning stage. Based on the measured anatomical change at treatment, the most appropriate plan which encompasses the change is delivered. More advanced strategies apply deformable registration algorithms to transfer contours and dose distributions between datasets, and automatic replanning is performed. A further advancement to in-room dose recalculation based on the imaged changed conditions of the patient to adapt the plan in real time is also under investigation.

In addition to the imaging modalities described above, ultrasound imaging (US) is also used in the context of IGRT and is gathering growing interest for ART: its two-dimensional (2D), three-dimensional (3D) and four-dimensional (4D) anatomical images allow interfraction motion and intrafraction motion estimation of soft tissues (i.e., ultrasound-guided radiotherapy (USgRT)). Furthermore, its functional and molecular imaging capability opens up the possibility of ultrasound based prognostic and predictive biomarkers. The next section provides more detail on why ultrasound can be considered an attractive imaging modality for radiotherapy guidance.

1.2 Rationale for using ultrasound guidance

Although ultrasound is mainly known as a diagnostic tool, for example, for foetal, heart or liver scanning, it has become increasingly popular for quantitative applications, especially for localisation and tracking of interventional structures or tools [15, 16]. Ultrasound acquisition is performed using a probe composed of transducers which create compressional ultrasound waves that propagate within the scanned media. Whenever an interface between different tissues or media is traversed by the wave, part of the wave energy is reflected back to the probe. From the time of flight and the speed of sound the position of the interface can be calculated. All the echo amplitudes are then converted to brightness values and plotted against the calculated depth, resulting in the traditional B-mode ultrasound image most people are familiar with. Until now only time of flight and amplitude have been used, but it should be noted that more data could potentially be extracted, such as that from spectral analysis of the ultrasound signal.

Ultrasound is unique in that images are provided in real time and it is a non-ionising modality. Moreover, most ultrasound systems are portable, often very compact (for example the Butterfly iQ (Butterfly Network Inc., Guildford, CT, USA), an ultrasound probe which can be used with a smartphone), and cost-effective, if compared to any other medical imaging modality. In terms of image quality ultrasound, among the other advantages, can offer virtually unlimited resolution capabilities, as they scale with frequency; and excellent soft tissue contrast, allowing visualisation of structures that for example cannot be identified on CT scans. The image formation process described above can easily be extended to 3D, and with continuous scanning over time, also 4D monitoring of tissues is achievable. This makes ultrasound the only volumetric real time imaging modality available for medical applications, especially in complex environments like a radiotherapy room or an operating theatre.

In the radiotherapy workflow, currently ultrasound is used to help set up the patient at treatment and to monitor target position during irradiation (figure 1.1). If the positions of the target tissues change with respect to the plan, an ultrasound image can be used to determine their new location and the patient setup can be corrected. It is also feasible that the information about the anatomy obtained by ultrasound can be used to recalculate the dose in the case of ART. Beyond this, other advanced ultrasound imaging modalities, such as elastography and contrast enhanced ultrasound (CEUS), and ultrasound tissue characterisation have the potential to inform on the status of target tissues prior to treatment and post-treatment in order to predict and measure the response of tumours to radiotherapy [17, 18].

As mentioned before, ultrasound is primarily used as a qualitative diagnostic tool (except for specific applications such as foetal measurements in obstetrics [19]), which relies on the operator skills and expertise. As a consequence, it has been often regarded as a user dependent modality, showing important inter-operator variability [20, 21]. Not only is this an obvious limitation on the reproducibility of ultrasound, it is also a practical problem for radiotherapy departments which usually do not have (a sufficient number of) operators with the necessary skills in their staff to cover the normal routine practice. Other specific problems include: possible tissue displacements caused by the ultrasound probe [22]; general image quality, especially when deep structures need to be visualised or when air and bone shield part of the field of view; possible interference with the treatment beam [23]; reliable acoustic coupling between the probe and the patient; speed of sound aberration [24] etc. Efforts have been made in recent years to improve these limitations introducing strict imaging protocols, enhanced image formation algorithms, speed of sound aberration correction algorithms [25], more advanced transducer technologies [26], robotic probe holders [27–29], viscous coupling gels and investigating automatic interpretation of images [30] and automatic probe positioning [31]. These innovations are discussed within this book. Ultrasound is well suited for ART applications, especially those that require real-time monitoring of structures. But it cannot provide physical density information, which is essential to calculate dose and hence to replan the treatment. Solutions have been proposed for this issue too, which involved deformable registration of the ultrasound with the simulation CT scan and using the density information from the latter [32] (see chapter 4).

Ultrasound has been used clinically in radiotherapy mainly for two cancer sites of interest: prostate [33] and breast [34]. But applications have been explored in several other cancer sites, including upper abdomen [35], pancreas [36], gallbladder [37], liver [38, 39], cervix [40], head and neck lymph nodes [41] and bladder [39].

It is noteworthy that while in traditional photon therapy the treatment is delivered to the patient over several fractions, other approaches using fewer fractions (hypofractionation) or different types of radiation (for example, protons) are becoming increasingly more widespread, because they are more convenient for the patient [42] or have the potential for improved therapeutic outcomes [43]. These treatments, though, require higher standards of accuracy in patient setup and target position monitoring than traditional strategies, which require soft tissue visualisation making ultrasound an excellent candidate for guidance. In particular, for proton therapies (and more in general hadron therapies) which are most likely to benefit paediatric patients, ultrasound does not impart concomitant radiation, it is expected that with the growth of proton therapy centres in the world there will be new and increased interest in ultrasound based guidance methods.

1.3 A brief history of ultrasound in radiotherapy

Publications on the use of ultrasound in radiotherapy date back to the early 1970s. In 1970, Smith and Holm presented the idea that ultrasound can be used to obtain 'true anatomical cross-sections of a tumour, surrounding normal tissues, and the external body contour' for the purpose of planning radiotherapy [44, 45]. Cohen and Hass reported on the use of ultrasound to aid the placement of treatment portals for abdominal tumours and may have been the first to propose that ultrasound can be used as a tool to monitor response to treatment [44, 45]. In 1974, Sanders proposed the use of ultrasound to localise the kidney, both at the time of planning but also as a localisation or image-guidance technique for use during radiotherapy delivery [46].

In general, the technology necessary for the use of ultrasound in the radiotherapy treatment room, which typically combines an ultrasound system with a means of locating the probe, was developed during the 1990s. Patents filed on this novel technology include the use of transrectal ultrasound for localisation of the prostate prior to surgery and radiotherapy [47], the use of ultrasound for localisation of individual lesions [48] or organs [49], apparatus to monitor the position of an ultrasound probe in treatment reference coordinates [50] and technology for correlating ultrasonic imaging data with radiological images [51].

During this time, early ultrasound guidance methods and apparatus were reported in the literature and were focussed on radiotherapy for prostate cancer. Troccaz *et al* [52] presented an ultrasound-based image-guided radiotherapy system, which used a transabdominal 2D ultrasound probe and infrared (IR) emitting light emitting diodes (LEDs) to localise the probe and software to automatically register CT and ultrasound images using user defined point-based registration of the prostate. This system was able to acquire volumetric images by manual manipulation of the probe (see section 2.3). Transrectal ultrasound combined with orthogonal radiographs at simulation to localise the prostate, rectum and bladder was investigated, and found to be useful for the positioning of blocks to shield the rectum [53]. This group also presented software for combining portal x-ray images with ultrasound. Later, algorithms for the registration of CT and ultrasound data for prostate radiotherapy were also developed [54]. During this time, the only other tumour site investigated was breast where the use of ultrasound to measure the depth of the surgical cavity for selection of boost electron energies was reported [55, 56]. The first commercial systems became available for use in radiotherapy clinics in the late 1990s to the early 2000s and are introduced in more detail in chapter 5.

1.4 Summary of the book structure

This book aims to comprehensively describe ultrasound guidance techniques and technologies in radiotherapy, with special attention on future directions, innovative applications and potential cross pollination from other clinical and research fields.

After this chapter, introducing the topic and giving a brief overview of the rationale for ultrasound guidance in radiotherapy and of its history, chapter 2 provides an overview of the physics of ultrasound imaging, and the technology currently used both clinically and in research is described. The first challenge encountered when introducing ultrasound into radiotherapy is described in chapter 3: localising the probe in the simulation suite and in the treatment room to enable comparison of the positions of anatomical structures at the two stages. The solutions available are introduced together with a detailed description and analysis of the sources of error and uncertainty. After the probe has been localised, the next steps are to evaluate if the image acquired is of sufficient quality and segment all the relevant structures of interest. In an ideal scenario, the whole procedure should be automatic, so in chapter 4 the tools currently available to perform these tasks automatically are reviewed. In chapter 5 the role of ultrasound in the first stage of the radiotherapy workflow, planning, is introduced: it can be used to identify the anatomical structures important for radiotherapy planning, in particular the treatment target. Practical challenges are highlighted, for example, how to acquire the simulation CT scan with the ultrasound probe in place avoiding CT imaging artefacts that would compromise the planning process. The treatment phase is discussed in chapter 6 and chapter 7. The former investigates USgRT for interfraction motion estimation. In this chapter the two main types of USgRT are introduced (inter- and intramodality), and the clinical applications reported in the literature for each of the anatomical sites are reviewed together with the potential errors in patient setup. In chapter 7 the use of ultrasound for intrafraction monitoring is described, including the different approaches, with corresponding requirements, and challenges. The information collected for the purpose of inter- and intrafraction motion estimation can then be used to adapt the treatment, when necessary: this is the topic of chapter 8, where adaptive radiotherapy applications using ultrasound are reviewed. The last four chapters focus on innovations and advanced technologies. In particular, chapter 9 highlights the autonomous and robotic technologies and their integration into the workflow described in the previous chapters, with potential benefits, challenges and risks. Chapter 10 explores the most recent and fascinating tools from the artificial intelligence (AI) world and their use in USgRT. Finally, chapter 11 introduces verification of the spatial distribution of proton or ion therapy dose delivery using ionacoustics, the detection of ultrasonic emissions generated by the deposition of the kinetic energy of particles (protons or ions). The last chapter, chapter 12, concludes with a vision on what the future directions will be, and explores the most recent and novel technologies not yet discussed in the other chapters.

References

[1] WHO 2018 www.who.int/cancer/PRGlobocanFinal.pdf

[2] Jonsson J H, Karlsson M G, Karlsson M and Nyholm T 2010 Treatment planning using MRI data: an analysis of the dose calculation accuracy for different treatment regions *Radiat. Oncol.* **5** 62

[3] Schewe J E, Balter J M, Lam K L and ten Haken R K 1996 Measurement of patient setup errors using port films and a computer-aided graphical alignment tool *Med. Dosim.* **21** 97–104

[4] Bel A, Vos P H, Rodrigus P T, Creutzberg C L, Visser A G and Stroom J C *et al* 1996 High-precision prostate cancer irradiation by clinical application of an offline patient setup verification procedure, using portal imaging *Int. J. Radiat. Oncol. Biol. Phys.* **35** 321–32

[5] Srinivasan K, Mohammadi M and Shepherd J 2014 Applications of linac-mounted kilo-voltage cone-beam computed tomography in modern radiation therapy: a review *Pol. J. Radiol.* **79** 181–93

[6] Verellen D, Soete G, Linthout N, Van Acker S, De Roover P and Vinh-Hung V *et al* 2003 Quality assurance of a system for improved target localization and patient set-up that combines real-time infrared tracking and stereoscopic x-ray imaging *Radiother. Oncol.* **67** 129–41

[7] O'Neill A G M, Jain S, Hounsell A R and O'Sullivan J M 2016 Fiducial marker guided prostate radiotherapy: a review *Br. J. Radiol.* **89** 20160296

[8] Willoughby T R, Kupelian P A, Pouliot J, Shinohara K, Aubin M and Roach M *et al* 2006 Target localization and real-time tracking using the Calypso 4D localization system in patients with localized prostate cancer *Int. J. Radiat. Oncol. Biol. Phys.* **65** 528–34
[9] Hall W A, Paulson E S, van der Heide U A, Fuller C D, Raaymakers B W and Lagendijk J J W *et al* 2019 The transformation of radiation oncology using real-time magnetic resonance guidance: a review *Eur. J. Cancer* **122** 42–52
[10] Ng J A, Booth J T, Poulsen P R, Fledelius W, Worm E S and Eade T *et al* 2012 Kilovoltage intrafraction monitoring for prostate intensity modulated arc therapy: first clinical results *Int. J. Radiat. Oncol. Biol. Phys.* **84** e655–61
[11] Covington E L, Fiveash J B, Wu X, Brezovich I, Willey C D and Riley K *et al* 2019 Optical surface guidance for submillimeter monitoring of patient position during frameless stereotactic radiotherapy *J. Appl. Clin. Med. Phys.* **20** 91–8
[12] Bertholet J, Knopf A, Eiben B, McClelland J, Grimwood A and Harris E *et al* 2019 Real-time intrafraction motion monitoring in external beam radiotherapy *Phys. Med. Biol.* **64** 15TR01
[13] Bourland J D (ed) 2012 *Image-Guided Radiation Therapy* (Boca Raton, FL: CRC Press) https://www.crcpress.com/Image-Guided-Radiation-Therapy/Bourland/p/book/9781439802731
[14] Li X A (ed) *Adaptive Radiation Therapy* (Boca Raton, FL: CRC Press) https://www.crcpress.com/Adaptive-Radiation-Therapy/Li/p/book/9781439816349
[15] Fontanarosa D, van der Meer S, Bamber J, Harris E, O'Shea T and Verhaegen F 2015 Review of ultrasound image guidance in external beam radiotherapy: I. Treatment planning and inter-fraction motion management *Phys. Med. Biol.* **60** R77–114
[16] Antico M, Sasazawa F, Wu L, Jaiprakash A, Roberts J and Crawford R *et al* 2019 Ultrasound guidance in minimally invasive robotic procedures *Med. Image Anal.* **54** 149–67
[17] Vlad R M, Brand S, Giles A, Kolios M C and Czarnota G J 2009 Quantitative ultrasound characterization of responses to radiotherapy in cancer mouse models *Clin. Cancer Res.* **15** 2067–75
[18] Sadeghi-Naini A, Falou O, Tadayyon H, Al-Mahrouki A, Tran W and Papanicolau N *et al* 2013 Conventional frequency ultrasonic biomarkers of cancer treatment response *in vivo* *Transl. Oncol.* **6** 234–43
[19] Issel E P, Prenzlau P, Bayer H, Lüder R, Schulte R and Wohlfahrth G *et al* 1975 The measurement of fetal growth during pregnancy by ultra-sound (B-scan) *J. Perinat. Med.* **3** 269–75
[20] Enke C, Ayyangar K, Saw C B, Zhen W, Thompson R B and Raman N V 2002 Inter-observer variation in prostate localization utilizing BAT *Int. J. Radiat. Oncol. Biol. Phys.* **54** 269
[21] Langen K M, Pouliot J, Anezinos C, Aubin M, Gottschalk A R and Hsu I C *et al* 2003 Evaluation of ultrasound-based prostate localization for image-guided radiotherapy *Int. J. Radiat. Oncol. Biol. Phys.* **57** 635–44
[22] Artignan X, Smitsmans M H P, Lebesque J V, Jaffray D A, van Her M and Bartelink H 2004 Online ultrasound image guidance for radiotherapy of prostate cancer: impact of image acquisition on prostate displacement *Int. J. Radiat. Oncol. Biol. Phys.* **59** 595–601
[23] Martyn M, O'Shea T P, Harris E, Bamber J, Gilroy S and Foley M J 2017 A Monte Carlo study of the effect of an ultrasound transducer on surface dose during intrafraction motion imaging for external beam radiation therapy *Med. Phys.* **44** 5020–33
[24] Fontanarosa D, van der Meer S, Bloemen-van Gurp E, Stroian G and Verhaegen F 2012 Magnitude of speed of sound aberration corrections for ultrasound image guided radiotherapy for prostate and other anatomical sites *Med. Phys.* **39** 5286–92

[25] Fontanarosa D, van der Meer S, Harris E and Verhaegen F A 2011 CT based correction method for speed of sound aberration for ultrasound based image guided radiotherapy *Med. Phys.* **38** 2665–73
[26] Schlosser J and Hristov D 2016 Radiolucent 4D ultrasound imaging: system design and application to radiotherapy guidance *IEEE Trans. Med. Imag.* **35** 2292–300
[27] Şen H T, Lediju Bell M A, Zhang Y, Ding K, Wong J and Iordachita I *et al* 2015 System integration and preliminary in-vivo experiments of a robot for ultrasound guidance and monitoring during radiotherapy *Proc. Int. Conf. Adv. Robot.* **2015** 53–9
[28] Schlosser J, Gong R H, Bruder R, Schweikard A, Jang S and Henrie J *et al* 2016 Robotic intrafractional US guidance for liver SABR: system design, beam avoidance, and clinical imaging *Med. Phys.* **43** 5951
[29] Gerlach S, Kuhlemann I, Jauer P, Bruder R, Ernst F and Fürweger C *et al* 2017 Robotic ultrasound-guided SBRT of the prostate: feasibility with respect to plan quality *Int. J. Comput. Assist. Radiol. Surg.* **12** 149–59
[30] Camps S M, Houben T, Carneiro G, Edwards C, Antico M and Dunnhofer M *et al* 2020 Automatic quality assessment of transperineal ultrasound images of the male pelvic region, using deep learning *Ultrasound Med. Biol.* **46** 445–54
[31] Camps S M, Verhaegen F, Vanneste B G L, de With P H N and Fontanarosa D 2018 Automated patient-specific transperineal ultrasound probe setups for prostate cancer patients undergoing radiotherapy *Med. Phys.* **45** 3185–95
[32] van der Meer S, Camps S M, van Elmpt W J C, Podesta M, Sanches P G and Vanneste B G L *et al* 2016 Simulation of pseudo-CT images based on deformable image registration of ultrasound images: a proof of concept for transabdominal ultrasound imaging of the prostate during radiotherapy *Med. Phys.* **43** 1913
[33] Camps S M, Fontanarosa D, de With P H N, Verhaegen F and Vanneste B G L 2018 The use of ultrasound imaging in the external beam radiotherapy workflow of prostate cancer patients *Biomed. Res. Int.* **2018** 7569590
[34] Fraser D J, Wong P, Sultanem K and Verhaegen F 2010 Dosimetric evolution of the breast electron boost target using 3D ultrasound imaging *Radiother. Oncol.* **96** 185–91
[35] Fuss M, Salter B J, Cavanaugh S X, Fuss C, Sadeghi A and Fuller C D *et al* 2004 Daily ultrasound-based image-guided targeting for radiotherapy of upper abdominal malignancies *Int. J. Radiat. Oncol. Biol. Phys.* **59** 1245–56
[36] Fuss M, Wong A, Fuller C D, Salter B J, Fuss C and Thomas C R 2007 Image-guided intensity-modulated radiotherapy for pancreatic carcinoma *Gastrointest. Cancer Res.* **1** 2–11
[37] Fuller C D, Thomas C R, Wong A, Cavanaugh S X, Salter B J and Herman T S *et al* 2006 Image-guided intensity-modulated radiation therapy for gallbladder carcinoma *Radiother. Oncol.* **81** 65–72
[38] Bloemen-van Gurp E, van der Meer S, Hendry J, Buijsen J, Visser P and Fontanarosa D *et al* 2013 Active breathing control in combination with ultrasound imaging: a feasibility study of image guidance in stereotactic body radiation therapy of liver lesions *Int. J. Radiat. Oncol. Biol. Phys.* **85** 1096–102
[39] McBain C A, Green M M, Stratford J, Davies J, McCarthy C and Taylor B *et al* 2009 Ultrasound imaging to assess inter- and intra-fraction motion during bladder radiotherapy and its potential as a verification tool *Clin. Oncol. (R Coll. Radiol.)* **21** 385–93

[40] Mason S A, O'Shea T P, White I M, Lalondrelle S, Downey K and Baker M *et al* 2017 Towards ultrasound-guided adaptive radiotherapy for cervical cancer: evaluation of Elekta's semiautomated uterine segmentation method on 3D ultrasound images *Med. Phys.* **44** 3630–8
[41] Fraser D, Fava P, Cury F, Vuong T, Falco T and Verhaegen F 2007 Evaluation of a prototype 3D ultrasound system for multimodality imaging of cervical nodes for adaptive radiation therapy *Medical Imaging 2007: Visualization and Image-Guided Procedures* ed K R Cleary and M I Miga (Bellingham, WA: SPIE) 65090Y
[42] Henderson D R, Tree A C and van As N J 2015 Stereotactic body radiotherapy for prostate cancer *Clin. Oncol. (R Coll. Radiol.)* **27** 270–9
[43] Mohan R and Grosshans D 2017 Proton therapy – present and future *Adv. Drug Deliv. Rev.* **109** 26–44
[44] Cohen W N and Hass A C 1971 The application of B-scan ultrasound in the planning of radiation therapy treatment ports *Am. J. Roentgenol. Radium Ther. Nucl. Med.* **111** 184–8
[45] Smith E H and Holm H H 1970 Ultrasonic scanning in radiotherapy treatment planning *Radiology* **96** 433–5
[46] Sanders R C, Hughes B and Hazra T A 1974 Ultrasound localization of kidneys for radiation therapy *Br. J. Radiol.* **47** 196–7
[47] US5810007A 2020 Ultrasound localization and image fusion for the treatment of prostate cancer. Google Patents [Internet]. [cited 2020 Mar 22]. Available from: https://patents.google.com/patent/US5810007A/en
[48] Carol M P 1995 Method and apparatus for patient positioning for radiation therapy *US Patent* US5411026A
[49] Cinquin P, Lavalle S, Dubois F, Troccaz J, Peris O and Mazier B 1995 Method for determining the position of an organ *US Patent* US5447154A
[50] Gronningsaeter A, Olstad B and Unsgaard G 2000 Method for ultrasound guidance during clinical procedures *US Patent* US6019724A
[51] Getzinger T W and Shmulewitz A 1997 Methods and apparatus for correlating ultrasonic image data and radiographic image data *US Patent* US5640956A
[52] Troccaz J, Laieb N, Vassal P, Menguy Y, Cinquin P and Bolla M *et al* 1995 Patient setup optimization for external conformal radiotherapy *Comp. Aided Surg.* **1** 113–20
[53] Holupka E J, Kaplan I D, Burdette E C and Svensson G K 1996 Ultrasound image fusion for external beam radiotherapy for prostate cancer *Int. J. Radiat. Oncol. Biol. Phys.* **35** 975–84
[54] Ionescu G, Lavallée S and Demongeot J 1999 Automated registration of ultrasound with CT images: application to computer assisted prostate radiotherapy and orthopedics *Medical Image Comuting and Computer-Assisted Intervention—MICCAI'99* ed C Taylor and A Colchester (Berlin, Heidelberg: Springer) pp 768–77
[55] Helyer S J, Moskovic E, Ashley S, Hastings L and Jr Y 1999 A study testing the routine use of ultrasound measurements when selecting the electron energy for breast boost radiotherapy *Clin. Oncol. (R Coll. Radiol.)* **11** 164–8
[56] Leonard C, Harlow C L, Coffin C, Drose J, Norton L and Kinzie J 1993 Use of ultrasound to guide radiation boost planning following lumpectomy for carcinoma of the breast *Int. J. Radiat. Oncol. Biol. Phys.* **27** 1193–7

Chapter 2

Ultrasound imaging physics and technology

Emma Harris

This chapter gives a brief overview of some of the fundamental physics of ultrasound imaging and the basic principles which underpin medical ultrasound technology. Section 2.1 describes how an ultrasound image is formed and reminds the reader of the physics of the propagation of ultrasound through matter. The acoustic characteristics of tissue that affect the formation and quality of ultrasound image are reviewed. Section 2.2 describes ultrasound probe technology, how ultrasound is focussed and the different types of arrays used in medical ultrasound. Section 2.3 gives an overview of three-dimensional (3D) ultrasound imaging—a technology highly pertinent to ultrasound-guided radiotherapy which often relies on volumetric images to localise tissues in three dimensions. Finally, section 2.4 reviews common ultrasound imaging parameters, most of which can be adjusted using scanner settings to optimise ultrasound image quality.

2.1 Basic physics of medical ultrasound

2.1.1 Medical ultrasound image formation

Medical ultrasound typically relies on the formation of 'B-mode' images, which are cross-sectional images that represent the internal organs or tissues of a patient. A B-mode image is formed by placing an ultrasound probe in contact with the skin and transmitting short bursts (pulses) of ultrasound waves into the patient. These ultrasound waves are compressional waves with a frequency usually in the range 1–50 MHz [1]. Only the ultrasound waves that are reflected or scattered back towards the probe can be detected by the probe and used to form the image. The reflection of ultrasound waves (echoes) occurs at tissue boundaries, and scattering occurs at small structures within tissue. The reflected or backscattered ultrasound is displayed at a point in the image, which represents the spatial position of its origin, i.e. where it was scattered or reflected from. The brightness of the image at that point

doi:10.1088/978-0-7503-2552-3ch2

is related to the amplitude of the reflection, which is the reason for the term B-mode or brightness-mode. To display the anatomical feature that reflects or scatters ultrasound in the correct position, the ultrasound imaging system needs to know (1) the distance (or depth into the patient) of the feature from the ultrasound probe and (2) the position and direction of the emitted ultrasound beam. The distance is determined using the pulse-echo principle which is demonstrated in figure 2.1. A short pulse of ultrasound emitted at time, $t = 0$, is transmitted through the body to an anatomical feature which reflects ultrasound back to the probe. If the speed of sound in the body is c_s and the distance of the feature from the probe is d, the time required for the return trip of the ultrasound pulse is

$$t = 2d/c_s \tag{2.1}$$

If we rearrange equation (2.1) the distance can be calculated using

$$d = c_s t/2 \tag{2.2}$$

where the system typically assumes a speed of sound in tissues of 1540 ms^{-1} and measures t. The ultrasound image is formed by multiple sequential ultrasound pulse-echo sequences, each of which forms one line in the image. These lines are referred to as A-lines (amplitude lines). The position and direction of an ultrasound beam which creates the A-line is known by the system and depends on the shape of the probe, the portion of the probe that is used to form the beam and if beam steering is applied. These factors are discussed in more detail below in section 2.2.2. The spatial

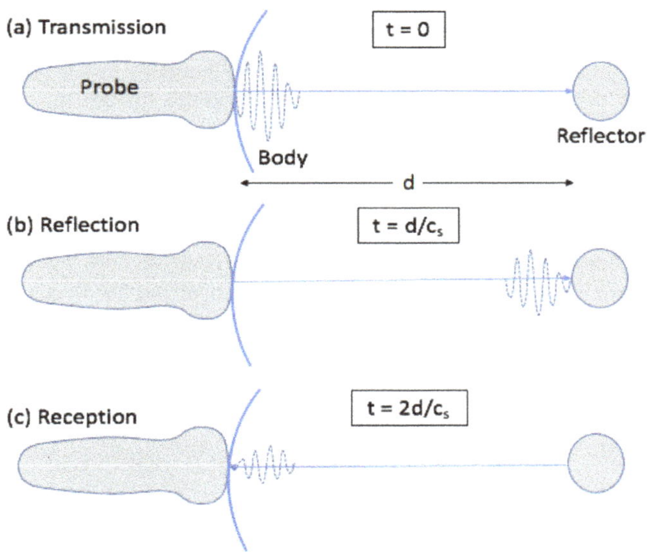

Figure 2.1. Measurement of the distance of a reflector from the probe using a pulse-echo sequence. An ultrasound pulse is transmitted into the body at time $t = 0$ in (a). The ultrasound propagates through the body at a speed of sound c_s, and reaches an anatomical feature situated a distance d from the probe in and is reflected back towards the probe (b) and received by the probe in (c). The distance d is calculated using equation (2.2).

resolution of an ultrasound imaging system is the minimum distance between two reflectors which allows them to be seen as separate features in the B-mode image. The spatial resolution of an ultrasound system is usually divided into three components which correspond to three directions: axial (the direction of the propagation of the ultrasound beam), lateral (perpendicular to the axial direction) and elevational (perpendicular to both the axial and lateral directions).

2.1.2 Speed of sound

The propagation of the ultrasound wave is governed by the elastic properties of the tissue as well as its mass density and the speed of sound c_s can be determined from the compressibility κ and the density ρ of a tissue and is given by:

$$c_s = \sqrt{\frac{1}{\kappa\rho}} \tag{2.3}$$

The compressibility κ is inversely related to the bulk modulus of tissue which is a measure of stiffness. Although diagnostic ultrasound scanners often assume $c_S = 1540\ \mathrm{ms}^{-1}$ through tissue to measure the distance of anatomical features, the speed of sound in the body can vary considerably (see table 2.1). Due to their high compressibility, sound speed is low in gases and therefore, lung tissue has a low speed of sound. Bone has a high speed of sound due to its high stiffness, or low compressibility. Variation of the speed of sound from 1540 ms^{-1} assumed by the scanner can lead to geometric distortions which are important in the context of ultrasound-guided radiotherapy, something which is discussed in detail in chapter 6. It should be noted that most soft tissues have a speed of sound within 5% of the 1540 ms^{-1}, which produces geometric distortions on the order of a few millimeters, and do not present significant problems in a diagnostic ultrasound imaging setting. Neither bone nor lung are commonly imaged using ultrasound for reasons that are discussed below.

Table 2.1. The speed of sound, attenuation coefficient and acoustic impedance of different tissues found in the body. Superscripts indicate sources where data was obtained. 1 = Zagzebski 1996 [2], 2 = Goss *et al* 1978 [3], 3 = Mast 2000 [4], 4 = Gonza *et al* 2004 [5]. Table reproduced from [6] with kind permission.

Material	Sound speed at 37 °C (m s^{-1})	Attenuation coefficient at 1 MHz (dB cm^{-1})	Impedance (kg m^{-2} s^{-1} × 10^6)
Air (lung)	334[4](600[1])	—	0.0004[1](0.18[1])
Fat	1478[3]	0.48[3]	1.34[1]
Kidney	1560[3]	1.0[3]	1.63[1]
Liver	1595[3]	0.50[3]	1.65[1]
Blood	1584[3]	0.20[3]	1.65[1]
Muscle	1580[3]	0.74[3]	1.71[1]
Skull bone	2840[2]	20[2]	7.8[1]

2.1.3 Reflection and refraction

When an ultrasound wave encounters an interface between two tissues of different acoustic impedance (Z), a fraction of the energy of the wave is reflected back into the first tissue and a fraction is transmitted into the second tissue. The specific acoustic impedance of a tissue can be determined by the tissue density ρ and the speed of sound c_s using:

$$Z = \rho c_s \tag{2.4}$$

It is an important property of tissues and the differences in acoustic impedance of tissues either side of a tissue boundary determines the amplitude of the reflected and transmitted ultrasound waves.

Reflection occurs at well-defined boundaries of a feature (or organ) where the size of the feature (or organ) is large compared to the wavelength of the US wave [7]. Reflection and transmission of ultrasound at a tissue boundary are illustrated in figure 2.2. If the direction of propagation of the incident ultrasound wave is not perpendicular to the boundary and c_s is different for the two tissues the transmitted wave is refracted, which means its direction of propagation is changed. The amount of refraction depends on the difference in c_s and can be predicted using Snell's law, which is given in equation (2.5) [7], where c_1 and c_2 are the sound speeds of tissue 1 and tissue 2, respectively, θ_i is the angle of the incident ultrasound wave, and θ_t is the angle of the transmitted ultrasound wave.

$$\frac{\sin \theta_i}{\sin \theta_t} = \frac{c_1}{c_2} \tag{2.5}$$

Reflection from a smooth boundary is referred to as specular reflection. The strength of the echo is dependent upon the orientation of the ultrasound transducer with

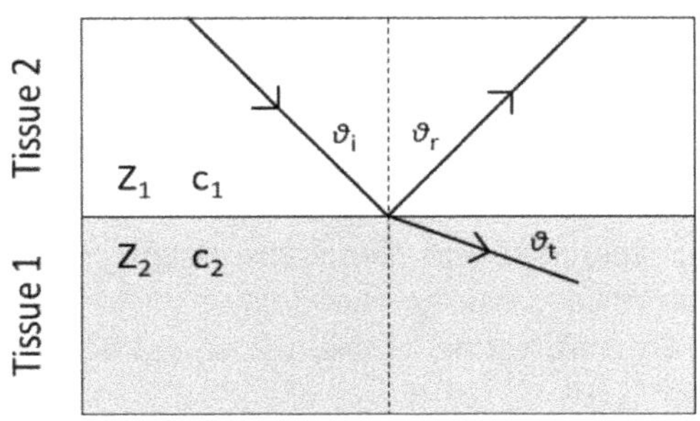

Figure 2.2. Schematic of ultrasound reflection and refraction. If ultrasound is incident on a boundary between two tissues with different sound speeds (c_1 and c_2) and acoustic impedances (Z_1 and Z_2) at an angle of incidence θ_i part of the wave is reflected at an angle θ_r (which is equal to θ_i), and part of it is transmitted through the tissue. In the case of non-perpendicular incidence, the transmitted wave is refracted and travels at angle θ_t (see equation (2.5)). The intensity of the reflected sound beam is determined by the intensity reflection coefficient, which can be calculated using equation (2.6).

respect to the reflector, with a perpendicular incidence yielding the strongest signal. The intensity of the reflected sound wave is given by the intensity reflection coefficient (R), which can be calculated using equation (2.6) [7], where Z_1 and Z_2 are the acoustic impedances of tissues 1 and 2 respectively, θ_i is the angle of the incident sound wave, and θ_t is the angle of the transmitted sound wave.

$$R = \left(\frac{Z_2\cos\theta_i - Z_1\cos\theta_t}{Z_2\cos\theta_i + Z_1\cos\theta_t}\right)^2 \tag{2.6}$$

Reflection from a rough boundary tends to become incoherent, but retains some of its directionality and therefore will also depend on the angle of incidence. Table 2.1 contains values for the acoustic impedance of tissues. Note that as the impedance mismatch between tissues increases, R also increases, thus reducing the intensity of the transmitted sound wave. This is observed when ultrasound is used to image the lung, the large mismatch between the acoustic impedance of lung (mostly air) and muscle means up to 99% of the acoustic energy is reflected, and the formation of images of lung tissue are extremely difficult. Lung ultrasound, however, is an active area of research [8] and has a proven role in emergency medicine [9] for the rapid diagnosis of pathologies which introduce fluid into the lungs. It is because of the high reflectivity of ultrasound at air interfaces, that air should be excluded from between the ultrasound probe and the patient's skin. Ultrasonic gel is commonly used as a coupling agent to more efficiently transmit ultrasound into the body.

2.1.4 Attenuation

Attenuation is defined as the reduction in the intensity of an ultrasound wave as it propagates through tissue. The reduction in intensity of an ultrasound beam is due to scattering of ultrasound out of the beam, divergence of the beam and absorption of ultrasound energy. Absorption is the process with which ultrasound energy is converted into heat and depends on the frequency of the ultrasound wave, with an increase in frequency resulting in poorer penetration into tissues [2]. Table 2.1 gives the attenuation coefficients of various materials in the body. Note the high attenuation of ultrasound by bone which means it is extremely difficult to use ultrasound to image the brain, or inside of bones, as little ultrasound energy can be transmitted through bone. Indeed, imaging tissues beyond bones is hampered by the formation of acoustic shadows, and therefore imaging upper abdominal organs which reside within the ribcage can be challenging.

Scattering refers to any redirection of the ultrasound wave away from its original direction, with different types of scattering phenomena occurring at different levels of tissue structure. Scattering includes reflection and refraction, and is responsible for the grainy appearance of tissues in B-mode images. This grainy pattern or texture is ultrasonic speckle and is discussed in more detail below. Ultrasound scattering occurs in one of three regions (Rayleigh, stochastic and geometric), which is influenced by the size of the scatterer and the wavelength of sound. At medical ultrasound frequencies the wavelength of sound is typically between 1.5 mm and 0.03 mm. Cellular structures (e.g. blood cells) which are smaller than the wavelength will scatter ultrasound in the

Rayleigh region. Structures that are larger than the wavelength (e.g., large vessels, tissue interfaces, bones, cysts etc) will scatter in the geometric region and structure that are approximately the same size of the wavelength will scatter in the stochastic region [7].

2.1.5 Ultrasonic speckle

The grainy appearance of some tissues on B-mode ultrasound images referred to as speckle is due to Rayleigh scattering which occurs at the smallest tissue structure, where the scatterers are smaller than the wavelength of the incident ultrasound wave. A single scatterer generates a coherent scattered wave [7]. Many of these small scatterers are present within the resolution cell of the scanner, which is the volume defined by the spatial resolution of the scanner. (The spatial resolution of the ultrasound imaging system is discussed in more detail below.) Coherent waves generated from each individual scatterer may interfere to create a resultant wave whose amplitude and phase depends strongly on the position, orientation, and frequency of the incident acoustic wave [7, 10]. The fluctuations in amplitude of the detected ultrasound signal caused by the interference of waves are responsible for ultrasonic speckle [11]. Figure 2.3 demonstrates how the appearance of an ultrasound image of homogeneous tissue changes with an increasing number of scatterers within the resolution cell.

In terms of image intensity, speckle can be quantified by the signal-to-noise ratio (abbreviated SNR, defined as the ratio of the mean grey level μ to the standard deviation σ) in a region within an ultrasound image with no resolvable structure [12].

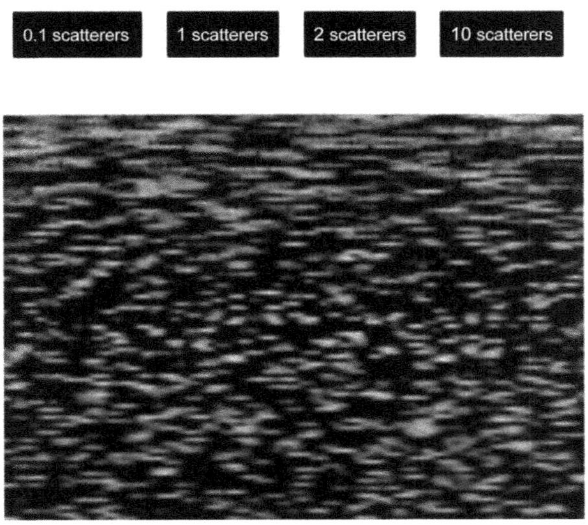

Figure 2.3. This interactive figure demonstrates the appearances of a homogeneous medium containing randomly distributed scatterers with different number of scatterers per resolutions cell. Note how, as the number of scatterers per resolutions cell increase, the individual scatterers are not resolved and the medium appears more homogeneous. The lateral focus is placed mid-depth (see section 2.2). Images were simulated using Field II [13] and are courtesty of George West. Animation available at https://iopscience.iop.org/book/978-0-7503-2552-3.

Speckle is useful for certain applications such as ultrasound elastography and more relevant to ultrasound-guided radiotherapy, motion tracking which is discussed in sections 7.2.1. In general diagnostic imaging, speckle is considered an artefact because it obscures small high-contrast targets, low contrast targets, and changes in the non-speckle component of image texture [11].

The speckle pattern in an ultrasound image changes depending on the orientation of the incident sound beam with respect to the scatterers; the smaller the angular overlap between image views, the greater the statistical independence of the underlying speckle patterns [13]. Spatial compounding (which is discussed in depth in chapter 4) is a technique that improves the SNR of ultrasound images by taking advantage of the speckle decorrelation achieved by imaging the same structure from different viewpoints but comes at the cost of reduced imaging frame rate.

2.2 Ultrasound probe technology

In this book we will refer to the ultrasound probe as the entire hand-held device used to acquire ultrasound images. The ultrasound probe consists of an outer casing that contains the ultrasound transducer and associated electronics required to operate the transducer. Other components include: a matching layer to reduce the effect of the mismatch in acoustic impedance between the transducer and the body; an acoustic lens which focuses the ultrasound beam in the elevational direction (discussed below); and a damping block which absorbs sound reflected from the matching layer/body interface (see figure 2.4) [14].

For some 3D imaging probes, electronic motors and mechanical parts to rotate or translate the transducer (see section 2.4) are also enclosed within the probe housing. The overall shape and size of the probe will be influenced by its intended medical use.

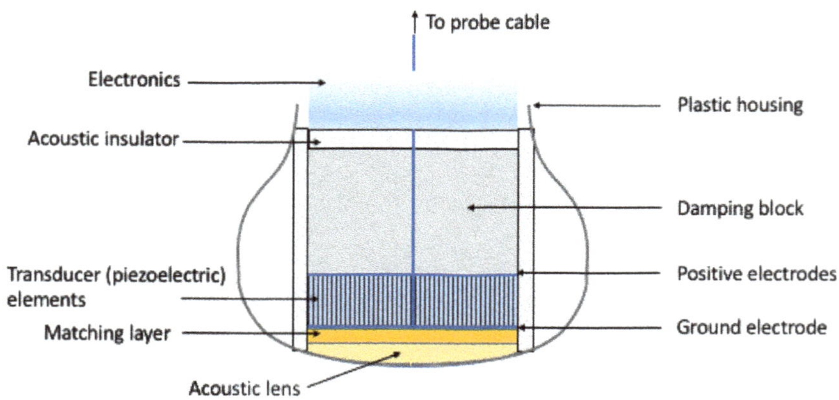

Figure 2.4. Schematic diagram of a cross-section through a typical ultrasound probe. The probe casing contains a linear array of ultrasound transducer elements, which are biased using a positive electrode. A matching layer is used to help transmit sound from the transducer into the subject, however, some acoustic energy is always reflected and therefore a damping block is used to absorb this reflected energy.

2.2.1 The ultrasound transducer element

The ultrasound transducer is fundamental to any ultrasound imaging system. An ultrasound transducer generates an ultrasound wave by converting electrical signal to pressure waves. See figure 2.4 for a schematic of the ultrasound probe structure. The transducer also receives ultrasound, converting incident pressure waves, reflected or scattered from the tissues within the body, to electrical signals. The design of the transducer determines the spatial resolution of the specific probe and how it varies within the field of view.

Transducers are most commonly made of piezoelectric elements. These elements are commonly cut from a ceramic (such as lead zirconate titanate, PZT) or a plastic (such as polyvinylidine difluoride, PVDF). In the last few years, capacitive micro-machined ultrasound transducers (CMUTs), which do not operate using piezo-electricity but instead use a change in capacitance to convert pressure waves to electrical signals, have become commercially available. CMUTs emit and receive ultrasound at a wider range of frequencies than their piezoelectric counterparts, which is advantageous for some advanced ultrasound imaging techniques such as contrast enhanced ultrasound and ultrasound tissue characterisation. For piezo-electric transducers, the fundamental resonance frequency is determined by the thickness of the element, and the speed of sound in the element. Transducers used in radiotherapy tend to operate at frequencies in the 2–8 MHz range to provide penetration depths in soft tissues of around 8–15 cm [15].

2.2.2 Multi-element arrays

For most medical imaging applications multiple element transducers are used for pulse-echo imaging. Multiple elements can increase the field of view and may be used for electronic beamforming. An ultrasound beam is typically formed by emission of ultrasound waves from many ultrasound elements. Beamforming determines the beam width, the lateral spatial resolution (beam focussing) and the direction of the beam (beam steering) and can be performed on both transmission and reception of ultrasound waves. The beam width is determined by the number of elements used to form the beam and the strength of lateral focussing. If ultrasound is emitted from all the elements simultaneously, the ultrasound beam is not focussed in the lateral direction and approximates a plane wave. Focussing and steering of the beam is achieved by applying short delays to the electronic pulses used to stimulate the transducer elements to emit ultrasound waves. The temporal and spatial pattern of the delays determine the strength and depth of the focus and the beam direction. These concepts are demonstrated in animated figure 2.5.

A single A-line of ultrasound data is acquired using a beam of ultrasound which is typically formed by multiple elements. The beam is laterally translated along the array of elements to form an image. This is illustrated in figure 2.6. Focussing of the beam in the lateral direction on transmission can only be done once per pulse-echo sequence and results in one beam focus at a fixed depth. In interactive figure 2.3, note how the scatterers appear less elongated at the central depth, in these simulations the lateral focus was placed at this mid-depth position. Some systems

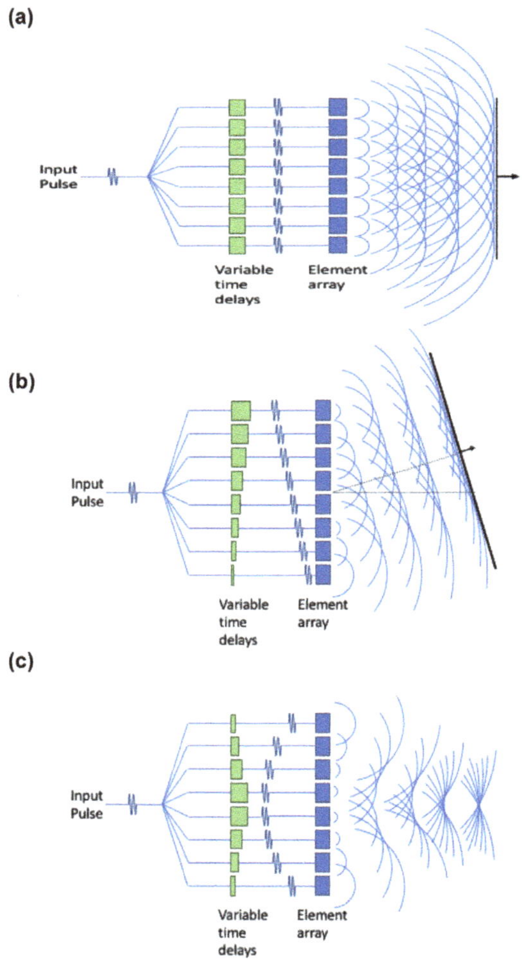

Figure 2.5. This animated figure provides animated illustrations of transmit beamforming to perform (a) plane waves imaging, (b) phased beam steering, and (c) focussing (lateral). ((b) Adapted from Chetvorno https://commons.wikimedia.org/w/index.php?curid=54005685). Animation available at https://iopscience.iop.org/book/978-0-7503-2552-3.

offer multiple lateral foci, which vary in depth, however, this is at the cost of a reduced frame rate as the final image will have to be built up from a number of pulses equal to the number of foci. The strength of the lateral focus, described by the *F-number* and therefore the lateral spatial resolution is dependent on the depth of focus, D and the width of the aperture (or number of elements), d, (see figure 2.6) and is given by:

$$F_{\text{number}} = \frac{D}{d} \tag{2.7}$$

Receive focussing, however, can be achieved at almost every depth along an A-line and can be performed during a single pulse-echo sequence. This is referred to as

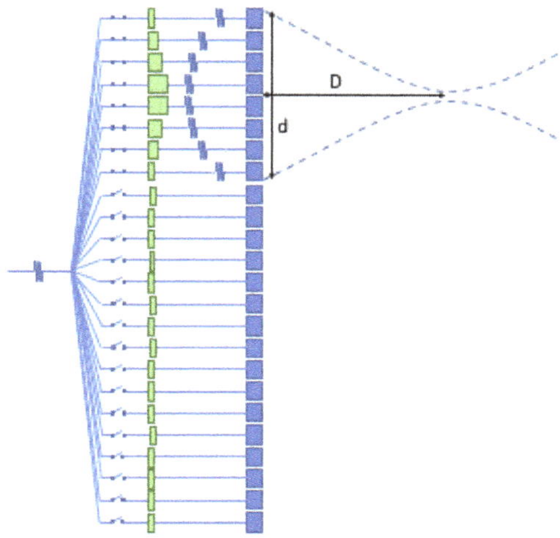

Figure 2.6. This animated figure illustrates how a 2D image is formed by lateral translation of the ultrasound beam by sequentially selecting a group of elements positioned at different lateral positions along the array. The strength of the focus, or F-number, is determined by the width of the aperture, *d*, (determined by the number of elements selected to form the beam), and the depth of the focus, *D*. Adapted from Chetvorno https://commons.wikimedia.org/w/index.php?curid=54005685. Animation available at https://iopscience.iop.org/book/978-0-7503-2552-3.

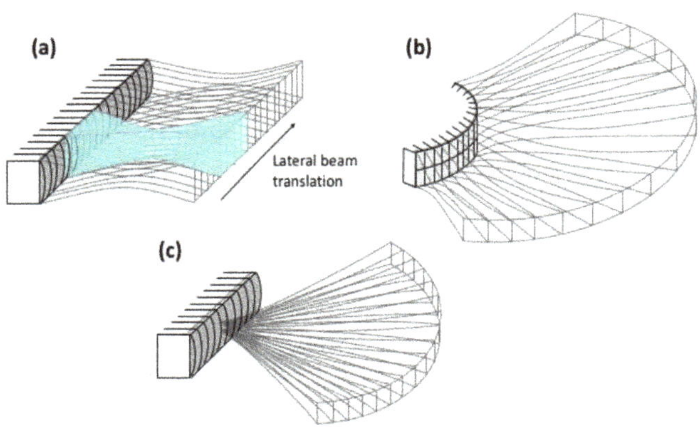

Figure 2.7. Illustration of (a) a linear array, (b) a curvilinear array and (c) a phased array.

dynamic receive focussing and is achieved by applying time delays to the received signals at each element before the signals are combined to form a line within the image.

There are several types of multi-element array configurations, those most relevant to the field of ultrasound-guided radiotherapy are most commonly found in diagnostic imaging: the linear array, the curvilinear array and the phased array. Linear (figure 2.7a) and curvilinear (figure 2.7b) arrays will allow beam translation (laterally along the array) and beam steering. A convex curvilinear array provides a sector scan format without the need for phased beam steering.

Phased arrays (see figure 2.7c) have a smaller array size but allow phased beam steering to generate a sector scan. They use every element to transmit and receive to form a single line of the image and build up the image using steering only (not translation). These arrays have been designed to image soft tissues that are deep inside the body and beyond a relatively small acoustic window, e.g., between the ribs. The disadvantage of phased arrays compared to linear or curvilinear arrays is the small field of view at shallow depths, poorer lateral spatial resolution due to the limited number of elements used to focus the beam and reduced lateral resolution at the edges of the field of view due to grating lobes. Grating lobes are beyond the scope of this chapter and the reader is referred to [16] for further details.

For 1D arrays the spatial resolution in the elevational direction is determined by the strength of the elevational focus and the length of the transducer element. For 1D arrays, the elevational focus is produced by mechanical focussing, typically a lens, and is the weakest focus. The spatial resolution in the elevational direction is greatest at the focus and reduces with distance from the probe due to beam divergence past the elevational focus. 2D arrays, or matrix arrays which are discussed below (see figure 2.8), permit electronic control of the elevational focus (in strength and depth) and can produce an elevational focus as strong as the lateral focus.

2.3 Three-dimensional ultrasound imaging

Radiotherapy image guidance requires a geometrically accurate description of the location of the boundaries of target tissues and organs at risk in three spatial dimensions. First generation ultrasound-guided radiotherapy (USgRT) systems used 2D imaging transducers (incorporating 1D transducer arrays) to acquire two

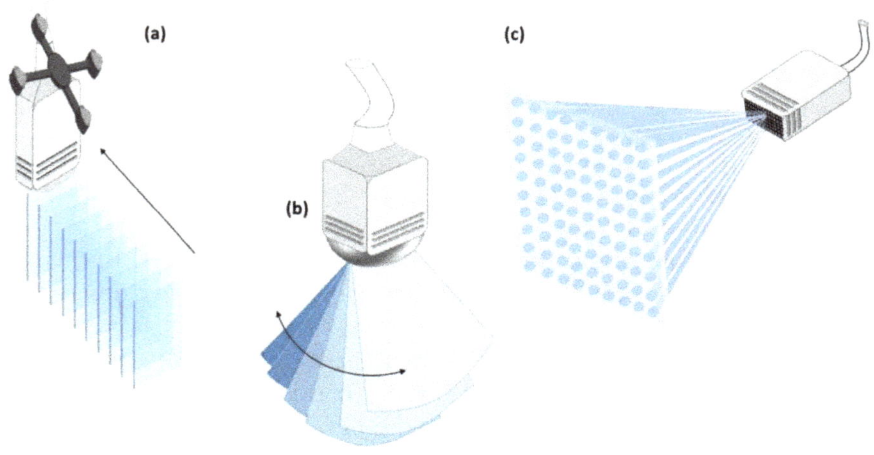

Figure 2.8. Illustration of three different techniques used for acquiring 3D images: (a) freehand scanning using a 1D transducer array (2D probe) the position of which is tracked using a tracking device or marker, (b) a 3D mechanically scanned probe in which the 1D transducer is tilted back and forth to sweep out a 3D volume, and (c) a matrix array probe with a 2D array of transducer elements.

orthogonal planes bisecting the target tissue. The disadvantage of this approach is that it only provides a limited amount of information with which to identify the position of the tissues. USgRT systems rely on the registration of images to estimate interfraction motion. The use of 2D images increases the likelihood of out-of-plane misregistration of images [17], which can occur when 2D ultrasound images of adjacent cross-sections of tissue appear similar. Volumetric, or 3D imaging, reduces the possibility of out-of-plane misregistrations and provides a greater amount of image information, thereby reducing registration uncertainty. Three major approaches can be used to acquire 3D ultrasound images: freehand scanning with position sensing, mechanical scanning and electronic scanning (see figure 2.8).

Freehand scanning

This approach typically requires that the transducer is used in conjunction with a tracking device which may be optical, mechanical or electromagnetic. Tracking device options are described in more detail in section 3.1. Briefly, the tracking device samples the position and orientation of the probe with respect to some external frame of reference, in the case of USgRT this is the radiation treatment room coordinate system, in real-time. Synchronisation of image acquisition with the position and orientation of the transducer allows each 2D image, which may be arbitrarily positioned and orientated, to be reconstructed onto a 3D Cartesian grid using interpolation. Whilst arbitrary scan planes can be stitched together, it is common for the operator to 'sweep' the transducer in the elevational direction whilst attempting to produce contiguous 2D images of a section of the patient. To achieve this, the operator must scan at a sufficiently slow speed, which is a function of the elevational beam width and the 2D frame rate; ideally, the sampling interval is less than half the elevational resolution [17]. Accurate synchronisation of the signal from the tracking device and the image acquisition time is important, any mismatch between probe position and image will introduce a geometrical bias [18].

If a tracking device is not used, generation of a 3D image relies upon image processing algorithms to calculate the relative position of the planes. An advantage of not using a tracking device is that no extra hardware is required, potentially allowing greater flexibility in the position and orientation of the probe. For example, when using an optical system, the camera has to have a clear 'line-of-sight' of a tracking tool or marker attached to the probe, limiting the range of motion of the probe. No commercial USgRT systems, however, have relied on image processing techniques alone to construct a 3D image from 2D images acquired freehand, possibly because they have typically lower geometrical accuracy compared to tracking [16].

Mechanical scanning

Mechanical scanning requires a motor to move the transducer. The motor is typically integrated within the probe housing and moves the transducer only inside the probe. To enable the transducer to move independently of the probe housing, whilst maintaining acoustic coupling with the housing, the transducer resides in an oil or water filled reservoir. The transducer is moved across the front face of the probe, which may either be made of a semi-flexible or rigid material, and can be

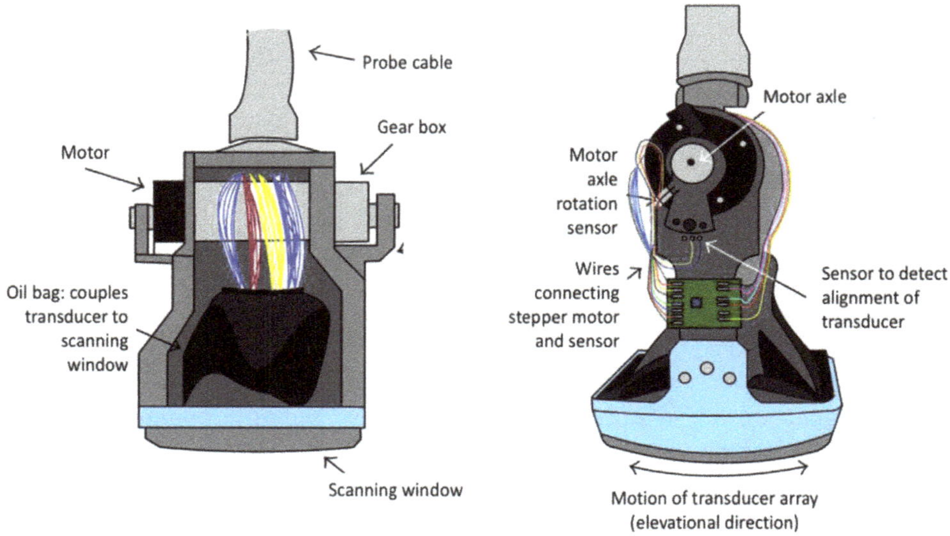

Figure 2.9. Internal components of a 3D mechanical ultrasound transducer. Adapted from Huang and Zeng 2017 [19] under Creative Commons Attribution license, courtesy of Hindawi.

moved in three ways: translational, tilting and rotational. Figure 2.9 shows the internal construction of a probe which uses mechanical scanning to form a 3D image by translating the probe across the front face of the transducer. Translational motion is typically employed using linear multi-element arrays. A set of 2D parallel and equally spaced 2D images are acquired as the transducer is translated back and forth in the elevational direction. The speed of the translation should be matched to the 2D frame rate to ensure that the sampling interval in elevational direction is less than half of the elevational resolution. As 2D frame rates are often variable, ideally the speed will be variable, however, many systems will have manufacturer defined parameters with limited options for variation. In the plane of the 2D images, the axial and lateral resolution is equivalent to that of the 2D images, in the elevational direction the resolution will be determined by the elevational resolution of the array provided the above spatial sampling criteria is met.

One benefit of mechanical scanning compared to freehand scanning is the geometry of the 2D imaging planes is predefined, less complex and allows for fast image reconstruction. A tilting motion will form a fan of radial images spaced at regular angular intervals about an axis which is parallel to the transducer face. This fan geometry allows a wide field of view to be imaged with a stationary probe. Reducing the total tilt angle may allow an increase in volume acquisition rate and increasing or decreasing the angular interval can decrease or increase the image quality of the reconstructed 3D image, respectively. Due to the fan arrangement of 2D images, the elevational resolution will decrease with radial distance (depth within the patient) due to the increase in sampling distance between image planes. Mechanical rotational motion of the transducer rotates the array around a fixed axis, which is perpendicular to the array face. Typically, rotational scanning is used for intracavitary imaging, i.e., using transrectal or transvaginal probes, and whilst commonly used to guide surgical biopsy, these types of probes have yet to be applied to USgRT.

Electronic scanning
Both freehand and mechanical scanning use 1D arrays to acquire a series of conventional 2D images. An alternative is to use a 2D transducer element array, often referred to as the '2D matrix array', which allows the user to acquire volumetric images at high volume rates because the beam is steered electronically rather than mechanically. The 2D array also eliminates the problems of mechanical components, and array localisation, and has the advantage that they are able to focus in both the lateral and elevational directions. 2D phased arrays with a pyramidal field of view which could be steered in two dimensions were developed as early as the late 1980s (see figure 2.8). The first devices were designed for application to 3D echocardiography [20, 21] and today their use is still predominantly for this application which requires a relatively small aperture size and fast volumetric imaging (> 20 Hz). Their development has been slowed by the high cost of the transducer arrays and the complexity and cost of interconnecting a large number of elements. Typically a linear array used for imaging relatively shallow and accessible tissues such as the breast will contain more than 128 elements providing a relatively large lateral field of view. To provide an equivalent 2D array requires over 16 000 elements and 16 000 electrical connections, which make the probe and its cable cumbersome and non-ergonomic. Manufacturers overcome this problem by including electronics to allow beam forming on the probe and multiplexing of the image data back to the scanner. Using this approach, cardiac probes with 64×64 (4096) elements, and more recently, larger arrays with over 9000 elements for general purpose applications (abdominal, obstetrics, foetal and gynaecological) have been manufactured and are now available [22].

2.4 Ultrasound imaging parameters

The array of knobs and sliders available on a diagnostic ultrasound scanner can be overwhelming for the inexperienced user of ultrasound (see figure 2.10). In general, to reduce this complexity, the array of functions available to the user are restricted by the manufacturers of ultrasound guidance equipment for radiotherapy, favouring instead the use of presets which automatically set the parameters. The following gives an overview of the principal imaging parameters that will affect image quality for both single and dynamic (cine) image acquisitions.

2.4.1 Ultrasound transmit frequency

Ultrasound imaging systems use pulse-echo sequences which were described above. An ultrasound element is excited with an electronic signal varying with frequency f, which results in the transmission of ultrasound waves. It is then switched to receive mode in order that it can detect reflected ultrasound waves until it is time for the next ultrasound pulse to be generated. The pulse length is measured in units of time and

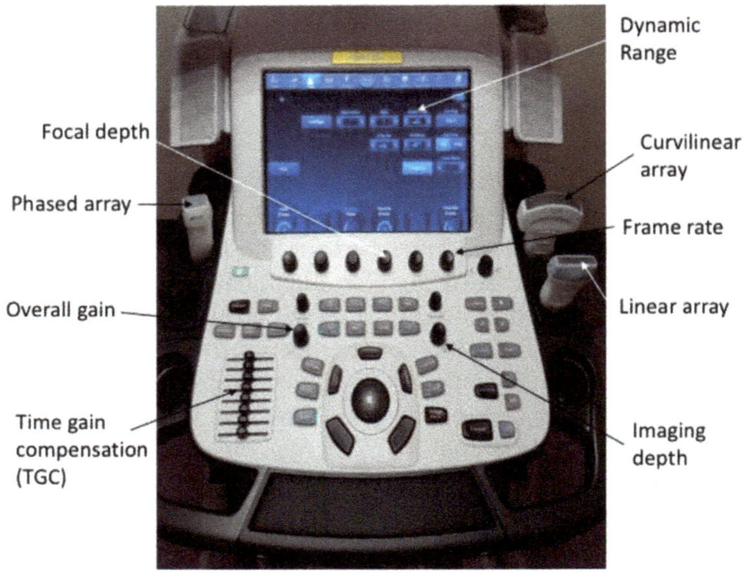

Figure 2.10. Photograph of a typical console of a diagnostic ultrasound scanner illustrating the large number of user controls available. This scanner is GE Vivid E95 scanner (GE Healthcare Inc., Chicago, IL, USA). Photograph courtesy of Mark O'Leary.

comprises a number of cycles of the electronic signal. The shorter the pulse length the greater the range of frequencies, or the greater the bandwidth of the emitted ultrasound waves. The use of a greater number of cycles reduces the axial resolution of the ultrasound imaging system. Typically, imaging systems use pulse-lengths of one or two cycles. The (input) frequency at which a probe has its peak operating efficiency is the resonant frequency of the elements and is referred to as the central frequency of the probe. Typically, the frequency of the transmitted ultrasound sound, and therefore the probe, is chosen to suit the clinical application and is a compromise between axial spatial resolution and depth of penetration. Spatial resolution in the axial direction is related to the frequency of sound ($1/\lambda$), and the number of cycles, n, by:

$$\text{Axial Resolution} = \frac{n\lambda}{2} \tag{2.8}$$

For abdominal organs, which tend to be deeper inside the body, for example, liver and uterus, the probes are operated at 3 MHz to 5 MHz. For superficial organs, such as the breast or thyroid, that do not require much depth of penetration, higher frequencies can be used, i.e., 8 MHz to 12 MHz, which provides superior imaging resolution.

2.4.2 Transmit power control

Most scanners will allow the user to increase the amplitude of the imaging pulse. The setting 0 dB refers to the maximum pulse amplitude and users can adjust the amplitude, normally in predefined steps, i.e. −3 dB, −6 dB. Increasing the pulse amplitude will increase the amplitude of echoes in the image and increase the depth at which there is sufficient SNR to detect echoes. Maximum pulse amplitude is limited by the scanner to ensure safe exposure levels of ultrasound.

2.4.3 Gain and time gain compensation

The amplitude of ultrasound echoes can be increased using two methods; overall gain and time gain compensation (TGC). An increase in overall gain will increase image brightness equally at all depths in the image. It should be noted that overall gain or TGC do not increase the penetration depth, to do this the transmit power must be increased or the frequency must be reduced. Increasing the overall gain can have the undesirable effect of saturating the image at shallow depths or at highly reflective boundaries, which can lead to loss of contrast and information. Overall gain also increases electronic noise, which can dominate low signals from deeper regions potentially reducing the benefit of applying gain. TGC overcomes this problem through the application of varying amounts of gain with imaging depth. Low voltage signals produced by the piezoelectric elements are amplified using a variable controlled amplifier (VCA) before being digitised using an analogue-to-digital convertor (ADC) [16]. The VCA gain profile, which is applied to the received signals, is a function of the time that signal is received. Since the signal strength typically decreases with time because it has travelled through, and is attenuated by, more tissues. The VCA gain profile can be adjusted using a group of controls on the scanner. This allows the user to fine tune the VCA setting to optimise the image brightness for different anatomies. For example, to reduce highly specular reflections at shallow depths due to layers of adipose tissues and increase gain at deeper depth to visualise highly attenuated echoes.

2.4.4 Imaging depth

Manufacturers will define a maximum possible imaging depth for a specific probe which is determined by several factors including the transmit frequency, aperture size, the typical ultrasound attenuation of the tissues found in the tissues to be imaged and the minimum (ultrasound) signal-to-(system) noise ratio that the manufacturer wishes to achieve. Whilst scanning, an imaging depth less than the maximum imaging depth can be set by the user. There are several advantages to adjusting the imaging depth to just beyond the tissues of interest. Less data per image is captured, i.e., the image size is smaller, allowing the image to be displayed at greater magnification and less data storage capacity is required. The time window in which ultrasound is received is also reduced as the sound has less far to travel as the imaging depth is shallower, allowing higher imaging frame rates to image moving tissues with greater temporal resolution.

2.4.5 Number and depth of foci

To achieve good spatial resolution the beam must be focussed in the lateral direction. The operator can set the depth of lateral focus on the scanner. Usually an arrow head alongside the image indicates the depth of focus. Multiple foci on transmission can be selected, however, as stated in section 2.2.2, this will increase the time required to form an image and decrease the frame rate. Typically, dynamic receive focussing is not controlled by the operator, as that requires automated adjustment of the receive focus depending on the time the echoes are received and is applied to all depths in the image.

2.4.6 Frame or volume rate

The frame rate or scanning speed can be defined as the number of times an image is formed. The higher the frame rate, the greater the ability to image fast moving structures and to overcome motion artefacts. This will obviously impact on the ability of an ultrasound-guided radiotherapy system to estimate intrafraction motion (see chapter 7). On some scanners the imaging frame rate is not directly adjusted by the user but is typically set automatically by the scanner according to the sector size, the imaging depth, the number of transmit foci, and the line density of the image, and for 3D probes, the elevational dimension of the imaging volume. Other scanners allow adjustment of the frame rate, for example the Vivid E95 shown in figure 2.10, adjusting the frame rate on this scanner will automatically adjust the line density and therefore lateral spatial resolution. To increase the frame or volume rate, there is a compromise between the ability to image objects moving at faster velocities and the field of view and the spatial resolution. If an increased frame rate is achieved by reducing the sector size, elevational dimension or imaging depth, there will be a decreased field of view and the user must ensure the tissues of interest are still captured within the image. Increasing the frame rate by reducing the number of transmit foci or the line density will reduce the lateral spatial resolution and the user must be aware of the impact of this reduced image quality on the ability to visualise or, for intrafraction motion estimation, track tissues.

2.4.7 Dynamic range

Ultrasound which is reflected from large scatterers (geometric region) can vary considerably in amplitude [14], with almost 100% of the ultrasound energy reflected backwards from an air–tissue interface. In the Rayleigh region, the reflected signal amplitude depends on scatterer size and the frequency of ultrasound but is typically much smaller than echoes received from larger interfaces. Indeed, the reflected echo amplitude from small scatterers such as blood cells or stromal components of tissue may be as much as −100 dB (on the order of 10^{-5}) lower than the signal amplitude reflected from an air–tissue interface. The dynamic range of signals received by the transducer is defined as the largest echo amplitude that does not cause signal saturation divided by the smallest signal that can be detected above noise. Both strong and weak echoes may contain important information, however, the range of signal amplitudes that can be displayed is typically in the order of 60 dB. Commonly, log compression is used to reduce the range of signals detected at the transducer to the range of signals that can be displayed to the user. If the gain is increased to display weak echoes, regions of strong echogenicity will become saturated in the image. Conversely, if the gain is increased to display the information in highly echogenic regions, weakly echogenic, typically parenchymal tissues, will be displayed as dark regions and characteristic parenchymal texture will not be visible. Some scanners will allow you to adjust the dynamic range and therefore the range of signals displayed, effectively highlighting or suppressing tissue parenchyma.

2.4.8 Tissue harmonic imaging

Tissue harmonic imaging (THI) exploits the non-linear propagation of ultrasound, which results in harmonics at higher frequencies (i.e., multiples of the fundamental frequency). THI exploits the second harmonic and has two main advantages. The first is that the harmonic signal initially builds up as it propagates through tissue and is therefore weaker closer to the surface of the patient, which is typically characterised by heterogeneous tissues such as layers of fat and/or muscle. The degree of beam distortion that occurs in these superficial tissues will be reduced in the second harmonic, improving SNR. The second advantage is that the second harmonic is preferentially generated along the beam axis. Harmonics which are generated due to side lobes, scattering and reverberations are less prominent and usually not detected by the transducer which increases lateral resolution and contrast-to-noise ratio. One drawback is that the axial resolution is not improved and may be worsened by a reduction in the pulse bandwidth required to perform THI [16]. For a full explanation please refer to [23] or [24].

Acknowledgements

The author gratefully acknowledges the input and contribution of table 1.2. (reproduced from [6]) from Sarah Mason.

Consolidation quiz

Q1: The speed of sound is:
- ○ greater in tissues with high compressibility
- ○ lower in tissues with low compressibility
- ○ greater in tissues with low stiffness

Q2: Ultrasound is attenuated most by:
- ○ the ribs
- ○ the liver
- ○ the breast

Q3: The depth of penetration of ultrasound:
- ○ increases with increasing pulse length
- ○ increases with increasing depth of focus
- ○ increases with decreasing ultrasound transmit frequency

Q4: The spatial resolution of ultrasound depends on:

- ○ the wavelength of ultrasound and the strength of the elevational focus
- ○ the wavelength of ultrasound, the pulse length, the strength of the lateral and elevational foci
- ○ the wavelength of ultrasound, the pulse length, the depth of the lateral and elevational foci

References

[1] McDicken W N and Anderson T 2011 Basic physics of medical ultrasound *Clinical Ultrasound* (Amsterdam: Elsevier) pp 3–15

[2] Zagzebski J A 1996 *The Essentials of Ultrasound Physics* (St Louis, MO: Mosby)

[3] Goss S A, Johnston R L and Dunn F 1978 Comprehensive compilation of empirical ultrasonic properties of mammalian tissues *J. Acoust. Soc. Am.* **64** 423–57

[4] Mast T D 2000 Empirical relationships between acoustic parameters in human soft tissues *ARLO* **1** 37–42

[5] Velasco S, Román F L, González A and White J A 2004 A computer-assisted experiment for the measurement of the temperature dependence of the speed of sound in air *Am. J. Phys.* **72** 276–9

[6] Mason S 2018 Ultrasound-guided radiotherapy for cervical cancer *Doctoral dissertation* University of London

[7] Bamber J C and Tristam M 1988 Diagnostic ultrasound *The Physics of Medical Imaging* ed S Webb (Boca Raton, FL: CRC Press) 319–88 p

[8] Patterson B and Miller D 2019 Measurements of ultrasound attenuation in human chest wall *J. Acoust. Soc. Am.* **146** 3071

[9] Cortellaro F, Colombo S, Coen D and Duca P G 2012 Lung ultrasound is an accurate diagnostic tool for the diagnosis of pneumonia in the emergency department *Emerg. Med. J.* **29** 19–23

[10] Burckhardt C B 1978 Speckle in ultrasound B mode scans *IEEE Trans. Sonics Ultrasonics* **25** 1–6

[11] Bamber J C 1993 Speckle reduction *Advances in Ultrasonic Techniques and Instrumentation* ed P N T Wells (London: Churchill Livingstone) pp 55–67

[12] Jensen J A and Nikolov I 2000 Fast simulation of ultrasound images *2000 IEEE Ultrasonics Symp. Proc. An Int. Symp. (Cat No00CH37121)* (IEEE) pp 1721–4

[13] Shankar P M 1986 Speckle reduction in ultrasound B-scans using weighted averaging in spatial compounding *IEEE Trans. Ultrason. Ferroelectr. Freq. Control* **33** 754–8

[14] Hoskins P R, Martin K and Thrush A (ed) 2019 *Diagnostic ultrasound: physics and equipment* 3rd edn (Boca Raton, FL: CRC Press)

[15] Fontanarosa D, van der Meer S, Bamber J, Harris E, O'Shea T and Verhaegen F 2015 Review of ultrasound image guidance in external beam radiotherapy: I. Treatment planning and inter-fraction motion management *Phys. Med. Biol.* **60** R77–114

[16] Bamber J, Miller N and Tristam M 2012 Diagnostic ultrasound *Webb's Physics of Medical Imaging* (Boca Raton, FL: CRC Press)

[17] Fenster A, Downey D B and Cardinal H N 2001 Three-dimensional ultrasound imaging *Phys. Med. Biol.* **46** R67–99

[18] Harris E J, Symonds-Taylor R, Treece G M, Gee A H, Prager R W and Brabants P *et al* 2009 Evaluation of a three-dimensional ultrasound localisation system incorporating probe pressure correction for use in partial breast irradiation *Br. J. Radiol.* **82** 839–46

[19] Huang Q and Zeng Z 2017 A review on real-time 3D ultrasound imaging technology *Biomed. Res. Int.* **2017** 6027029
[20] von Ramm O T and Smith S W 1990 Real time volumetric ultrasound imaging system *J. Digit. Imag.* **3** 261–6
[21] Smith S W, Pavy H R and von Ramm O T 1991 High-speed ultrasound volumetric imaging system. I. Transducer design and beam steering *IEEE Trans. Ultrason. Ferroelectr. Freq. Control* **38** 100–8
[22] Acar P, Battle L, Dulac Y, Peyre M, Dubourdieu H and Hascoet S *et al* 2014 Real-time three-dimensional foetal echocardiography using a new transabdominal xMATRIX array transducer *Arch. Cardiovasc. Dis.* **107** 4–9
[23] Desser T S and Jeffrey R B 2001 Tissue harmonic imaging techniques: physical principles and clinical applications *Semin. Ultrasound CT MRI.* **22** 1–10
[24] Whittingham T A 1999 Tissue harmonic imaging *Eur. Radiol.* **9** 323–6

IOP Publishing

Chapter 3

Registration of ultrasound with radiotherapy room coordinates

Davide Fontanarosa, Saskia Camps and Svenja Ipsen

Image guided-radiotherapy relies on imaging technologies to localise internal target tissues, or surrogates for target tissues, in the radiation treatment room. This chapter describes how tissues visualised in the ultrasound image can be accurately located within the frame of reference, or coordinate system, associated with the radiotherapy delivery. Key to this localisation are methods to locate the probe in the treatment room, these methods are described in section 3.1. The mathematical methods used to determine the spatial calibration which relate the ultrasound coordinate system to the radiotherapy coordinate system are described in section 3.2. Section 3.2 also includes a description of the tools required to determine the spatial calibration and how the spatial calibration may be validated. Finally, the sources of geometrical error in the localisation of target tissues in the radiotherapy delivery room are discussed in section 3.3.

3.1 Methods for localising the ultrasound probe

When ultrasound systems are used for image guidance, the position of each pixel (or voxel) in the images (or volumes) must be known in the same system of coordinates as the one used for treatment planning and delivery. To this end, the position of the pixel in the ultrasound image coordinates must be first transformed to the ultrasound guidance system coordinates defined by the relative position of the image frame to a tracking marker (or beacon) used to localise the probe; then to the tracking system coordinates; then to the room system coordinates. Typically these transformations are implemented with a calibration procedure performed using a specific calibration phantom which is aligned to known reference points in the room (for example the treatment isocentre indicated by room lasers) and contains

doi:10.1088/978-0-7503-2552-3ch3

structures in known positions. These calibration procedures will be described in detail in section 3.2.

The techniques that can be used to track the position and orientation of the probe include optical, electromagnetic (EM), mechanical, x-ray and robotic tracking. Table 3.1 taken from Western *et al* [1] provides an overview of typical spatial resolution and acquisition rates as well as specific characteristics such as the need for ionising radiation of these techniques.

For optical tracking, a marker (or combination of markers) is rigidly connected to the ultrasound probe and localised by cameras in the linac coordinate system. Optical or infrared stereoscopic cameras are used on the currently commercially available systems, with reflective passive markers mounted on the ultrasound probe. Other camera systems in the visual optical band have been proposed for this purpose, for example a system using dot patterns on a surface as the tracking marker [2] or the now discontinued I-Beam system (Computerised Medical Systems Inc. MD, USA) used a grid pattern that was situated in the head of the linac and viewed by a camera which was mounted on the probe [3]. Similar solutions are already commercially available in other fields, as for example the OptiTrack system (Corvallis, OR, USA) or the Vantage system (Vicon Motion Systems Ltd, Centennial, CO, USA), but currently this is the only application reported in radiotherapy. Optical tracking allows high spatial and temporal resolution, but relies on direct view of the trackers from the cameras which may be a limitation in some applications.

Ultrasound probe holders, both mechanical or robotic, can also be used to localise the probe, as long as each of the joints' angles is known and an accurate geometric description of the device is available. This approach has been followed by the first version of the B-mode Acquisition and Targeting system (BAT, NOMOS Corporation, Sewickly, PA, USA) which implemented a high precision mechanical arm between the ultrasound workstation and the patient [4, 5]. Robotic arms, instead, have been proposed in literature, but are currently not implemented in any commercial system. Examples include the telerobotic system proposed by [6] and the

Table 3.1. Overview of techniques that can be used for tracking the position and orientation of an ultrasound probe with corresponding characteristics such as the presence of ionising radiation or the possibility for metal interferences. Adapted from [1] under Creative Commons Attribution License CC-BY-3.0.

	Optical	Electromagnetic	Mechanical	X-ray
Typical spatial resolution	0.2–0.4 mm	0.5–0.8 mm	0.1–5.0 mm	0.2 mm
Typical acquisition rate	20–60 Hz	20–200+ Hz	300–1000 Hz	<0.2 Hz. Limited by safety considerations
Line of sight issues?	Yes	Yes for some materials	No	Yes for some materials
Metal interference?	None	High	None	None
Ionising radiation?	No	No	No	Yes

robotic placement method investigated by [7]; the cooperatively controlled robot by [8]. These systems need high precision manufacturing and high quality materials and design to achieve the required accuracy. They do not present line of sight issues, but they need to be carefully evaluated for use in the radiotherapy clinic to ensure impact risks with the moving inac, the patient and beam interference are minimised. Robotic systems are discussed in detail in chapter 9.

EM tracking systems are also potentially available for ultrasound probe tracking [9]. In other fields, such as ultrasound-guided biopsy [10] or ultrasound-guided surgery [11] electromagnetic tracking has been explored but the limited sensitive volume and the susceptibility to the presence of magnetic objects have prevented these from being implemented in commercial ultrasound guidance products. In particular, there is evidence in literature that the magnetic field might be specifically distorted by the probe thus possibly generating significant errors in the localisation [12].

Another group [13] has investigated using the Cyberknife stereo x-ray cameras with x-ray markers to localise the ultrasound probe for cardiac radiosurgery. This approach produces accurate localisations, but relies on x-ray imaging which delivers extra dose to the patient.

3.2 Spatial calibration

3.2.1 Setup and transformations

Integration of image guidance into the radiotherapy workflow generally requires target localisation in absolute coordinates of the reference coordinate system, for example of the linac. Consequently, ultrasound image coordinates need to be transformed into treatment room coordinates. Since ultrasound imaging relies on direct contact between ultrasound probe and patient, the target position in the image will change if the probe is moving. It is therefore necessary to decouple external probe motion and internal target motion by continuously localising the target in the image data as well as the probe itself within the treatment room.

Transformations from one coordinate system to another can be described with translation and rotation combined in a single 4×4 matrix. Figure 3.1 illustrates the system components and coordinate systems relevant for ultrasound guidance in radiotherapy. Following the respective transformations indicated by arrows, it can be seen that

$$^{\mathrm{W}}T_{\mathrm{M},i}\,^{\mathrm{M}}T_{\mathrm{US}}\,^{\mathrm{US}}T_{\mathrm{Target},i} = {}^{\mathrm{W}}T_{\mathrm{Target},i} \tag{3.1}$$

where $^{W}T_{M,i}$ describes the transform at time point i from the optical tracking system W to the optical tracking marker M attached to the probe, $^{\mathrm{M}}T_{\mathrm{US}}$ points from M to the ultrasound image space *ultrasound*, $^{\mathrm{US}}T_{\mathrm{Target},\,i}$ refers to the target position within the ultrasound image at time point i, while $^{\mathrm{W}}T_{\mathrm{Target},i}$ is the desired transformation from W to the current target position. The transformations $^{\mathrm{W}}T_{\mathrm{M},i}$ and $^{\mathrm{US}}T_{\mathrm{Target},i}$ can be determined via optical tracking and target localisation within the ultrasound data, respectively, so that the only missing component is the unknown $^{\mathrm{M}}T_{\mathrm{US}}$.

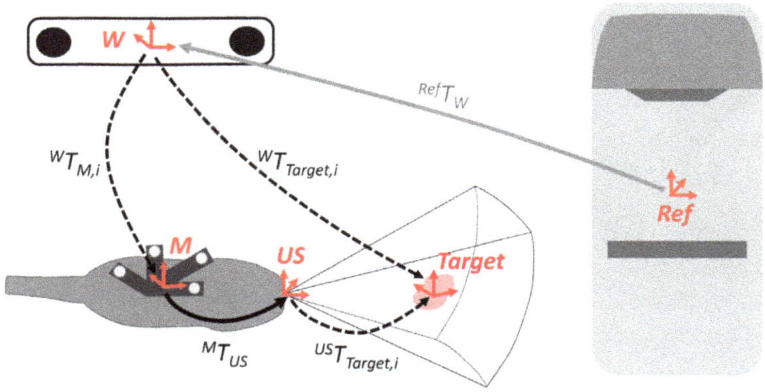

Figure 3.1. Coordinate systems and transformation matrices required for registration of the ultrasound images 'US' to the treatment room 'Ref' via a pre-calibrated optical tracking system 'W'. Dashed lines refer to transformations that change over time (i.e. with probe or target position) while solid lines describe fixed relationships that remain static.

For motion compensation with treatment adaptation, it is usually necessary to express ${}^{W}T_{\text{Target},i}$ relative to the world reference frame Ref in treatment coordinates. This is realised by multiplying equation (3.1) with ${}^{\text{Ref}}T_{\text{W}}$, i.e. the alignment of the optical tracking system within the treatment room, so that the final target position can be calculated as

$$ {}^{\text{Ref}}T_{\text{Target},i} = {}^{\text{Ref}}T_{\text{W}}\, {}^{\text{W}}T_{\text{Target},i}. \tag{3.2} $$

3.2.2 Calibration methods and phantoms

Spatial calibration describes the geometric alignment of different coordinate systems and is a common procedure, especially in robotics and computer vision tasks. In an ultrasound guidance context, two calibration steps are usually performed to determine the unknown transformations ${}^{\text{Ref}}T_{\text{W}}$ and ${}^{\text{M}}T_{\text{US}}$ illustrated in figure 3.1. To determine the alignment of the probe tracking system within the treatment room ${}^{\text{Ref}}T_{\text{W}}$, a calibration pose with known absolute coordinates (e.g. the isocentre and main treatment axes) is measured. For mechanical tracking, the calibration pose can be recorded relative to the linac using a fixed holder attached to the gantry to bring the mechanical arm into a predefined configuration. Optical tracking systems are commonly used in radiotherapy and can be calibrated with a predefined marker geometry, e.g. shown in figure 3.2, placed at the isocentre using the room lasers for alignment with the treatment room coordinate system.

The transformation from the attached probe holder (mechanical tracking) or marker geometry (optical tracking) to ultrasound image space ${}^{\text{M}}T_{\text{US}}$ is estimated with probe calibration. Depending on the ultrasound probe type (2D versus 3D) and the type of calibration phantom used (see figure 3.2), two different approaches can generally be chosen: defined phantom (DP) or hand-eye (HE) calibration [14]. For DP calibration, customised phantoms with internal structures of known geometry and attached tracking markers are used to define a fixed reference coordinate system.

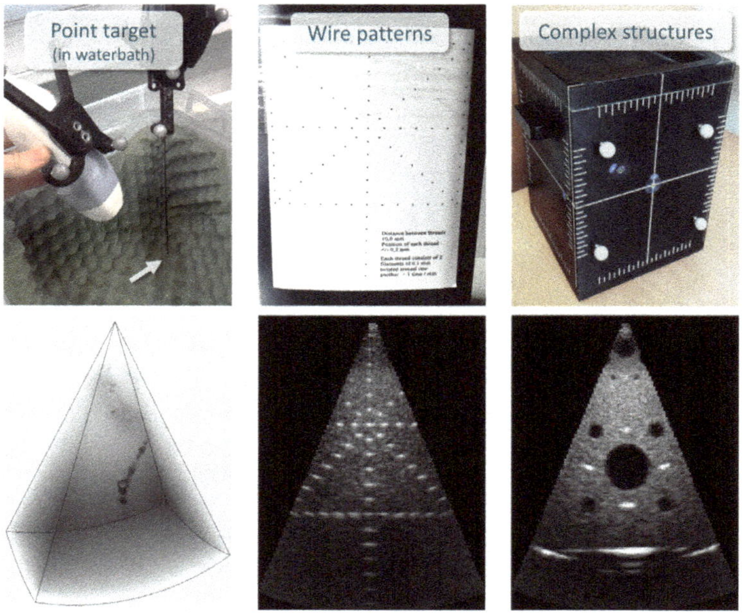

Figure 3.2. Different phantom types for ultrasound probe calibration: single target/stylus with optical markers (left), nylon wires (centre) and complex structures with optical markers and markings for laser-based positioning (right).

The goal of the calibration is then to estimate the transformation between the ultrasound image coordinates and the corresponding points in the phantom's reference coordinate system by acquiring ultrasound images of the phantom structures and extracting them using image processing or manual annotation. To determine ${}^{M}T_{US}$, multiple poses of the US probe relative to the phantom, and thus different values for ${}^{W}T_{M,i}$ and ${}^{US}T_{\text{Target},i}$, are recorded as shown in interactive figure 3.3. From these measurements, the components of ${}^{M}T_{US}$ can be approximated using a least-squares minimisation of the distances between the transformed image coordinates and the known phantom structures in the reference coordinate system. Different types of phantoms can be chosen for this approach, e.g. containing a single target, multiple wires in X- or Z-shapes or complex objects [15], illustrated in figure 3.2. DP calibration can be performed for both 2D and 3D ultrasound probes. Due to its reliance on a well-defined reference frame for accurate calibration results, DP approaches require high-precision manufacturing and stability of the phantom.

In robotics, HE calibration is the most common approach to determine the transformation between a sensor and a tracked manipulator. In the case of optical tracking, the ultrasound probe serves as the sensor and the optical marker M as the manipulator. Many HE calibration approaches have been proposed to date, using either separable solutions that first solve the rotational part and then the translation (e.g. Tsai and Lenz [16]), simultaneous solutions that solve both at the same time (e.g. Horaud and Dornaika [17]), or non-linear approaches [18]. The HE approach is based on measuring relative changes between probe poses and therefore does not

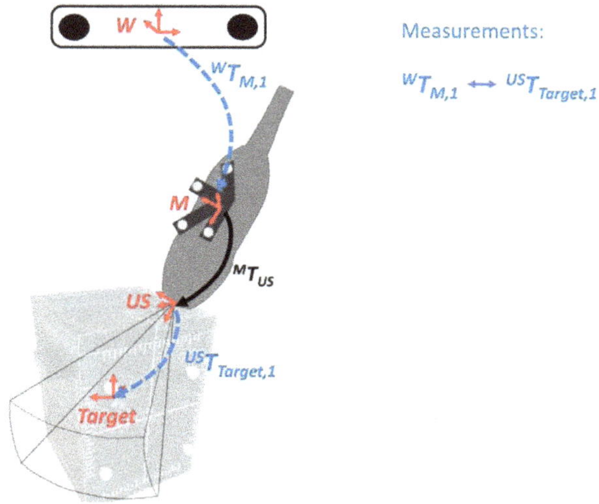

Figure 3.3. Iterative acquisition of calibration measurements using optical tracking of the probe position and target localisation within the ultrasound volume to determine the relevant transformations frame by frame. To solve the linear system of equations, multiple measurements from different viewing angles are usually required. Animation available at https://iopscience.iop.org/book/978-0-7503-2552-3.

inherently rely on a phantom defining an absolute reference coordinate system. It requires at least three measurements from distinct perspectives to solve for ${}^{M}T_{US}$ and some approaches can even solve for ${}^{Ref}T_{W}$ simultaneously. Combined with automatic feature detection, HE calibration offers the practical advantage of not requiring an accurately manufactured calibration phantom or manual localisation of phantom points. At the same time, typical HE approaches require position data with six DOF, i.e. translation and rotation, which can only be achieved using 3D ultrasound probes. Schlosser *et al* [19] presented a solution to the HE problem using automatic image registration between ultrasound volumes, thus not relying on handcrafted landmarks or features. Ernst *et al* [20] presented an HE approach that can still provide a full solution for ${}^{M}T_{US}$ and a partial solution for ${}^{Ref}T_{W}$ using ultrasound data with only three DOF (translation only). Since volume registration in ultrasound can be time-consuming and prone to errors due to speckle and artefacts, localisation of a simple point target with three DOF could potentially be possible with higher accuracy and can also be measured with 2D ultrasound.

DP and HE approaches each have their characteristic strengths and weaknesses and no clear tendency towards higher accuracy or superior robustness has been reported for a specific group of algorithms to date. Studies comparing both approaches in an ultrasound context also yielded rather inconclusive results, with one study favouring HE [14] and another DP [21]. A comprehensive review of calibration techniques for ultrasound probes can be found in Mercier *et al* [22].

3.2.3 Validation

After successful calibration, the ultrasound images can be transformed into treatment room coordinates using equation (3.1). A calibration phantom placed at the

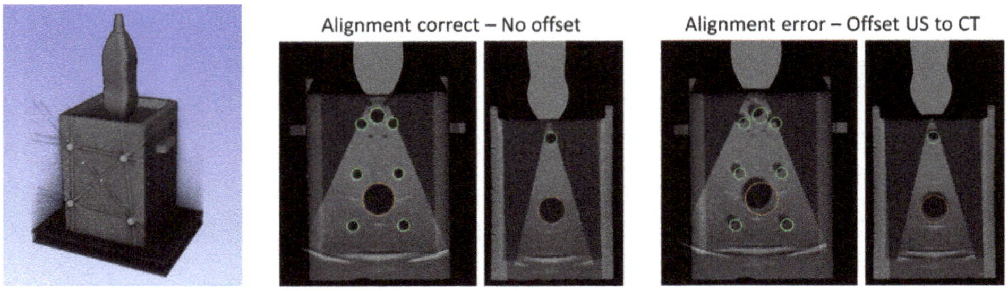

Figure 3.4. Phantom aligned with the reference coordinate system for accuracy validation. If the spatial calibration is accurate, the structures in the ultrasound scan are aligned with the contours from the CT scan (orange and green circles) of the optically tracked phantom. Discrepancies, e.g. caused by calibration errors, will lead to a misalignment of the structures and indicate the need for recalibration.

isocentre, e.g. by using the pre-calibrated room lasers, can be used to assess the accuracy of the solutions for ${}^{\mathrm{M}}T_{\mathrm{US}}$ and ${}^{\mathrm{Ref}}T_{\mathrm{W}}$. In a first step, the in-room alignment of the probe tracking system relative to the reference coordinate system should be verified separately. If an offset above a certain acceptance threshold is detected, the mechanical arm or the optical tracking camera must be recalibrated using the method described above.

In a second step, probe calibration must be validated using an optically tracked ultrasound phantom with an internal geometry known from manufacturing or from a CT scan. If ${}^{\mathrm{M}}T_{\mathrm{US}}$ has been calculated correctly, the structures in the calibrated ultrasound image will align with the structures extracted from CT as depicted in figure 3.4. An error in the calibration causes a mismatch between the ultrasound image and the CT model of the phantom that, if exceeded, demands a recalibration of the probe. Since even a slight change of the marker position on the probe will lead to a different transformation matrix ${}^{\mathrm{M}}T_{\mathrm{US}}$, probe calibration accuracy should be verified before every treatment.

3.3 Uncertainties and technical limitations

3.3.1 In-room alignment and tracking

The previous section focussed on the theoretical framework and methods for in-room registration of the ultrasound image coordinates to the treatment reference frame. To date, several studies have investigated the achievable accuracy for realistic calibration scenarios of ultrasound probes. Early studies on DP calibration using mechanical 3D probes, specially designed wire phantoms and manual or semi-automatic feature segmentation, reported accuracies between 1.5 mm [15] and 3.4 mm [14]. Schwaab *et al* [23] demonstrated an accuracy of 4.8 mm was measured using a 'pseudo-3D' cross-plane probe with a wire phantom. Studies using HE calibration with automatic intramodality registration between subsequent ultrasound volumes achieved accuracies from 2.4 mm [24] to less than 1.5 mm [19, 25].

The reported calibration accuracies are the overall errors between an absolute target position in reference coordinates and a reconstructed position measured in the ultrasound image data. However, all calibration steps are affected by errors from different sources that can accumulate along the chain of transformations, from the probe tracking system to the target localisation within the ultrasound data. For example, mechanical tracking systems can measure displacements with an accuracy between 0.1 mm and 5.0 mm depending on their design and intended purpose [1], while optical tracking systems usually yield a relatively high spatial resolution of 0.2 mm to 0.4 mm. The in-room alignment of the probe tracking system can also be affected by errors due to the manual placement of the calibration phantom at the isocentre, usually guided by the room lasers or x-ray imaging. However, when performed with care, these errors are typically small. Especially for DP approaches, the accuracy of the phantom geometry itself also directly influences the calibration errors as it is used to define the reference frame. Another source of errors is the localisation of phantom structures within the ultrasound image data. Typical target localisation errors in 2D and 3D ultrasound are in a range of 1–2 mm (see also chapters 6 and 7 on inter- and intrafractional ultrasound guidance). It should be noted that many studies on ultrasound-guided motion compensation have been based on retrospective analysis of previously acquired image data (e.g. De Luca *et al* [26, 27]), assessing only errors in image space and not in absolute coordinates, therefore not considering the errors typically introduced by in-room calibration.

3.3.2 Speed of sound errors

Speed of sound (SOS) is the property of the tissues used by pulse echo ultrasound systems to calculate the depth of the reflecting structures from the time of flight (TOF) (see section 2.1.1). As described in chapter 2, SOS values can vary significantly in human soft tissues, from 1450 m s^{-1} in fat to 1613 m s^{-1} in connective tissue (at body temperature, 37 °C) [28]. Most ultrasound systems, though, assume a fixed value for SOS of 1540 m s^{-1} [29], because it is impossible to know *a priori* the SOS distribution in the tissues that are being scanned. When the tissues have an SOS which is known to differ significantly from 1540 m s^{-1}, as for example when the breast or liver is imaged, mitigation can be introduced by altering the assumed SOS value in the ultrasound system [30]. More recently, manufacturers have implemented an option to change the SOS assumed by the scanner, resulting in better image quality and improved diagnostic reliability (for example the RS85 Prestige scanner from Samsung Healthcare). For quantitative applications, such as in radiotherapy, where accuracy in localisation, volume and distance measurement is essential, the discrepancy between the assumed and the real SOS values can produce significant errors. For example, for deep-seated structures in the liver (SOS value of 1600 m s^{-1}), localisation errors potentially as large as 7 mm have been reported in literature [31] (see figure 3.5). In general, SOS aberration is a well reported problem in literature (see for example Salter *et al* [32]), for which few solutions have been proposed [33].

For intramodality systems, which compare a reference ultrasound image acquired at planning to ultrasound images acquired prior to treatment delivery, such as Clarity, uncertainties due to this type of aberration should be limited. When similar scanning procedures are used to acquire the two images, both should be affected by

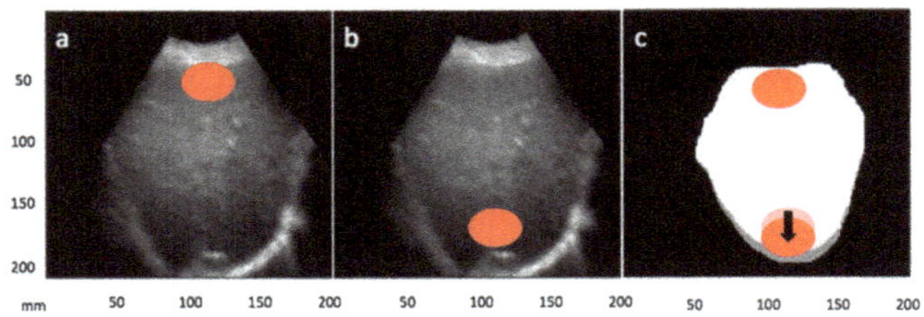

Figure 3.5. Different impact of SOS aberration on a shallow (a) or deep (b) structure inside the liver: the apparent volume of the liver before (white in image c) and after (grey in image c) SOS correction shows a shift of more than 7 mm of the distal wall (and hence a similar estimated error on the position of the deep structure), while the position of the proximal wall (and of the shallow structure) are unaltered [31].

the SOS aberration in the same way [34]. There are examples in the literature of discrepancies in the measurement of setup errors possibly due to SOS aberrations also with intramodality systems. For example in the context of prostate radiotherapy, Li *et al* [35] report a significant −1.9 mm mean with a 2.3 mm standard deviation in the differences in setup errors in the longitudinal direction measured using 3DUS and seed-match in CBCT. The authors ascribed these differences to a deviation in the calibration of the ultrasound system due to SOS aberration. The reason would be that the intramodality approach can compensate for the aberration, as mentioned previously, but only if the tissues are imaged in the same configuration at simulation and at treatment. If major anatomical changes occur, for example because of bladder filling, the compensation is not effective anymore. This issue has been investigated more in depth by Fontanarosa *et al* [36], who concluded that in some cases SOS aberration correction might be necessary even for intramodality workflows. When intermodality systems, which compare ultrasound images acquired prior to radiation delivery with the planning CT, are used, it is important to be aware that the registration between ultrasound and CT scans using the spatial calibration described above might generate discrepancies in the position of the structure. An average difference in localisation of structures inside the liver between ultrasound and CT, was reported to be 3.5 mm [37]. In these cases, manual correction of the registration may have to be introduced, but then it is also important to consider potential operator dependent variability.

3.3.3 Probe pressure

To enable the acquisition of ultrasound images with good quality, it is important to ensure that the acoustic coupling between the skin of the patient and the ultrasound probe is sufficient. Acoustic coupling is typically established using ultrasound gel which acts to eliminate air from in between the probe and the skin. In addition, the operator can apply pressure on the ultrasound probe to further improve the coupling and the ultrasound image quality. Pressure can also reduce the imaging depth of the tissues of interest, displacing other tissues so they are no longer in the path of the ultrasound beam, as demonstrated in figure 3.6.

The application of ultrasound probe pressure is a concern during ultrasound-guided radiotherapy (USgRT) workflows, as this pressure could result in displacement and/or

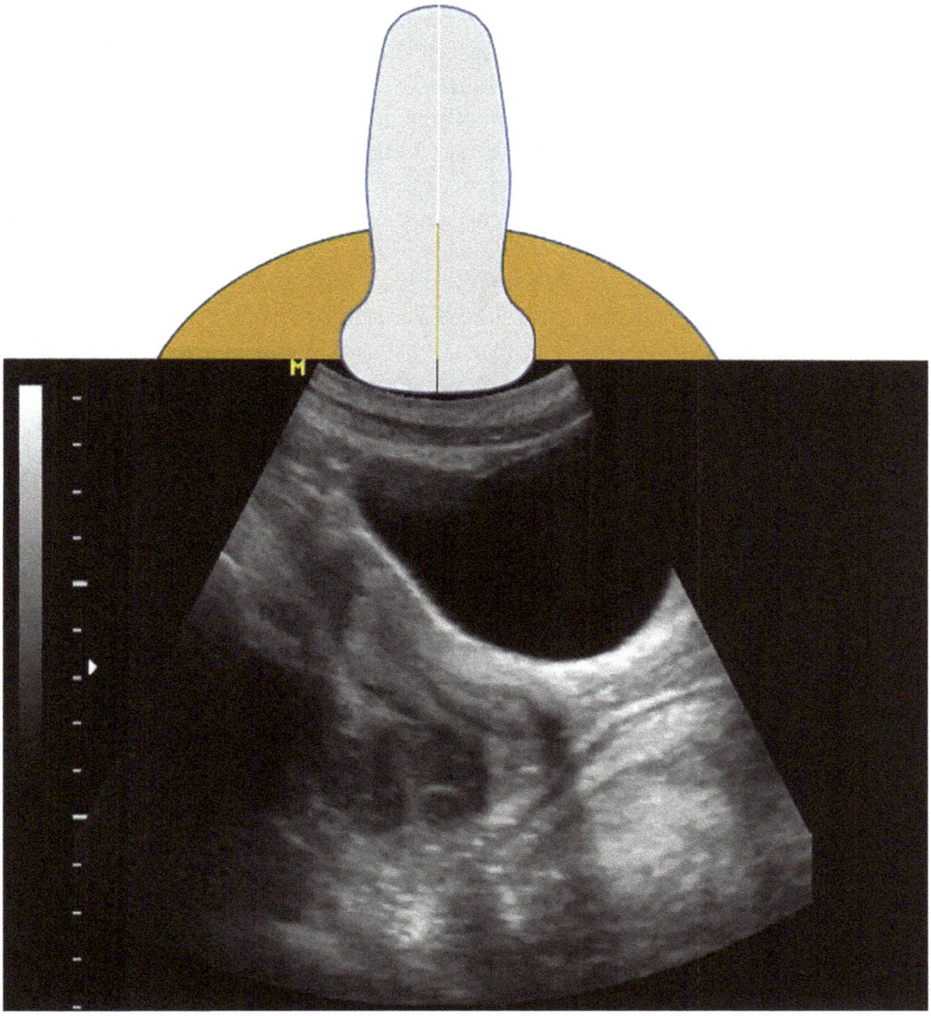

Figure 3.6. Animated schematic demonstrating how the application of probe pressure can push overlying tissues out of the tissue out of the field of view and decrease the length of the acoustic path to the target tissues. In this case, the lower bowel which typically contains air is obstructing the ultrasound beam and is pushed aside with probe pressure. Animation available at https://iopscience.iop.org/book/978-0-7503-2552-3.

deformation of the anatomical structures. In a scenario where ultrasound imaging is used only for interfraction patient setup (described in chapter 6), the ultrasound probe is positioned on the body of the patient to acquire ultrasound images and align the patient accordingly. Subsequently, the probe has to be removed to start the treatment. If the anatomical structures were displaced due to ultrasound probe pressure, the structures will most probably displace again when the probe is removed. This would result in a new tissue distribution and therefore the need of a re-alignment of the patient making the just performed alignment suboptimal or even wrong.

The effects of probe pressure are most profound for anatomical structures that are not inside the ribcage, such as the structures in the pelvic region. In addition, also the geometry of the probe makes a difference in the need for probe pressure. For example, if a convex probe is used for imaging with almost no probe pressure, only a small part of the probe will be in contact with the skin. This will degrade the ultrasound image quality and field of view unless a very thick layer of gel is used to improve the acoustic coupling with the remaining parts of the probe and the patient's skin [38].

The probe pressure effect in radiotherapy workflows has been most extensively described for the prostate. Most studies used a relative method to assess the prostate displacement. This means that a reference ultrasound image was acquired with zero/low probe pressure and subsequent images acquired at a medium and high pressure were compared to this reference situation. Following this approach, mean displacement vectors of the prostate of 2.5 mm [39] and 3 mm [34] were found for transabdominal ultrasound imaging and 2–4 mm [40] for transperineal ultrasound imaging. Baker and Behrens [41] used a different approach in which transperineal ultrasound imaging was used to measure the prostate displacement due to transabdominal ultrasound probe pressure. This resulted in a mean displacement vector for the prostate of 1.3 mm.

In addition to the displacement of the prostate, the effect of pressure of a transperineal probe on the penile bulb has been investigated [42]. Due to probe pressure, the penile bulb can be pushed towards the high dose region, which could result in increased dose to the penile bulb, which has been associated with erectile dysfunction [43]. Ideally, every time ultrasound images are acquired the same amount of pressure should be applied on the same anatomical structures. In this way, the anatomical structure displacement should be the same and so predictable. Some groups have investigated the possibility to replace a human operator with a robot, which could potentially result in more stable ultrasound probe pressure [6, 25, 44]. In chapter 9 of this book an extensive description of the use of robotics for ultrasound imaging is provided.

Consolidation quiz

Q1: Optical tracking devices require that the following condition must be met:

- ○ The line of sight between the optical marker on the probe and the camera must not be obstructed
- ○ The ultrasound probe must be acquiring images.
- ○ There must be no operators in the treatment room

Q2: Spatial calibration describes the geometric alignment of different coordinate systems. Which two approaches are generally used to calibrate ultrasound image coordinates to room coordinates?

- ○ Optical tracking and mechanical tracking
- ○ Defined phantom (DP) and hand-eye (HE)
- ○ Six degrees of freedom (6 DOF) and three degrees of freedom (3 DOF)

Q3: Calibration accuracy is affected by cumulative uncertainties from a range of sources, including phantom alignment and tracking accuracy. Some sources are ultrasound-specific and affect the registration accuracy of:
- ○ Intermodality ultrasound guidance systems only
- ○ Intramodality ultrasound guidance systems only
- ○ Both inter- and intramodality ultrasound guidance systems

Q4: What is a possible effect of the application of ultrasound probe pressure on the skin of the patient?
- ○ Anatomical structure displacement
- ○ Anatomical structure deformation
- ○ Anatomical structure displacement and deformation

References

[1] Western C, Hristov D and Schlosser J 2015 Ultrasound imaging in radiation therapy: from interfractional to intrafractional guidance *Cureus.* **7** e280

[2] Camps S, Costa M, Stevens E, Sanches P G, Fonseca G P and Bellezzo M *et al* 2017 Evaluation of optical localization in the visible band for ultrasound guidance in radiotherapy using a robotic arm *J. Cancer Control Treat.* **30** 319–29

[3] Molloy J A 2012 Ultrasound-guided radiation therapy *Image-Guided Radiation Therapy* ed J D Bourland (Boca Raton, FL: CRC Press) p 13–26

[4] Lattanzi J, McNeeley S, Pinover W, Horwitz E, Das I and Schultheiss T E *et al* 1999 A comparison of daily CT localization to a daily ultrasound-based system in prostate cancer *Int. J. Radiat. Oncol. Biol. Phys.* **43** 719–25

[5] Lattanzi J, McNeeley S, Donnelly S, Palacio E, Hanlon A and Schultheiss T E *et al* 2000 Ultrasound-based stereotactic guidance in prostate cancer—quantification of organ motion and set-up errors in external beam radiation therapy *Comput. Aided Surg.* **5** 289–95

[6] Schlosser J, Salisbury K and Hristov D 2010 Telerobotic system concept for real-time soft-tissue imaging during radiotherapy beam delivery *Med. Phys.* **37** 6357–67

[7] Kuhlemann I, Jauer P, Schweikard A and Ernst F 2016 SU-G-JeP3-08: robotic system for ultrasound tracking in radiation therapy *Med. Phys.* **43** 3672

[8] Şen H T, Lediju Bell M A, Iordachita I, Wong J and Kazanzides P 2013 A cooperatively controlled robot for ultrasound monitoring of radiation therapy *2013 IEEE/RSJ Int. Conf. on Intelligent Robots and Systems (Tokyo)* (IEEE) **2013** 3071–6

[9] Franz A M, Haidegger T, Birkfellner W, Cleary K, Peters T M and Maier-Hein L 2014 Electromagnetic tracking in medicine—a review of technology, validation, and applications *IEEE Trans. Med. Imaging* **33** 1702–25

[10] Buckner C A, Venkatesan A, Locklin J K and Wood B J 2011 Real-time sonography with electromagnetic tracking navigation for biopsy of a hepatic neoplasm seen only on arterial phase computed tomography *J. Ultrasound Med.* **30** 253–6

[11] Franz A M, März K, Hummel J, Birkfellner W, Bendl R and Delorme S *et al* 2012 Electromagnetic tracking for US-guided interventions: standardized assessment of a new compact field generator *Int. J. Comput. Assist. Radiol. Surg.* **7** 813–8

[12] Hastenteufel M, Vetter M, Meinzer H-P and Wolf I 2006 Effect of 3D ultrasound probes on the accuracy of electromagnetic tracking systems *Ultrasound Med. Biol.* **32** 1359–68

[13] Ipsen S, Bruder R, Jauer P, Ernst F, Blanck O and Schweikard A 2016 An improved tracking framework for ultrasound probe localization in image-guided radiosurgery *Curr. Dir. Biomed. Eng.* **2** 409–13
[14] Lange T and Eulenstein S 2002 Calibration of swept-volume 3-D ultrasound *Proc. of Medical Image Understanding and Analysis, MIUA (Portsmouth, UK)* pp 29–32
[15] Poon T C and Rohling R N 2005 Comparison of calibration methods for spatial tracking of a 3-D ultrasound probe *Ultrasound Med. Biol.* **31** 1095–108
[16] Tsai R Y and Lenz R K 1989 A new technique for fully autonomous and efficient 3D robotics hand/eye calibration *IEEE Trans. Robot. Automat.* **5** 345–58
[17] Horaud R and Dornaika F 1995 Hand-Eye Calibration *Int. J. Rob. Res.* **14** 195–210
[18] Zhuang H and Shiu Y C 1992 A noise tolerant algorithm for wrist-mounted robotic sensor calibration with or without sensor orientation measurement *Proc. of the IEEE/RSJ Int. Conf. on Intelligent Robots and Systems* (IEEE) pp 1095–100
[19] Schlosser J, Kirmizibayrak C, Shamdasani V, Metz S and Hristov D 2013 Automatic 3D ultrasound calibration for image guided therapy using intramodality image registration *Phys. Med. Biol.* **58** 7481–96
[20] Ernst F, Richter L, Matthäus L, Martens V, Bruder R and Schlaefer A *et al* 2012 Non-orthogonal tool/flange and robot/world calibration *Int. J. Med. Robot.* **8** 407–20
[21] Bergmeir C, Seitel M, Frank C, De Simone R, Meinzer H P and Wolf I 2009 Comparing calibration approaches for 3D ultrasound probes *Int. J. Comput. Assist. Radiol. Surg.* **4** 203–13
[22] Mercier L, Langø T, Lindseth F and Collins D L 2005 A review of calibration techniques for freehand 3-D ultrasound systems *Ultrasound Med. Biol.* **31** 449–71
[23] Schwaab J, Kurz C, Sarti C, Bongers A, Schoenahl F and Bert C *et al* 2015 First steps toward ultrasound-based motion compensation for imaging and therapy: calibration with an optical system and 4D PET imaging *Front. Oncol.* **5** 258
[24] Huang X, Gutierrez L F, Stanton D, Kim P C W and Jain A 2010 Image registration based 3D TEE-EM calibration *2010 IEEE Int. Symp. on Biomedical Imaging: From Nano to Macro* (IEEE) pp 1209–12
[25] Ipsen S, Bruder R, Kuhlemann I, Jauer P, Motisi L and Cremers F *et al* 2018 A visual probe positioning tool for 4D ultrasound-guided radiotherapy *Conf. Proc. IEEE Eng. Med. Biol. Soc.* **2018** 883–6
[26] De Luca V, Benz T, Kondo S, König L, Lübke D and Rothlübbers S *et al* 2015 The 2014 liver ultrasound tracking benchmark *Phys. Med. Biol.* **60** 5571–99
[27] De Luca V, Banerjee J, Hallack A, Kondo S, Makhinya M and Nouri D *et al* 2018 Evaluation of 2D and 3D ultrasound tracking algorithms and impact on ultrasound-guided liver radiotherapy margins *Med. Phys.* **45** 4986–5003
[28] Mast T D 2000 Empirical relationships between acoustic parameters in human soft tissues *ARLO.* **1** 37–42
[29] Carson P L 1978 Biomedical ultrasonics. By P.N.T. Wells, PhD, Academic Press, Inc. London, Copyright 1977. 635 pages. $46.90 *J. Clin. Ultrasound* **6** 126–7 (book review)
[30] Barr R G, Rim A, Graham R, Berg W and Grajo J 2009 Speed of sound imaging: improved image quality in breast sonography *Ultrasound Q.* **25** 141–4
[31] Fontanarosa D, van der Meer S, Bloemen-van Gurp E, Stroian G and Verhaegen F 2012 Magnitude of speed of sound aberration corrections for ultrasound image guided radiotherapy for prostate and other anatomical sites *Med. Phys.* **39** 5286–92

[32] Salter B J, Wang B, Szegedi M W, Rassiah-Szegedi P, Shrieve D C and Cheng R *et al* 2008 Evaluation of alignment error due to a speed artifact in stereotactic ultrasound image guidance *Phys. Med. Biol.* **53** N437–45

[33] Fontanarosa D, van der Meer S, Harris E and Verhaegen F A 2011 CT based correction method for speed of sound aberration for ultrasound based image guided radiotherapy *Med. Phys.* **38** 2665–73

[34] van der Meer S, Bloemen-van Gurp E, Hermans J, Voncken R, Heuvelmans D and Gubbels C *et al* 2013 Critical assessment of intramodality 3D ultrasound imaging for prostate IGRT compared to fiducial markers *Med. Phys.* **40** 071707

[35] Li M, Ballhausen H, Hegemann N-S, Ganswindt U, Manapov F and Tritschler S *et al* 2015 A comparative assessment of prostate positioning guided by three-dimensional ultrasound and cone beam CT *Radiat Oncol.* **10** 82

[36] Fontanarosa D, van der Meer S and Verhaegen F 2012 On the significance of density-induced speed of sound variations on US-guided radiotherapy *Med. Phys.* **39** 6316–23

[37] Bloemen-van Gurp E, van der Meer S, Hendry J, Buijsen J, Visser P and Fontanarosa D *et al* 2013 Active breathing control in combination with ultrasound imaging: a feasibility study of image guidance in stereotactic body radiation therapy of liver lesions *Int. J. Radiat. Oncol. Biol. Phys.* **85** 1096–102

[38] Molloy J A, Chan G, Markovic A, McNeeley S, Pfeiffer D and Salter B *et al* 2011 Quality assurance of U.S.-guided external beam radiotherapy for prostate cancer: report of AAPM Task Group 154 *Med. Phys.* **38** 857–71

[39] Fargier-Voiron M, Presles B, Pommier P, Rit S, Munoz A and Liebgott H *et al* 2014 Impact of probe pressure variability on prostate localization for ultrasound-based image-guided radiotherapy *Radiother. Oncol.* **111** 132–7

[40] Li M, Hegemann N-S, Manapov F, Kolberg A, Thum P D and Ganswindt U *et al* 2017 Prefraction displacement and intrafraction drift of the prostate due to perineal ultrasound probe pressure *Strahlenther. Onkol.* **193** 459–65

[41] Baker M and Behrens C F 2015 Prostate displacement during transabdominal ultrasound image-guided radiotherapy assessed by real-time four-dimensional transperineal monitoring *Acta Oncol.* **54** 1508–14

[42] Mantel F, Richter A, Groh C, Lawrenz I, Weick S and Polat B *et al* 2016 Changes in penile bulb dose when using the clarity transperineal ultrasound probe: a planning study. Pract *Radiat Oncol.* **6** e337–44

[43] Mangar S A, Sydes M R, Tucker H L, Coffey J, Sohaib S A and Gianolini S *et al* 2006 Evaluating the relationship between erectile dysfunction and dose received by the penile bulb: using data from a randomised controlled trial of conformal radiotherapy in prostate cancer (MRC RT01, ISRCTN47772397) *Radiother. Oncol.* **80** 355–62

[44] Lediju Bell M A, Şen H T, Iordachita I, Kazanzides P and Wong J 2014 *In vivo* reproducibility of robotic probe placement for a novel ultrasound-guided radiation therapy system *J. Med. Imag.* **1** 025001

Chapter 4

Ultrasound probe setup and image quality

Saskia Camps, Alexander Grimwood and Sarah Mason

The ability of an operator to find a suitable acoustic viewing window that allows for visualisation of the anatomical structures of interest with sufficient image quality is crucial for the usability of the ultrasound images during radiotherapy workflows. This chapter describes clinical image quality requirements for radiotherapy purposes as well as general ultrasound quality conventions, such as spatial resolution, and how artefacts can affect image quality. In addition to the more traditional visual inspection of the images, it also explores automatic quality assessment of ultrasound images. The final part of the chapter focuses on the improvement of ultrasound image quality. Image quality can be improved by, for example, assisting the operator to find a suitable acoustic viewing window or performing spatial compounding of ultrasound images acquired from several viewing angles.

4.1 Introduction

Despite the many advantages of ultrasound, which were outlined in chapter 1, the use of ultrasound imaging is presently not widespread in clinical radiotherapy workflows. This can be mainly attributed to the need for a highly trained operator to perform the ultrasound image acquisition and interpret the images afterwards.

In current clinical practice, ultrasound imaging is primarily used for diagnostic purposes [1]. During diagnostic imaging, an operator has to manually position the ultrasound probe on or close to the patient's body part of interest, which enables the collection of a live stream of ultrasound images of the internal anatomy. While moving the ultrasound probe on the patient's body, the operator has to continuously assess the quality of the ultrasound images in this live stream and verify if the correct anatomical structures are visualised. This is crucial in order to find a suitable (acoustic) viewing window for this patient. Also, when the viewing window is found, ultrasound image quality has to be monitored continuously, as small motion of the patient or changes in

doi:10.1088/978-0-7503-2552-3ch4

anatomical structures can (heavily) compromise image quality. This quality deterioration can result from, for example, a loss of acoustic coupling and/or a sudden appearance of shadowing artefacts.

As described in chapters 6 and 7, ultrasound imaging can be used for interfraction and intrafraction motion monitoring by the acquisition of images both during simulation and treatment. The ultrasound image acquisition workflow during these stages is similar to the diagnostic workflow described in the previous paragraph. At the simulation stage, the ultrasound images are typically acquired immediately before or after the computed tomography (CT) scan in the CT room [2]. This usually takes up to 10 minutes during which the ultrasound operator is present in the CT room. The technicians who are responsible for the acquisition of the simulation CT scan and the radiation delivery are not trained for ultrasound image acquisition of various body parts. This implies that either these technicians need to complete sonography training, which has a steep learning curve associated with it, or that a trained sonographer needs to be present at simulation in addition to these technicians.

Also at treatment stage, an operator with ultrasound training needs to position the ultrasound probe on the body of the patient. However, in the case of intrafraction motion monitoring, the operator has to leave the treatment room after the probe is positioned and before the irradiation starts. For this reason, the ultrasound probe cannot be held manually by the operator and a device, such as a holder [3], mechanical arm [4], or robotic arm [5] has to be used to fix the probe instead (chapter 9). During the radiation delivery, small motions of the patient or changes in anatomical structures, as described in the diagnostic workflow, can occur. For this reason, the ultrasound image quality has to be assessed continuously during the treatment to promptly identify quality loss and, if necessary, take appropriate action. Also, this continuous assessment would need to be performed by a trained operator or a specifically trained technician.

Automatic assessment of the ultrasound image quality can be of great help during several steps in the above described workflows. It can provide guidance to less experienced ultrasound operators, allowing them to acquire good quality ultrasound images that can be used for inter- and intrafraction motion monitoring. This could result in less operator dependence. In addition, the quality of the ultrasound images could be automatically assessed during treatment and the technician would only need to take appropriate action when a quality warning is issued, instead of continuously monitoring the images visually.

4.2 Clinical requirements for ultrasound image quality in radiotherapy

Some of the image quality requirements to be fulfilled by an ultrasound image used in a radiotherapy workflow are the same as for diagnostic ultrasound imaging. Such a requirement is, for example, related to the initial ultrasound probe setup on the body of the patient. For each individual patient, a viewing window needs to be found that allows the visualisation of the anatomical structures of interest. To further improve structure visualisation, every ultrasound device allows a number of scan parameters to be varied, which can significantly alter the ultrasound image visualisation and/or acquisition approach. These parameters, which are described in detail in chapter 2, influence the imaging depth, frame rate, width of the ultrasound sector, gain, dynamic range and many other image attributes [6]. A possible metric for ultrasound image quality could be based on the ability of an expert to localise relevant anatomical structures on the ultrasound image during visual inspection [7].

To allow for interfraction motion monitoring, the shape and absolute position of the anatomical structure of interest at both simulation stage and prior to each treatment fraction need to be compared [1] (see chapter 6). The ultrasound image quality metric could also be based on the ability of an expert to contour the relevant anatomical structure on the ultrasound image.

For intrafraction monitoring, typically an initial contour has to be input into a tracking algorithm (for example, [3]) that subsequently tracks the motion of the corresponding anatomical structure during radiation delivery (chapter 7). This initial contour can be provided by the segmentation generated for interfraction motion monitoring (see previous paragraph). However, the quality of the ultrasound images acquired during the treatment delivery has to be sufficient to follow the position of the anatomical structure of interest over time. Therefore, the ultrasound image quality metric could also be based on the ability of an algorithm to track the relevant anatomical structures over time based only on acquired ultrasound images.

A big difference between ultrasound imaging for diagnostic purposes and ultrasound imaging for motion monitoring during radiotherapy is related to the ultrasound probe pressure. In order to acquire an ultrasound image with good quality, the application of pressure on the probe is sometimes required. However, this pressure might result in a deformation and/or displacement of the anatomical structures of interest [8–11] (see chapter 3). To allow for absolute motion monitoring this pressure has to be reduced as much as possible or has to be reproduced from one imaging session to the next ([8–11]). Therefore, the ultrasound image quality metric could also be based on the occurrences of anatomical structure displacements or deformations due to probe pressure.

4.3 Ultrasound image quality conventions

Before the introduction of automatic quality assessment approaches, ultrasound image quality was primarily assessed using visual inspection and the calculation of a number of basic metrics which involves manual labour from an expert. The aim of this section is to give a brief overview of these visual inspection and metric calculation techniques. More detailed information regarding this topic can be found in the literature (see chapter 2 and e.g. [12]).

One of the traditional ways to assess the ultrasound image quality is by assessing the spatial resolution [13]. This metric gives information on the ability to distinguish two closely spaced objects in the ultrasound image. The spatial resolution can be determined in several directions: axial resolution (parallel to the ultrasound beam), lateral resolution (perpendicular to the ultrasound beam) and elevational resolution (perpendicular to the imaging plane). In addition to the spatial resolution, also the contrast resolution [13] can be used to assess the ultrasound image quality. This resolution metric refers to the ability to differentiate between tissues with different characteristics using contrast in the images. Typically, the spatial resolution and contrast resolution of an imaging system (ultrasound device and ultrasound probe combination) are assessed using phantoms (e.g. CIRS model 054GS) of which an example is given in figure 4.1. This initial assessment is done by a trained operator who performs a visual inspection of the images. In the end, this initial assessment can be confirmed by visual inspection of ultrasound images of human subjects.

The nature of ultrasound imaging can result in a variety of different image artefacts that find their origin in different aspects of the physics that is involved in the image acquisition [14]. Some artefacts can have a positive effect on the image perception, like speckle, which may allow the observer to distinguish adjacent tissues (see section 2.1.2), others can cause the ultrasound image quality to significantly deteriorate. For example, acoustic shadowing artefacts can occur below anatomical structures that strongly absorb or reflect the ultrasound waves. This and overall attenuation of ultrasound with depth results in reduced visualisation of the structures located deeper in the tissue (see figures 4.2(a) and (b)). On the other hand, this artefact can also be used for, for example, the detection of kidney stones. Conversely, below weekly attenuating tissues, i.e., the bladder, artificially brighter bands of image intensity may lead to the misinterpretation of images [15].

Artefacts can also occur due to assumptions made about the propagation path of the ultrasound waves [14]. For example, if the ultrasound waves encounter an interface between two tissues at a non-perpendicular angle, the difference in acoustic impedance of both tissues can cause refraction (described in section 2.1.3). The refracted portion of the wave could then encounter a reflector and cause an echo which is received by the transducer. As ultrasound devices make the assumption that all echoes have traveled a direct path, this would result in a display of this reflector at a wrong location. Reverberation artefacts occur when sound is reflected multiple times between boundaries. Image formation also assumes that sound is reflected back towards the transducer once and when this assumption is violated, reverberation, ring-down, comet-tails and mirror images may appear below the boundary

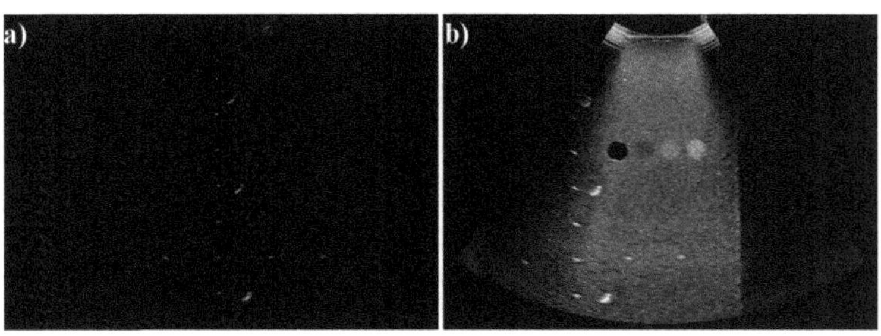

Figure 4.1. Example of an ultrasound quality assessment phantom scanned with a curvilinear probe, where: (a) acquisition parameters have been adjusted to suppress background and measure resolution targets; (b) acquisition parameters have been optimised to enable characterisation of one anechoic target and three contrast targets.

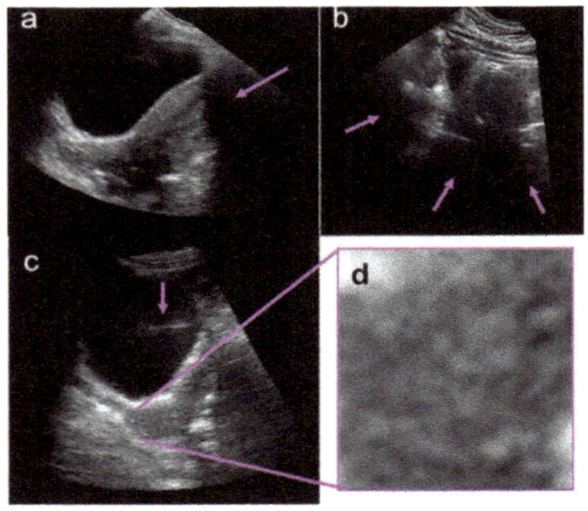

Figure 4.2. Example of artefacts observed in abdominal ultrasound images of the uterus. In (a), the fundus of the uterus is obscured by acoustic shadowing which is likely to be caused by gas in the overlying bowel. In general, the ultrasound image signal-to-noise will be attenuated as it propagates further through tissue and as demonstrated in (b), the useful imaging depth is limited. Reverberations from strongly reflecting boundaries can be observed at depths beneath the boundary, in the case of (c), a strongly reflecting boundary is present near or at the skin surface. Speckle, depicted in (d) can be considered useful for differentiating different tissues, however, some observers consider it distracting and therefore spatial compounding techniques (discussed in section 4.5.2) are used to reduce speckle. Image courtesy of Sarah Mason.

from which the sound is reflected [16] (see figure 4.2(c)). These artefacts are typically recognized visually by a trained operator during manual acquisition of the ultrasound images and can be reduced, or in some cases eliminated, by a skilled operator.

Artefacts may arise from the probe itself, for example element drop out will result in dark lines in the image where elements have either lost sensitivity or are completely functionless. Finally, artefacts can also arise from side lobes and grating lobes [14]. When detected echoes do not originate from the main beam, i.e. from side or grating lobes, they may appear to originate from other structures and be mistaken for tissue boundaries [15]. These types of artefacts can be picked up by a good ultrasound quality assurance protocol, which is an essential part of maintaining USgRT equipment.

4.4 Automatic quality assessment

In the literature a few papers can be found that explore automatic ultrasound image quality assessment (e.g. [17–20]). Even though the majority of these papers focus on diagnostic use of ultrasound imaging, the quality assessment approaches described in these papers are potentially also applicable to radiotherapy workflows. In principle, some of the ultrasound image quality conventions described in the previous paragraph can also be of use for automatic quality assessment.

One of the automatic quality assessment strategies reported in the literature involves manual crafting of features that give an indication of the image quality. These features are then used to train an algorithm such that it can assess the ultrasound image quality. This approach has been deployed by Schwaab *et al* [18]. In this work, an automatic image quality assessment system has been proposed for the assessment of automated breast ultrasound images. The aim was to train an algorithm to identify ultrasound images that contain specific artefacts in the images, such as a shadow caused by the nipple. In total three types of artefacts were investigated and for each of them a number of features, like the absolute nipple position, was manually crafted. Schwaab *et al* showed that even though the sensitivity of the algorithm trained using these features was only moderate, the specificity was 99% which made the algorithm useful in clinical practice. The approach described in this work could potentially be used in a breast cancer radiotherapy scenario without many modifications. A drawback of the manual feature crafting strategy is, however, that it requires a substantial amount of time from operators and it is heavily application specific.

Another strategy that can be found in the literature does not require any manual feature crafting, but instead involves the use of a deep learning algorithm that can generate its own features to distinguish between good and poor quality images. Camps *et al* [7, 20] published a deep learning strategy to perform automatic image quality assessment of 2D ultrasound images out of a 3D volume of the male pelvic region. In order to provide the deep learning algorithm with labeled images for training, a quality score was assigned to each image in the available database indicating the usability of this image during a prostate cancer radiotherapy workflow. If the prostate could be identified by an operator, the ultrasound image was classified as a good quality image, while if the prostate could not be identified the image quality was considered poor. Subsequently, in the same study a deep learning algorithm based on a DenseNet [21] and Gaussian Processes [22] was trained on this labeled data to perform the quality score assignment task automatically. In the end, the performance of the deep learning algorithm was compared with visual classification by three experts and it was shown that this algorithm performs at least as well as the worst performing expert.

In obstetrics, papers have been published (e.g. [17] and [23]) in which the ability to automatically segment specific anatomical structures in the ultrasound images, like foetal head or stomach bubble, gives an indication of the ultrasound image quality. The algorithm used to automatically segment the anatomical structures could be based on both manually and automatically determined features. In the USgRT field, papers have been published on automatic segmentation of anatomical structures (see chapters 5 and 10 and [24]), however, the performance of these algorithms has not been linked to image quality assessment yet.

Quality assessment of image registrations have also been implemented for both interfraction ultrasound guidance and intrafraction motion monitoring. In its simplest form, the value of a cost function used to find the optimal spatial transformation between fixed and moving images can be used to assess registration quality. This has proved problematic, because the cost function is also susceptible to changes in the inherent properties of an image, such as contrast-to-noise ratio (CNR), or variations in the appearance of anatomical features caused by changes to the insonation angle (figure 4.3). This is a common occurrence in interfraction matching, where the probe position tends to vary for each scan. Registration assessment of intrafraction image sequences has proved more successful. The Elekta Clarity system incorporates a classification-based machine learning approach to

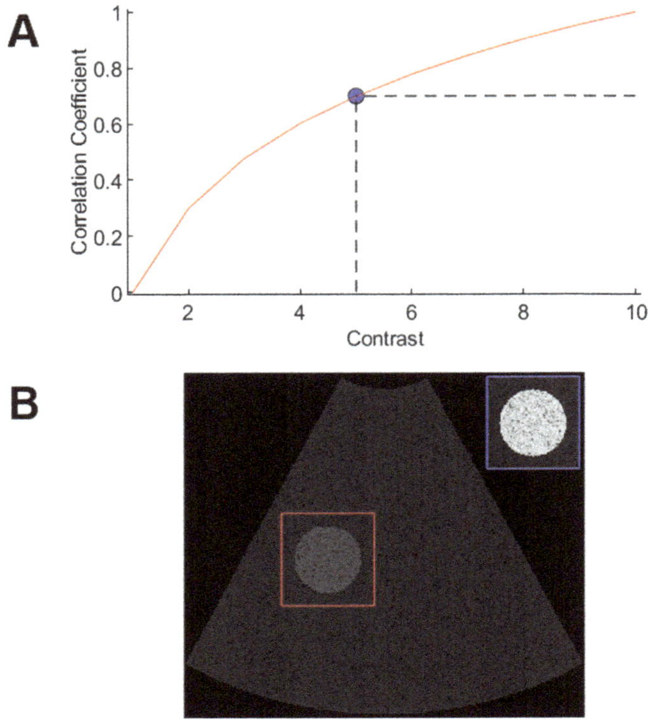

Figure 4.3. This interactive figure shows a plot of registration quality metric, correlation coefficient, as a function of image contrast (A), for a simulated ultrasound image (B). The reference feature is shown in the blue box and the registration location is denoted by the red box. Animation available at https://iopscience.iop.org/book/978-0-7503-2552-3.

predict the quality of prostate intrafraction motion estimates. Features derived from the scan data and cost function are used to predict the reliability of motion estimates [25]. A study assessing registration quality metrics on an intrafraction prostate ultrasound dataset identified the distinctiveness of the optimum cost function value as a significant indicator, along with the peak cross correlation value [26].

4.5 Methods for image quality improvement

4.5.1 Automated probe set up and operator assistance

Ultrasound-guided radiotherapy is possible only if adequate image quality can be achieved. Optimising image quality is further complicated by a lack of staff with sonography experience and by a need to scan patients continuously without staff present in the treatment room. To address these particular constraints, commercial ultrasound guidance systems incorporate adaptations designed to assist the operator when setting up the probe. These adaptations aid the process of consistently positioning the probe and optimising scan parameters during patient setup.

Probe set up can be defined by three tasks: the probe must be suitably positioned to ensure adequate field of view coverage of the relevant anatomical site; image

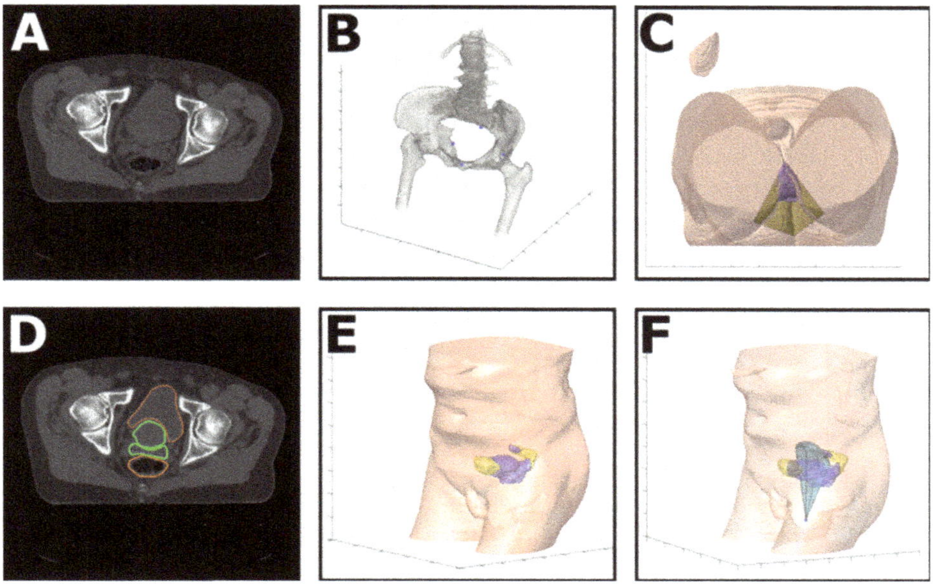

Figure 4.4. Method for patient-specific probe setup proposition. (A) Simulation CT scan; (B) binary bone mask with internal perineum boundaries indicated with blue dots; (C) total perineal surface (yellow) with the perineal skin accessible for probe setup in blue; (D) CT scan with anatomical target delineations in green and organs at risk in orange; (E) 3D representation of the anatomical structures with structures required in the field of view of the ultrasound in blue and the optional structures in yellow; (F) field of view of a possible patient-specific ultrasound probe setup.

quality must be optimised; finally, the overall system configuration must be consistent and repeatable across scan sessions.

Both Elekta Clarity (Elekta AB, Sweden) and NOMOS BATCAM (Best NOMOS, USA) systems optically track the ultrasound probe, as described in chapter 3. This enables the display of probe position information to an operator. For example, on treatment, Clarity displays a pair of trapezoidal symbols during patient setup. One symbol represents the probe field of view position at simulation and the other shows the current position in real time. This helps users to qualitatively assess the repeatability of probe positioning relative to the room laser isocentre.

In addition to the commercial solutions, Camps *et al* [4] have introduced a method that proposes a patient-specific transperineal ultrasound probe setup based on the simulation CT scan and corresponding anatomical structure delineations (see figure 4.4). The first step of this method was to extract a binary bone mask from the CT scan, which was then used to identify internal perineum boundaries (figure 4.4(B)). Subsequently, the perineum surface was constructed, projected to the skin and the perineal skin which was accessible for probe positioning was identified (see figure 4.4(C)). After segmentation of the target and the organs at risk, a decision was made regarding what anatomical structures are required in the ultrasound field of view (figures 4.4(D) and 4.4(E)). Finally, an algorithm evaluated all possible ultrasound probe setups to identify which configurations were most suited to the patient (figure 4.4(F)). The algorithm enabled visualisation of all required anatomical structures, assuming the proposed setup could be reproduced on the patient.

The range and complexity of possible scan parameters presents a challenge to any ultrasound user. As such, predefined scan protocols are routinely used to assist operators. Even within these protocols, on a typical diagnostic scanner, the sonographer is provided a high degree of control over scan settings. A clear difference between USgRT and diagnostic systems is the limited number of available protocols and the restrictions on operators to alter settings. These measures are intended to increase reliance on predefined scan parameters and promote consistency between operators and scan sessions.

4.5.2 Improving image quality through spatial compounding

Low probe-pressure scanning (see section 3.3.3 on probe pressure), operator and observer inexperience, a limited field of view and imaging artefacts including speckle can all contribute to the degradation of ultrasound image quality. Mason *et al* [27] proposed that the loss of image quality due to such factors may be partially restored by using 3D extended aperture (EA) spatial compounding. 3D-EA spatial compounding involves overlapping and mosaicking 3D ultrasound images acquired at multiple probe positions and orientations into a single 3D image. It was proposed that 3D-EA spatial compounding could decrease image noise (through speckle reduction), enhance the echo amplitude from tissue boundaries, and increase the field of view, thereby providing a better overall visualisation of the uterus. This approach is made possible by the optical tracking technology used for registration of ultrasound images with the radiotherapy room coordinate system (see chapter 3). Here we will provide a theoretical explanation of the benefits of conventional image compounding and discuss the advantages, in terms of image quality, of 3D-EA spatial compounding.

Spatial compounding is a well-established technique in 2D ultrasound imaging that insonates a region of tissue from different orientations [28–30]. As illustrated in figure 4.5, compounding can be achieved using different approaches. Common approaches include (i) 'multi-angle compound imaging' technique pioneered by

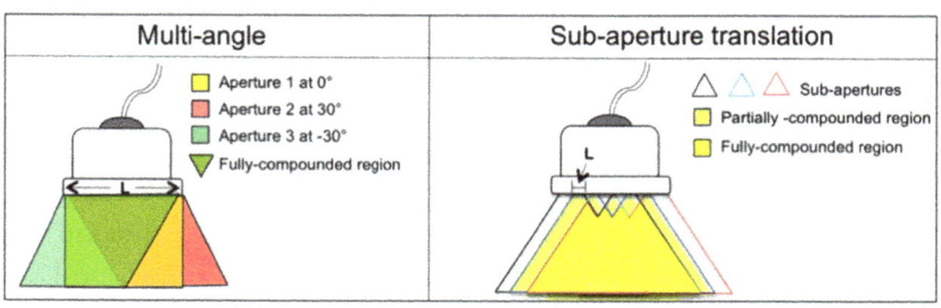

Figure 4.5. Schematic illustration of two conventional 2D spatial compounding approaches. Left: multi-angle compound imaging [30] using three apertures of length '*L*' to generate beams at 0°, 30°, and −30°. The fully compounded region is smaller than the total field of view and decreases with increasing imaging depth. Right: sub-aperture translation using six sub-apertures of length '*L*'. The fully-compounded region is larger and '*L*' is smaller compared with multi-angle compounding.

Jespersen *et al* [30], which generates ultrasound beams at different angles by activating the elements on a 1D transducer steering the sound beam in different directions, forming a sequence of simple linear-scan images with slightly different but overlapping fields of view, and (ii) by translating a sub-aperture of size 'L' across the length of the full array, forming a sequence of simple sector scans with overlapping fields of view.

Spatial compounding involves imaging the same structure from various angles and, therefore, boundary enhancement may be achieved by increasing the proportion of tissue boundaries that are oriented perpendicularly to (or nearly perpendicularly to) the incident sound wave, and thus the strongest echoes are reflected [30]. See section 2.1.3 for more discussion of ultrasound reflection. Spatial compounding reduces speckle because the speckle pattern changes when the angle of incidence of the sound beam changes. Therefore, averaging over multiple angles of incidence will reduce the speckle variance (σ^2) in intensity values of a homogeneous background region (i.e. a region with no resolvable structures) within an ultrasound image. Reducing speckle improves image quality, as both the signal-to-noise ratio (SNR) and contrast-to-noise ratio (CNR) increase with decreasing σ, as demonstrated in equations 4.1 and 4.2.

$$SNR = \frac{\mu_b}{\sigma_b} \tag{4.1}$$

where:

μ_b: is the mean intensity of a homogenous background region;

σ_b: is the standard deviation of the intensities of a homogenous background region.

$$CNR = \frac{\left|\mu_f - \mu_b\right|}{\sqrt{\sigma_f^2 + \sigma_b^2}} \tag{4.2}$$

where:

μ_f: is the mean intensity of a homogenous foreground region;

σ_f: is the standard deviation of the intensities of a homogenous foreground region.

Spatial compounding has the potential to improve the SNR by a factor of $\sqrt{N}$ (where N is the number of individual images included in the image compound) provided the speckle pattern from each image is statistically independent [31]. To achieve statistically independent speckle, it is favourable to have small sub-apertures to provide a greater number of independent viewpoints. However, as demonstrated by equation 4.3 [32], there is a trade-off between aperture size (L) and lateral resolution: the smaller L is, the worse the lateral resolution.

$$LR = \frac{n\lambda F}{L} \tag{4.3}$$

where:

LR: is the lateral resolution of the ultrasound system;
n: is a constant depending on the measurement technique;
λ: is the ultrasound wavelength;
F: is the focal depth;
L: is the length of the aperture.

In the case of multi-angle compounding, lateral resolution is mostly preserved as *L* spans the whole width of the transducer for each aperture, however, the whole field of view (FOV) of the ultrasound image is not fully compounded, as the area of overlap between different viewpoints decreases with increasing imaging depth, as shown in figure 4.4. Though the sub-aperture translation approach provides a larger fully-compounded region at large depth, the small sub-aperture size required substantially degrades lateral resolution. Furthermore, it is often not possible to steer the ultrasound beam from a fixed array such that every portion of a tissue boundary is perpendicularly insonated (or insonated at all), especially for large structures such as the uterus. This not only restricts the potential for enhancing tissue boundaries, but also severely limits the field of view of the ultrasound system.

4.5.3 Improvements offered by 3D-extended aperture spatial compounding

To overcome the limitations of conventional 2D compounding, there is an opportunity for the optical-tracking technology of the USgRT system to be used to perform 3D-extended aperture spatial compounding. With knowledge of the spatial location of individual 3D ultrasound volume images, it is possible to combine them into one larger image; this not only provides a means by which to extend the field of view, but overlapping regions between different volumes may provide additional information and increase both the CNR and SNR without reducing the aperture length. This method will result in an extension of the aperture compared to a single ultrasound volume image. It should be noted here, however, that an increase in aperture in this case cannot result in an improvement in the lateral resolution of the systems as the ultrasound echoes used to form neighboring 3D ultrasound volumes are not focussed at the same point and are not summed coherently.

Mason and colleagues [27] showed that 3D-extended aperture (3D-EA) spatial compounding using the Clarity system has the potential to improve ultrasound imaging in gynaecological radiotherapy. They proposed that a large number of ultrasound image volumes could be acquired at low probe pressure by a relatively inexperienced operator and combined to provide a large FOV, high contrast view of the uterus during treatment. Using 3D ultrasound images acquired from healthy volunteers and patients, Mason *et al* asked observers to rank the image quality of an original single 3D ultrasound image and several 3D-EA compounded images of the uterus. 3D-EA images consisted of an increasing number of single 3D ultrasound images acquired with a hand-held 3D ultrasound mechanically swept probe and the Elekta Clarity system at slightly varying positions and orientations on the abdomen.

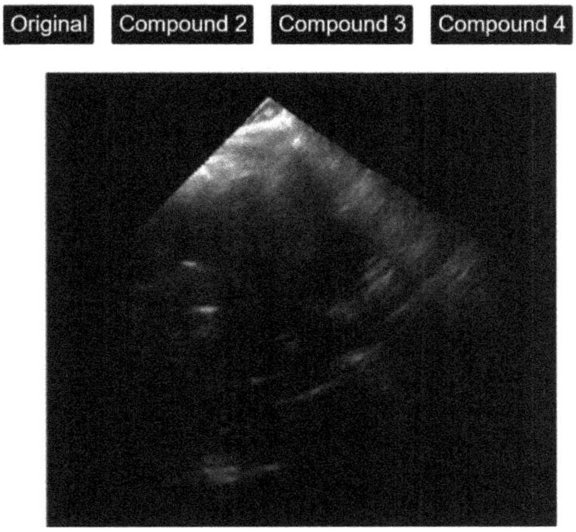

Figure 4.6. This interactive figure demonstrates how 3D extended aperture compounding can be used to improve image quality of an original image that can be considered. The buttons allow for a selection of a number of transabdominal ultrasound images to be included in the image compound of the uterus. Note, how the uterus is not visible in the original poor quality image and after the addition of three images acquired at alternative views, the boundary of the uterus can be discerned. Animation available at https://iopscience.iop.org/book/978-0-7503-2552-3.

Images were compounded using spatial averaging. Observers were blind to the number of images used to make the compounded image. This study showed that the image quality ranking statistically significantly improved as the number of images comprising the compounded image was increased. Image quality increased with up to three images and five images for patient and volunteer data, respectively. This is illustrated in figure 4.6. Mason *et al* argued that 3D-EA can improve image quality for a small time penalty; additional images took less than a minute to acquire and a similar time was required to compound the images. This approach has so far only been tested in the context of cervical cancer, but could be applied to any cancer site in the abdomen.

Consolidation quiz

Q1: Ultrasound probe setup and image quality assessment are predominantly manual tasks. Why are these tasks particularly challenging in a radiotherapy environment?

- ○ Ultrasound scanners cannot acquire images during radiotherapy delivery
- ○ Radiotherapy staff typically has limited experience with ultrasonography
- ○ The ultrasound probe must never be held by the operator

Q2: The clinical requirements of ultrasound in radiotherapy are similar to those of diagnostic ultrasound. One important difference in ultrasound image guidance is the need to maintain a consistently small probe pressure. Why?

- ○ To ensure the patient remains relaxed at all times

- To ensure the patient geometry at each treatment session is consistent
- To avoid annoying the radiotherapy oncologist

Q3: Which of these is not a common ultrasound imaging artifact?

- Shadowing
- Reverberation
- Cavitation

Q4: Why is automated quality assessment important?

- Automated quality assessment can reduce interobserver variation and improve image guidance accuracy
- Automated quality assessment improves ultrasound acquisition frame rates
- Manually assessing image quality is physically impossible

Q5: Peak detection, minimum detection and averaging are all methods of what?

- Combining regions of overlap from multiple ultrasound images
- Measuring lateral resolution in spatially compounded images
- Calculating sub-aperture translations for spatial compounding

References

[1] Fontanarosa D, van der Meer S, Bamber J, Harris E, O'Shea T and Verhaegen F 2015 Review of ultrasound image guidance in external beam radiotherapy: I. Treatment planning and inter-fraction motion management *Phys. Med. Biol.* **60** R77–114

[2] Grimwood A, McNair H A, O'Shea T P, Gilroy S, Thomas K and Bamber J C *et al* 2018 *In Vivo* validation of Elekta's clarity autoscan for ultrasound-based intrafraction motion estimation of the prostate during radiation therapy *Int. J. Radiat. Oncol. Biol. Phys.* **102** 912–21

[3] Lachaine M and Falco T 2013 Intrafractional prostate motion management with the clarity Autoscan system *Med. Phys. Int.* **1** 72–80

[4] Camps S, Verhaegen F, Vanneste B G L, de With P H N and Fontanarosa D 2018 Automated patient-specific transperineal ultrasound probe setups for prostate cancer patients undergoing radiotherapy *Med. Phys.* **45** 3185–95

[5] Schlosser J, Salisbury K and Hristov D 2010 Telerobotic system concept for real-time soft-tissue imaging during radiotherapy beam delivery *Med. Phys.* **37** 6357–67

[6] El-Zehiry N, Yan M, Good S, Fang T, Zhou S K and Grady L 2013 Learning the manifold of quality ultrasound acquisition *Med. Image Comput. Comput. Assist. Interv.* **16** 122–30

[7] Camps S M, Houben T, Fontanarosa D, Edwards C, Antico M and Dunnhofer M *et al* 2018 One-class Gaussian process regressor for quality assessment of transperineal ultrasound images *Proceedings of the 1st International Conference on Medical Imaging with Deep Learning 2018* ed I Isgum, C Sanchez and G Litjens (Netherlands: Medical Imaging with Deep Learning Conference Committee) pp 1–10

[8] van der Meer S, Bloemen-van Gurp E, Hermans J, Voncken R, Heuvelmans D and Gubbels C *et al* 2013 Critical assessment of intramodality 3D ultrasound imaging for prostate IGRT compared to fiducial markers *Med. Phys.* **40** 071707

[9] Fargier-Voiron M, Presles B, Pommier P, Rit S, Munoz A and Liebgott H *et al* 2014 Impact of probe pressure variability on prostate localization for ultrasound-based image-guided radiotherapy *Radiother. Oncol.* **111** 132–7

[10] Baker M and Behrens C F 2015 Prostate displacement during transabdominal ultrasound image-guided radiotherapy assessed by real-time four-dimensional transperineal monitoring *Acta Oncol.* **54** 1508–14
[11] Li M, Hegemann N-S, Manapov F, Kolberg A, Thum P D and Ganswindt U *et al* 2017 Prefraction displacement and intrafraction drift of the prostate due to perineal ultrasound probe pressure *Strahlenther. Onkol.* **193** 459–65
[12] Hill C R, Bamber J C and ter Haar G R 2004 *Physical Principles of Medical Ultrasonics* (Chichester: Wiley)
[13] Ng A and Swanevelder J 2011 Resolution in ultrasound imaging *Contin. Educ. Anaesth. Crit. Care Pain* **11** 186–92
[14] Kremkau F W and Taylor K J 1986 Artifacts in ultrasound imaging *J. Ultrasound Med.* **5** 227–37
[15] Meiburger K M, Acharya U R and Molinari F 2018 Automated localization and segmentation techniques for B-mode ultrasound images: a review *Comput. Biol. Med.* **92** 210–35
[16] Zagzebski J A 1996 *The Essentials of Ultrasound Physics* (St Louis, MO: Mosby)
[17] Rahmatullah B, Sarris I, Papageorghiou A and Noble J A 2011 Quality control of fetal ultrasound images: detection of abdomen anatomical landmarks using AdaBoost *2011 IEEE Int. Symp. on Biomedical Imaging: From Nano to Macro* (IEEE) p 6–9
[18] Schwaab J, Diez Y, Oliver A, Martí R, Zelst J and van Gubern-Mérida A *et al* 2016 Automated quality assessment in three-dimensional breast ultrasound images *J. Med. Imag.* **3** 027002
[19] Abdi A H, Luong C, Tsang T, Allan G, Nouranian S and Jue J *et al* 2017 Automatic quality assessment of echocardiograms using convolutional neural networks: feasibility on the apical four-chamber view *IEEE Trans. Med. Imag.* **36** 1221–30
[20] Camps S M, Houben T, Carneiro G, Edwards C, Antico M and Dunnhofer M *et al* 2020 Automatic quality assessment of transperineal ultrasound images of the male pelvic region, using deep learning *Ultrasound Med. Biol.* **46** 445–54
[21] Huang G, Liu Z, Maaten L and van der Weinberger K Q 2017 Densely connected convolutional networks *2017 IEEE Conf. on Computer Vision and Pattern Recognition (CVPR)* (Piscataway, NJ: IEEE) pp 2261–9
[22] Kemmler M, Rodner E, Wacker E-S and Denzler J 2013 One-class classification with Gaussian processes *Pattern Recognit.* **46** 3507–18
[23] Zhang L, Dudley N J, Lambrou T, Allinson N and Ye X 2017 Automatic image quality assessment and measurement of fetal head in two-dimensional ultrasound image *J Med. Imag.* **4** 024001
[24] Mason S A, O'Shea T P, White I M, Lalondrelle S, Downey K and Baker M *et al* 2017 Towards ultrasound-guided adaptive radiotherapy for cervical cancer: evaluation of Elekta's semiautomated uterine segmentation method on 3D ultrasound images *Med. Phys.* **44** 3630–8
[25] Brooks R 2017 System and method for target tracking using a quality indicator during radiation therapy *US Patent* WO/2017/001920
[26] Shams R, Xiao Y, Hebert F, Abramowitz M, Brooks R and Rivaz H 2018 Assessment of rigid registration quality measures in ultrasound-guided radiotherapy *IEEE Trans. Med. Imag.* **37** 428–37

[27] Mason S A, White I M, O'Shea T P, Lalondrelle S, Bamber J C and Harris E J 2018 Development of 3D extended-aperture spatial compounding to improve ultrasound-based localization of the uterus for radiotherapy treatment *2018 IEEE Int. Ultrasonics Symp. (IUS)* (Piscataway, NJ: IEEE) pp 1–4
[28] Behar V, Adam D and Friedman Z 2003 A new method of spatial compounding imaging *Ultrasonics* **41** 377–84
[29] Burckhardt C B 1978 Speckle in ultrasound B-mode scans *IEEE Trans. Son. Ultrason.* **25** 1–6
[30] Jespersen S K, Wilhjelm J E and Sillesen H 1998 Multi-angle compound imaging *Ultrason. Imaging* **20** 81–102
[31] Shankar P M 1986 Speckle reduction in ultrasound B-scans using weighted averaging in spatial compounding *IEEE Trans. Ultrason. Ferroelectr. Freq. Control* **33** 754–8
[32] Alomari Z, Harput S, Hyder S and Freear S 2015 The Effect of the transducer parameters on spatial resolution in plane-wave imaging *2015 IEEE Int. Ultrasonics Symp. (IUS)* (Piscataway, NJ: IEEE) pp 1–4

IOP Publishing

Modern Applications of 3D/4D Ultrasound Imaging in Radiotherapy

Emma Harris, Davide Fontanarosa, Saskia Camps and Frank Verhaegen

Chapter 5

Ultrasound in the radiotherapy planning process

Davide Fontanarosa, Emma Harris and Alexander Schlaefer

Ultrasound imaging can contribute to several different stages in the radiotherapy workflow. After a brief introduction to the chapter, the potential role of ultrasound in the definition of treatment targets at the treatment planning stage is presented in section 5.2. For the most advanced planning and treatment strategies, automatic processes are vital, in particular for segmentation of the structures of interest: in section 5.3 the main image processing based methods proposed in literature are reported with particular attention paid to the two currently most clinically relevant organs, the prostate (section 5.3.1) and the uterus (section 5.3.2). In section 5.4, the problem, unique to ultrasound based guidance of radiotherapy, of planning and treating the patient with the presence of a probe in place is discussed; in section 5.4.1 the integration with the other imaging modalities used for planning is presented, while in section 5.4.2 the possible strategies to account for the presence of the probe are introduced.

5.1 Introduction

With ultrasound imaging it is typically possible to visualise soft tissues with a quality superior to computed tomography (CT), both in terms of spatial resolution and contrast. This has led researchers to propose this imaging modality for target and organs at risk segmentation for radiotherapy planning purposes [1, 2]. An example is the identification of the interface between the bladder and the prostate. There are important limitations to this application, though, which have reduced the practical implementation of ultrasound based segmentation in the radiotherapy workflow at planning stage: firstly, ultrasound cannot be used to calculate dose, because it does not provide physical density information, so a CT scan, or more recently a pseudo-CT scan generated from an MR scan [3] is always necessary. Secondly, the field of view (FOV) of ultrasound images or volumes does not include the entire cross section of the patient, but only a portion of it, so it cannot be used to segment all the

doi:10.1088/978-0-7503-2552-3ch5

structures of interest. Even for the structures present in the FOV, it is often difficult to have a complete view of the whole region of interest (ROI), because they may be larger than the FOV or because imaging artefacts may reduce visibility. Finally, co-registration of ultrasound and CT scans is not trivial: even if the scans are performed at the same time point and with the same coordinate system, the two imaging modalities often show the structures with a different appearance, because of the different physics underlying them. For example, contouring the prostate on CT systematically produces volumes which are on average larger than the same organ segmented on ultrasound [4]; therefore, for planning purposes, usually only the CT scan is used to outline the target.

At treatment stage, usually there is no CT scan available; in most cases only a cone beam CT (CBCT) scan is taken of the patient, which has worse quality than CT and is often insufficient to properly segment all the tissues of interest. If an efficient segmentation algorithm is available, an ultrasound guidance system can become valuable not only to set up the patient but also to adapt the treatment (see chapter 8). In particular, for real-time adaptation strategies (see for example [5]), at the time this book is being written, ultrasound is the only viable option, as it is the only volumetric real-time imaging modality compatible with a radiotherapy clinical environment. While at simulation stage automation in contouring is not essential, because planning is performed off-line, at treatment it increases accuracy and speed for interfraction applications and it becomes absolutely vital for intrafraction applications.

5.2 Ultrasound for target volume definition

Several groups have investigated the use of ultrasound to assist with the delineation of the radiotherapy target volume in a number of tumour sites. The majority of work in this area focuses on use of ultrasound to define the breast surgical cavity, which is the target for a boost of radiation using photon or electron external beam radiotherapy. Breast ultrasound plays an important role in the diagnostic pathway as it is commonly used to guide breast biopsy of suspicious lesions and can be considered a natural choice for the localisation of the surgical cavity (or tumour bed) to guide electron boost post lumpectomy [6–9]. Studies of ultrasound localisation of the surgical cavity predate the wide use of CT for planning, however, once CT was introduced it was found that the surgical cavity was not well visualised on CT, with fibroglandular, seroma and scar tissues displayed with similar Hounsfield units. Typically, the surgical cavity was localised on CT by placing a wire on the scar at the skin surface, which was found to be a poor guide because the internal breast tissue could be deformed during surgery and the wire provided no information regarding the depth of the cavity. Using ultrasound the position of the surgical cavity could be identified by seroma (a pocket of blood plasma and inflammatory fluids), which appears as a hypoechogenic region on ultrasound. The localisation of the breast cavity to guide photon boosts and partial breast radiotherapy using 3D ultrasound was proposed by several groups [10–14]. Example 3D ultrasound images of the surgical cavity are shown in figure 5.1. Coles *et al* reported a statistically significant

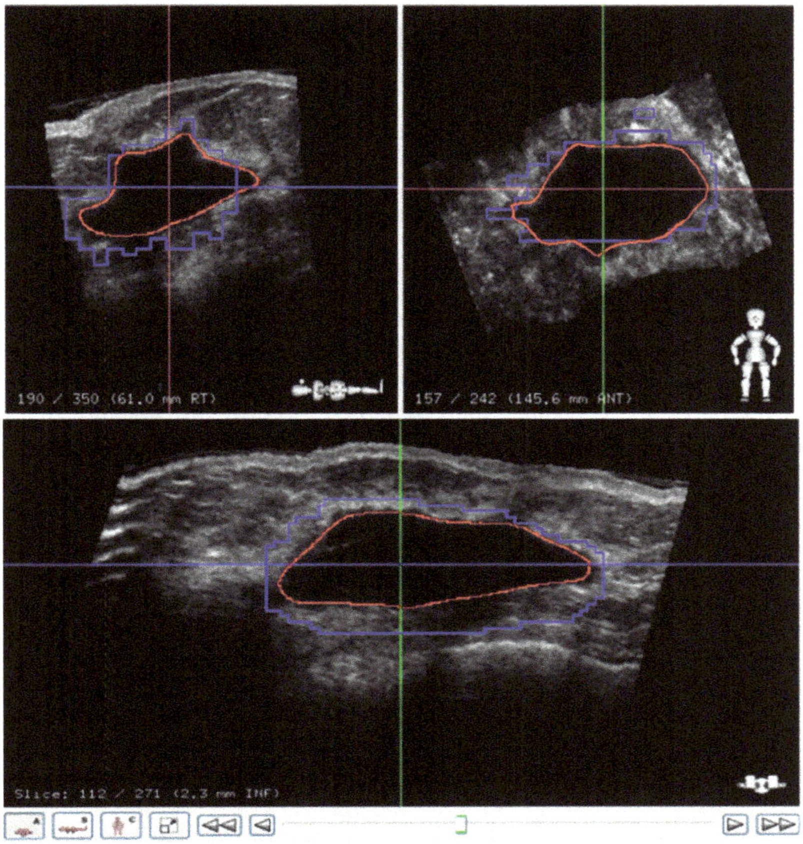

Figure 5.1. Example ultrasound central 2D images in the sagittal (top left), coronal (top right) and axial (bottom) planes sampled from a 3D ultrasound volume. The red contours show clinician outlining of the surgical cavity on ultrasound and the blue contours show outlining of the surgical cavity on CT. On ultrasound the surgical cavity is identified by seroma which is hypoechoic. Reproduced from [14] under Creative Commons Attribution Licence.

improvement in localisation accuracy with 3D ultrasound compared to 2D ultrasound. The use of ultrasound has subsequently been superseded by the use of surgical clips [15] which can be visualised on CT and their routine insertion is now recommended [16]. Comparative studies of the surgical cavity volumes defined using 3D ultrasound and clips have found that ultrasound defines a smaller volume than using clips visualised on CT [10] which results in clinically significant dosimetric differences. In some patients, clip defined volumes on CT were underdosed if ultrasound was used for volume definition. [17–19]. The discrepancy in volume may be explained by the reliance of ultrasound on seroma only to visualise the surgical cavity. In contemporary surgical practice, the cavity is sutured in a way which minimises the accumulation of seroma and the extent of the seroma will be smaller than the extent of the cavity resulting in a systematic underestimation of the extent of the cavity when using ultrasound.

Lymph nodes have little CT contrast and therefore definition of the lymph nodes typically relies on the identification of bony landmarks, however, ultrasound is routinely used to visualise lymph nodes to guide needle biopsies. In the context of head and neck radiotherapy, freehand 2D B-mode ultrasound and a tracking marker on the probe has been used to obtain 3D (stitched together) images of the entire neck region, in particular the regions containing lymph nodes [20]. Here, the registration of ultrasound and the planning CT was achieved by first using registration of the strongly reflecting skin surface depicted in each of the 2D ultrasound images with the body outline depicted on the CT. The surface registration was reviewed by a clinician, using anatomical landmarks visible in both CT and ultrasound to adjust the position if necessary. The final stage of registration used an intensity-based image registration algorithm, however, this was enabled using an intermediate step of processing cut-plane CT slices such that they resemble ultrasound images [21].

For gynaecological applications (endometrial or cervical cancer), if the bladder is full, (a full bladder is a typical requirement for patients undergoing radiotherapy) the uterus, cervix and vagina can be more easily visualised using ultrasound. Whilst ultrasound is not currently used to define the target volume for external beam RT (EBRT) for gynaecological cancers, transabdominal ultrasound has been used for the purposes of brachytherapy planning [22, 23]. In addition, recent work by Mason *et al* [24] has shown that the uterocervix can be better visualised on CBCT and ultrasound images fused together compared to CBCT alone (see chapter 8).

In the context of prostate cancer, target definition on CT only is routine if the target is the whole tumour and seminal vesicles. For a boost of external beam radiotherapy to the dominant intraprostatic lesion, magnetic resonance imaging (MRI) has been found to be a useful tool [25]. Recent work by Wildeboer *et al* has combined conventional B-mode and shear-wave elastography for the detection of prostate cancer [26]. If proven to have equal sensitivity and specificity to MRI, these ultrasound techniques could form an attractive (cheaper and more convenient) alternative to MRI.

Upper abdominal organs are subject to respiratory motion, which is discussed in more detail in chapter 7. Common approaches to account for respiratory motion during radiotherapy are the internal target volume or mid-ventilation volumes. Both methods require an assessment of the target motion as part of the radiotherapy planning process. Four-dimensional (4D) CT can be used to assess motion, however, it captures motion only over a limited time period and imparts additional dose to the patient. As ultrasound is a real-time imaging modality there is an opportunity to measure abdominal organ motion of, for example, the kidneys or the liver. Earlier studies have shown that motion assessment with ultrasound is feasible [27–30] and more recently the use of this data to construct target volume planning margins has been demonstrated for liver [31].

5.3 Automated segmentation of tissues on ultrasound images

The manual delineation of target tissues and organs at risk for radiotherapy planning is a time-consuming process and is subject to observer variation [32]. To maximise hospital resources and increase precision, there has been significant research into automated and semi-automated algorithms for segmentation of tissue on CT and MR images which aim to speed up the process and reduce uncertainty.

In the context of adaptive radiotherapy, several approaches have been proposed. They are (1) selection of the most appropriate treatment plan from a library of predetermined plan, (2) triggered adaptation or (3) on-line adaptation and are discussed in detail in chapter 8. All three approaches require a greater amount of delineation compared to conventional (non-adapted) radiotherapy, i.e., replanning is performed. The latter two approaches require that tissues be segmented to replan on significantly shorter timescales than those employed in the conventional workflow when planning is performed once prior to the start of therapy. Triggered replans are typically generated within 24 hours in time for the next fraction, and online replanning is, in principle, performed whilst the patient waits on the couch, i.e., in a matter of minutes. More recently, dynamic replanning has been proposed, which uses volumetric images acquired during radiation delivery to adapt and deliver the plan dynamically on the order of a few seconds. Automated or semi-automated segmentation algorithms are necessary to meet the increased demands of adaptive radiotherapy, both in terms of the increased number of delineations and the shorter timescales in which they are required.

Segmentation algorithms can be broadly classified as fully automated or semi-automated. Fully automated algorithms are able to segment tissue with no user input at the time of segmentation. Note this does not exclude user input at the time of algorithm development or training. Semi-automated algorithms rely on user input, often referred to as user initialisation. Manual initialisation requires users to provide (1) the approximate location of the tissues or even the boundary of the tissues, by outlining on one or maybe a few image planes; or (2) using so-called 'hint points' which may identify important anatomical features or landmarks in the image. Ideally, initialisation is simple and quick to perform, however, in the context of replanning on timescales such as minutes or seconds, user initialisation is not desirable, nor even feasible.

Segmentation of tissues on medical images is challenging because the form or shape, size, position and orientation, as well as the contrast or image texture of tissues can vary from patient to patient and between image acquisition time-points. Furthermore, different imaging modalities have their own set of characteristics that can change the appearance of tissues, degrade contrast, or introduce image artefacts. In particular, for ultrasound imaging, various characteristics and artefacts can obscure tissue boundaries, create artificial boundaries, reduce soft tissue contrast and alter the image texture of tissues [33]. Developing an algorithm for accurate segmentation of tissues on ultrasound images can be a challenging task. A variety of solutions are proposed in the literature [33, 34]. Commonly, image pixel intensity-based (also known as region-based methods [35]) segmentation algorithms can be formulated as force or energy minimisation functions. Image features such as intensity gradients and or texture features (i.e., statistical parameters which describe the spatial distribution of pixel intensities) can be used as one set of force/energy terms; and boundary regularisation constraints, such as contour curvature, can be used as another set of force/energy terms. Adjustment of weights of the force/energy terms achieves the optimal balance between sensitivity of the algorithm to image features and contour rigidity. These algorithms include active contouring [36], level sets [37], discrete dynamic contouring [38], and GrowCut [39]. With the exception of the requirement for initialisation, these algorithms require no prior knowledge of the target tissues and can be adapted to a variety of segmentation tasks. Prior to their use, images are typically preprocessed to enhance particular image features. Examples of preprocessing are edge enhancement obtained by applying an image gradient operator [40] or despeckling using image filters [41].

Force or energy minimisation functions can be susceptible to errors due to image artefacts, unclear definition of boundaries, spurious boundaries, or nearby tissues with well-defined boundaries. An alternative approach is the use of prior knowledge of the target intensity, contrast, size or shape. Shape-based constraints will assist in cases where the target tissues may be only partially visible, or help to exclude spurious boundaries. Two common approaches are statistical shape models and parametric shape models. The former uses point distribution models and includes active shape models [42] and active appearance models. These approaches are successful when the shape is relatively consistent, but tend to fail when tissues are subject to large deformations such as daily shape changes of the uterus [43]. The latter, parametric shape models, can be used to represent target structures using variable shapes that are defined using a combination of parameters that define simple shapes such as circles, ellipses, or polygons etc. Statistical shape models often require a large number of input shapes derived from images as training data which is not the case for parametric models. Another advantage of parametric models is that they can be independent of size and orientation, making them more applicable to situations where the exact shape is not explicitly represented in the training data.

The type of prior knowledge used for image segmentation varies according to the algorithm employed; however, it is worth noting that longitudinal imaging performed during the radiotherapy workflow lends itself to the generation of prior knowledge, at the initial planning stage. For example, contours generated either manually or automatically from CT or ultrasound images can be employed at later stages to aide tissue segmentation from treatment images, for example as shape priors.

Other segmentation methods include classification methods which can be supervised or unsupervised. Typically, they use the statistical properties of the small regions of the image to differentiate them into distinct tissue types. Each pixel or region may be allocated a number of properties, referred to as features which are contained within a feature vector. The aim is then to identify pixels or regions as belonging to a particular class, which could correspond to a number of tissue types, or simply target and background. Partitioning can be achieved using a classifier or clustering methods (figure 5.2). Classifiers use training data with labelled regions or structures to build up a predictor which can label unseen future image pixels or regions. Clustering methods identify groups of pixels or regions that are similar and proximity measures are used to group data into similar types [35]. Finally, a large body of research is now dedicated to the development of image segmentation algorithms based on convolutional neural networks. This is discussed in more detail in chapter 9.

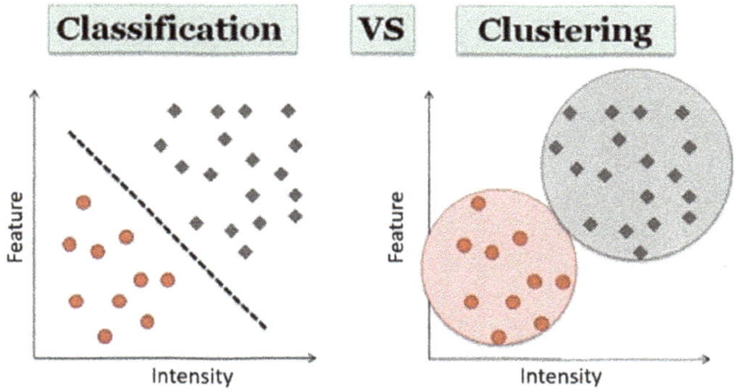

Figure 5.2. Difference between classifying and clustering approaches. In classifiers the target is seen as a prediction problem; in clustering the purpose is to determine intrinsic grouping in sets of data based on some metric. Reproduced with kind persmission of Martin Lachaine.

5.3.1 Automatic segmentation of the prostate

Prostate segmentation in radiotherapy traditionally is based on three imaging modalities: CT, MRI, and (for brachytherapy) transrectal ultrasound (TRUS). Contours based on the latter, in particular, are used to determine the prostate volume for follow-up and for multimodality fusion to localise tumours [44]. For TRUS several automatic contouring algorithms have been developed, comprehensively reported by [35]. In particular, the authors classified the most common methods into the following categories: contour- and shape-based methods; region-based methods; supervised and unsupervised classification methods; and hybrid methods. These techniques were developed for brachytherapy treatments, and are not used in EBRT because of its invasiveness and because the probe would likely be positioned in the treatment beam [44]. A potential application of TRUS in EBRT has yet to be fully explored, in particular in terms of possible impact on rectal dose.

Most of these algorithms work on 2D images [45, 46], and also when applied to 3D ultrasound volumes the segmentation is performed on single slices. This is a limitation on the use of the whole volumetric information, and might introduce errors when the 2D information is used to produce 3D results. Solutions have been proposed where contours are propagated and adapted between contiguous slices [47], where even small errors at each step may generate significant errors in the propagation. Real 3D methods have been proposed by [48] based on active shape and appearance models, then merged with feature learning by [49].

In terms of utilization in the clinical workflow, ultrasound based segmentation of the prostate has been implemented in cases where the target was not visible due to, for example, artefacts generated by the presence of hip prostheses [50]. With the introduction of ultrasound guidance in EBRT, semi-automatic segmentation algorithms have been implemented for transabdominal ultrasound (TAUS) on commercial systems (Clarity, Elekta), where a manual initialisation with four seed points in the slide corresponding to the midplane of the prostate was used by the algorithm to outline the whole organ on the 3D volume. The use of this solution has

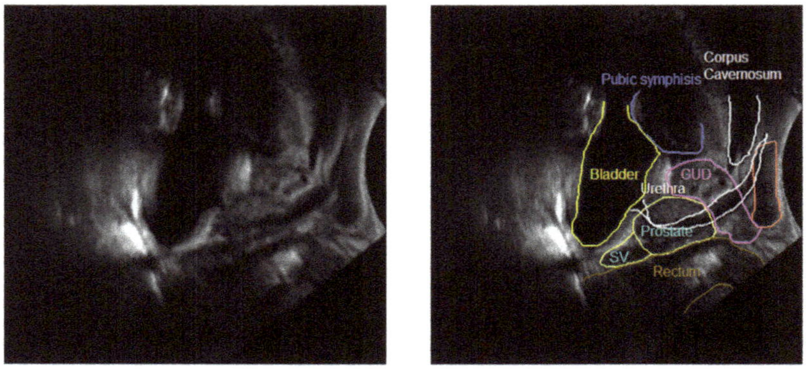

Figure 5.3. Illustration of the prostate and organs at risk on datasets acquired using the Elekta Autoscan system, which could potentially be automatically segmented.

not been reported in literature by the users, who instead in general seem to prefer importing the clinical target volume (CTV) and the planning target volume (PTV) from the co-registered CT scan to draw the Positioning Reference Volume (PRV) on ultrasound (see for example [51]). The more recent Autoscan system (Autoscan, Elekta. Stockholm, Sweden) adopts transperineal ultrasound (TPUS) scanning. Segmentation of the prostate at the simulation stage is done manually, as for the Clarity system. But since the Autoscan provides intrafraction monitoring it must allow for real-time automatic identification of the target (and potentially also of the critical structures, see figure 5.3) during treatment. Instead of fast segmentation, a rigid registration algorithm, based on normalised cross-correlation as the cost function, calculates the rotation-translation matrix between the simulation and the current ultrasound volumes. The transformation is then applied also to the planning contours and the new contours are used for comparison [52]. Among the few research works in EBRT in this field, Ermacora *et al* [53] proposed using the combined information from ultrasound and CT to increase contouring accuracy. In this study, the authors proved that their algorithm can optimally combine the characteristics of both imaging modalities to identify and automatically contour the prostate.

5.3.2 Automatic segmentation of the uterus

In the context of EBRT for cervical cancer, CT and MR are the established imaging modalities used for contouring of the uterocervix to define the treatment target volume and CBCT has become a common method for treatment verification. Uterine automated segmentation algorithms which combine level sets deformable models with a statistical shape prior [54] or active contouring [55] have been proposed in the literature for use with MRI and demonstrated reasonable agreement with manual segmentations. Fallahi *et al* [56] and Militello *et al* [57] investigated fully automatic Fuzzy C-Mean clustering (an unsupervised clustering method that uses distance, connectivity and intensity to cluster pixels, with the possibility of each pixel belonging to more than one cluster) combined with a series of morphological operations to segment the uterus on 2D MR images. Deformable image registration with multiple atlases has also been applied to segmentation of the bladder and uterus from CBCT images [58], although the authors reported that neither the bladder nor the uterus segmentations were accurate enough to fully represent the boundaries of these structures during treatment.

Studies of the segmentation of the uterus from ultrasound images are limited to a few. Gong *et al* [59] demonstrated high contour concordance between manual contours and contours generated using active contours with manual initialisation in six cases when segmenting the uterus on 2D laparoscopic ultrasound images. More recently, Lee *et al* [60] used region-guided adversarial learning to localise anatomical landmarks in the uterus (i.e. the fundus and endometrium) on transvaginal ultrasound images. Although some of these techniques have shown promise, the use of laparoscopic and trasnvaginal probes limits the relevance of these findings to 3DUS guided radiotherapy applications which use transabdominal imaging, i.e. the contrast between organs and well-defined boundaries may not be consistent between the different imaging views.

Ultrasound image quality degradation can obscure true organ boundaries, or even create pseudo boundaries that make it challenging for algorithms to segment the structure of interest (see section 4.3). It may be possible to overcome poor image quality by combining prior knowledge of the expected structure shape, contrast, and/or texture with features (such as edges or neighbourhoods) making algorithms less susceptible to errors arising from imaging imperfections. This approach was adopted by Elekta (Elekta Ltd, Crawley, UK) who base their Assisted Gyne Segmentation (AGS) algorithm, available as part of the Elekta Clarity system, on prior knowledge of the shape of the uterus and the size of the uterus which is indicated by a user positioning hint points. The AGS tool uses a discrete dynamic contouring (DDC) algorithm, adapted from Ladak *et al* [38, 61], Hu *et al* [38, 61], and Ghanei *et al* [62]. The AGS algorithm is demonstrated in figure 5.4.

Mason and colleagues [63] evaluated the use of AGS for the purpose of off-line segmentation of the uterus. This study found that the AGS algorithm performed

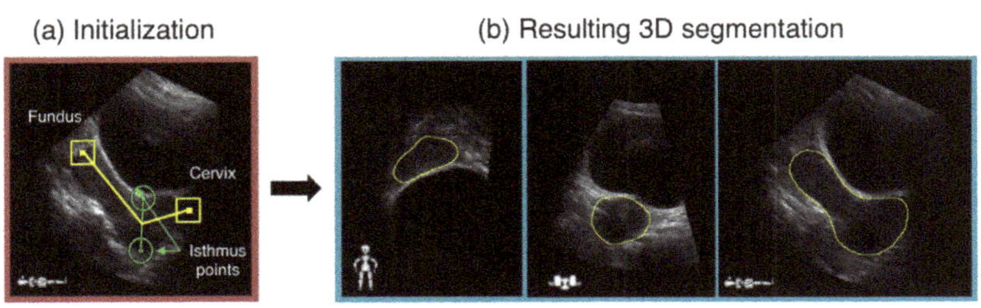

Figure 5.4. (a) Snapshot of AGS tool user interface and (b) resulting segmentation, where the placement of four anatomical hint points is required to initialise AGS segmentation. The hint points are the uterine fundus and base of the cervix (squares), and the anterior and posterior isthmus points (circles). The resulting segmentation is shown on three slices from the coronal, transversal, and sagittal planes, respectively. Reproduced from [63] under Creative Commons Attribution License (BY CC 2.0). Copyright 2017 John Wiley & Sons Ltd.

better on higher quality ultrasound images (images were rated for quality by observers) than images that were considered low quality. AGS was unable to return a result in 19% of images, which was attributed to partially obscured uterine boundaries in these images. The segmentations that were returned had a median (interquartile range) Dice Similarity Coefficient (DSC) 0.77 (0.14), which was considered to be acceptable when compared with the DSC commonly accepted in the literature (> 0.75). Mason *et al* also proposed their own semi-automated algorithm for uterine segmentation; the stacked-ellipse algorithm was based on a parametric shape model; it combined conventional boundary detection with prior knowledge about the uterus being hypoechoic compared to surrounding tissues and that the uterus can be represented as a series of stacked ellipses [43]. This algorithm performed only slightly better than the AGS with median (interquartile range) DSC 0.8 (0.03) but importantly returned a result for 100% of images.

5.4 Planning with the probe in place

Intrafraction motion monitoring requires that the ultrasound probe remain in the treatment room and in contact with the patient throughout radiation delivery. Careful consideration of probe position and orientation is necessary to ensure that radiation delivery is not compromised in terms of the dose received by both the target volume and normal tissues. The only commercially available solution for intrafraction motion estimation is the Autoscan system, which uses a probe positioned against the perineum to monitor the motion of the prostate. Not only does this configuration offer a better acoustic window to the prostate compared to a transabdominal approach, it also removes the probe from the radiation beam paths of common delivery strategies such as intensity modulated radiotherapy or arc therapy. One study established an increase skin dose arising from radiation scattered by the Autoscan transducer of up to 20% but this was considered clinically insignificant as the perineum can receive much higher doses of radiation from the primary radiation, and/or scattered radiation from the treatment volume [64]. This section considers the challenges associated with integrating the probe into the radiotherapy workflow for non-transperineal imaging configurations.

5.4.1 Integration of the probe with imaging for planning

It is not always possible to perform ultrasound scanning without deforming tissues close to the probe, and possibly at depth (see section 3.3.3 which discusses probe pressure in detail). Deformation due to probe pressure, combined with any abnormal deformation or displacement of soft tissue arising from the treatment pose, should be captured on planning images, and therefore, the probe should be present during simulation. CT images of ultrasound probes are typically subject to metal artefacts. Piezoelectric crystals have relatively high atomic number and hence high x-ray attenuation. Figure 5.5 demonstrates the extent of the CT artefacts that can be observed with a 2D matrix array placed in the plane of the axial CT scan image. Three-dimensional swept array probes containing a motor with metallic parts to support the motion of the array which will also highly attenuate x-rays.

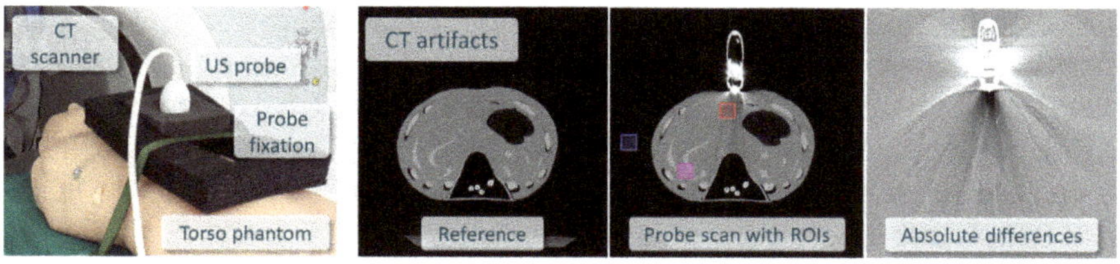

Figure 5.5. From Left to right: A 2D matrix array ultrasound probe positioned on the abdomen of a torso phantom. An axial CT image of the chest phantom alone (reference). A CT axial image with the probe (test). The absolute difference in hounsfield units between the test and reference images illustrating the extent of the artefacts caused by the probe. Adapted from [65] under Creative Commons Attribution License with permission of De Gruyter.

In addition, the probe has to be supported using mechanical, and possibly robotic supports. The parts of these supports that are contained within the field of view of the CT scanner will need to be manufactured using materials that are compatible with CT. For example, carbon fibre components can be used for integration with CT scanning. Ideally, the probe should be positioned so that it is not contained within the axial slices required for treatment planning; however, it may not be possible to obtain an adequate image of the target tissues if the probe is positioned too far from the target tissues, because of the attenuation of ultrasound or acoustic obstructions. Schlosser *et al* designed a 'radiolucent probe' which was a single-element transducer mechanically swept back and forth to generate 2D or 3D images [66]. This approach reduces the amount of material with high x-ray attenuation considerably; however, sweeping a single-element transducer in two dimensions would increase the volume acquisition time and the likelihood of image artefacts due to the relative motion between the tissues and transducer [67]. To our knowledge such a system has yet to be commercially exploited.

There is an increasing trend in the number of centres using magnetic resonance images rather than CT for planning [68] and consideration needs to be given to the integration of ultrasound with MRI. Although it is possible to use a diagnostic ultrasound probe [69] within the bore of a MRI scanner, there are several considerations that need to be taken into account such as electromagnetic interference from the radio frequency transmitters of the MRI scanner transmitters with the ultrasound signal, anchoring of the scanner to ensure it is not propelled towards the magnet and the distortion of the magnetic field and subsequently the MRI image due to the presence of the probe. These factors, combined with several other practical issues, such as moving an ultrasound scanner to an MR unit, hinder the use of ultrasound and MRI simultaneously. A dedicated MRI-compatible 2D matrix array transducer and ultrasound scanning system is currently under development by GE Healthcare Inc. [70]. The inventors propose to use the 4D probe to simultaneously acquire images of the liver whilst the patient is in the MRI scanner and breathing freely. This approach is similar to that proposed by Preiswerk *et al* [69], the ultrasound and MR images will be used to build a correlation model of liver motion detected on ultrasound and the motion of the radiotherapy target detected on MRI. Treatment is then performed on conventional linacs using 4D ultrasound and the model to predict target motion for the implementation of motion management strategies such as gated radiation delivery or tracking the radiation beam. During the acquisition of ultrasound and MRI images, the probe has to be supported using MRI compatible devices. The MRI compatible ultrasound probe developed by General Electric has a low profile and can be strapped to the body of the patient to allow it to be used in the bore of the MRI scanner where there is limited space.

Day-to-day variation in probe pressure during treatment should be minimised to ensure reproduction of the spatial distribution of soft tissues depicted on planning CT or MRI. This poses a further challenge: how to reproduce the position of the probe and the force exerted on the patient. One solution to the problems associated with integrating the probe with CT or MR described above is the use of a dummy probe made of a low atomic number or non ferromagnetic material. This relies on accurate positioning of the dummy probe in the same position as the ultrasound probe and also reproducing the pressure applied to the patient. Bell *et al* [71] explored the use of a robotic placement of a dummy probe for use during CT scanning guiding the robot by either position control or force control. The latter used a proportional-integral-derivative controller to reproduce the contact force normal to the probe. This work found that position control resulted in less positional uncertainty of the target tissues (less than 2 mm) compared to force control (between 4 and 6 mm) in canine liver and pancreas. The same group went on to develop an approach that also used the ultrasound image to guide the placement of the probe during therapy. Preliminary evidence of the superiority of the localisation of markers in the prostate, liver and kidneys using the position, force and image-based control is reported in [72].

A group based in Manheim, Germany was the first group to integrate ultrasound in the radiotherapy workflow for patients with liver cancer in research studies, i.e., to keep the probe in place during CT scanning and treatment [73]. This group used a research version of the Elekta Clarity system and a 3D swept array probe supported by an articulated arm to image lesions in the liver during inhalation breath hold. To ensure that probe pressure was not an issue the probe was positioned against the rib cage. Vogel *et al* [73] reported that by positioning the probe a suitable distance from the target tissues the artefacts in both CT and CBCT on treatment could be tolerated for the majority of patients.

5.4.2 Challenges with creating clinically acceptable treatment plans that account for the probe

Different approaches have been proposed to account for the probe interfering with the beam delivery. As with lower energy x-rays used to generate CT scans, therapeutic x-ray beams passing through the probe will be subject to additional attenuation and scattering, which complicates dosimetry. This has been illustrated by Bazalova-Carter *et al* [74], who performed Monte Carlo simulations for dose delivery through actual probes and concluded that beams intersecting the probe should be avoided. Moreover, the probe is typically placed on the skin in soft tissue regions. Hence, small patient motions as well as the need to maintain contact and to apply a certain force when holding the probe imply that the probe may move slightly during treatment. While the radiotranslucent ultrasound probe design described above allows beams to pass through [66], it would generally be preferable to avoid such beams completely and to account for potential probe and patient movements.

Noting that the inverse planning problem typically has multiple solutions corresponding to different clinically acceptable dose distributions, treatment planning itself can be used to minimise the impact of ultrasound imaging on the beam delivery. However, as the ultrasound probe will often be close to the PTV, the probe and the arm holding it will typically block a rather large solid angle. Moreover, a shorter distance between probe and PTV will be preferable with respect to image quality but also means that potentially efficient beam directions are blocked. Therefore, depending on the actual placement of the ultrasound probe the effect on the plan quality may be rather substantial.

One approach for identifying a suitable ultrasound probe pose would be a manual step in the planning workflow where a simulation environment is used to identify potential interference with beams and the delivery systems. This has been proposed by Schlosser *et al* [75] and demonstrated for linac based treatments. Another approach would be to extend the treatment planning problem to also optimise the pose of the ultrasound probe and the arm holding it. Schlüter *et al* [76] proposed a general search strategy to identify optimal configurations for a robot arm holding an ultrasound probe during treatment. Yet, the possible ultrasound image windows will typically allow for different probe poses (compare chapter 9) and hence the search space may become rather large and impractical for clinical treatment planning. However, Gerlach *et al* [77] illustrated that generally preferable configurations for an ultrasound probe carried by a robot can be identified. For prostate treatments the difference in the plan quality compared to planning without the ultrasound probe was a minor drop in coverage of 1 percentage point.

In the context of radiation beam tracking to mitigate for motion, another issue is the uncertainty with respect to the potential motion of beams and ultrasound probe. While the latter needs to be approximated depending on the probe placement, e.g., with active force control by a robot arm (see chapter 9), the motion of beams depends on the type of treatment delivery. If gating is employed to address cyclic motion, the beams will generally not move. However, ultrasound guidance would be particularly interesting to identify spontaneous motion, e.g., of the prostate. Here the beams would be re-targeted accordingly, potentially moving towards the ultrasound probe. Moreover, when active motion compensation is used, both spontaneous and cyclic movements of the target would result in respective beam motion. Again, the amount of this motion should be estimated before initial treatment planning. As typical for planning it can be represented by adding a safety margin, in this case around the ultrasound probe and the arm holding it, as proposed by Gerlach *et al* [77]. The general idea is illustrated in interactive figure 5.6, where a ray-tracing method is used to detect the robot's shadow with respect to a given beam direction (blue) and a distance transform is then used to add a safety margin (red lines at the perimeter). Note that collision avoidance can be performed in a similar way by computing the projection of a beam and checking for overlap.

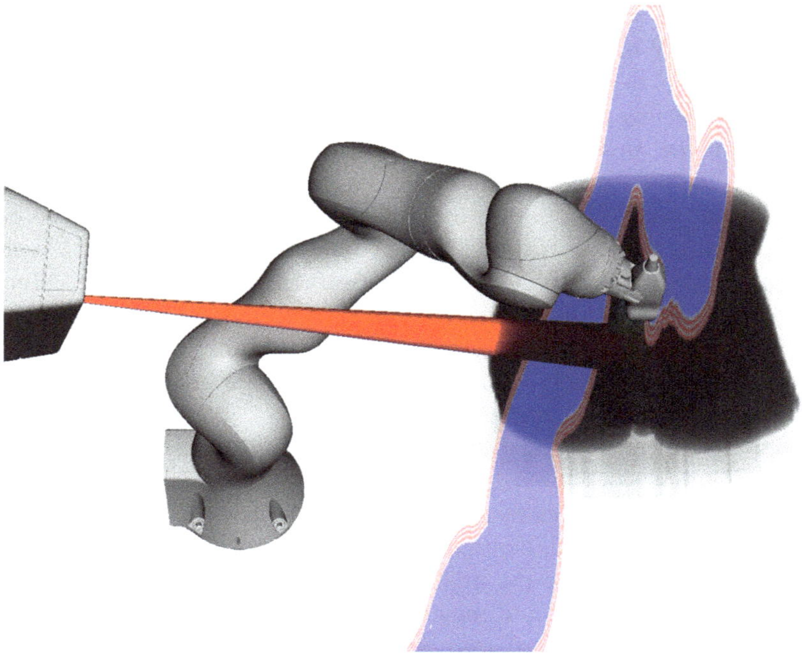

Figure 5.6. This interactive figure illustrates how the robot pose can be adjusted to ensure that the beam is not blocked. The pose is adapted using a ray-tracing method to detect the robots' shadow with respect to a given beam direction (blue) and a distance transform is then used to add a safety margin (red lines at the perimeter). (This figure was developed with the help of Stefan Gerlach, Hamburg University of Technology). Animation available at https://iopscience.iop.org/book/978-0-7503-2552-3.

Depending on the target region and the general setup, a substantial part of the beam blocking will be caused by the arm holding the ultrasound probe. Typically, robotic arms are considered for this purpose, particularly to maintain probe contact throughout treatment. In principle it is possible to build robotic arms without dense material. For example, Schlosser *et al* [75] proposed a specific robot design with cable driven wrist to reduce the impact on x-ray imaging and beam delivery. This design is optimised for gantry based beam delivery and targets in the lower abdomen. Another approach would be to use more conventional and readily available robotic arms with more than six degrees of freedom (DOF). The kinematic redundancy of such robots is often preferred in collaborative scenarios. For example, the 7-DOF KUKA LWR MED (KUKA GmbH, Augsburg, Germany) is designed as a platform for medical robotics and allows rotating the elbow while maintaining the same pose of its end-effector. Hence, this robot can hold an ultrasound probe in place while at the same time moving its elbow to avoid blocking beams. Gerlach *et al* [78] have demonstrated that this can substantially reduce the amount of beam blocking caused by the robot, and that the plan quality can be further improved.

Consolidation quiz

Q1: Why is it not possible to create a radiotherapy treatment plan based on ultrasound images?

- The field of view of a typical ultrasound image is too limited
- The ultrasound images do not provide physical density information, which makes it impossible to calculate radiation dose
- Soft-tissue interfaces are poorly visible on ultrasound images

Q2: Why should beams passing the ultrasound probe be avoided?

- The beams would destroy the ultrasound probe
- Attenuation and scattering may impact the delivered dose
- The US image quality would degrade

Q3: How can the impact of ultrasound probe blocking beams be mitigated?

- The ultrasound probe must be removed before each beam delivery
- Only ultrasound probe positions from lateral viewports are used
- Inverse planning can be used to identify preferable ultrasound probe positions

Q4: Why is it important to consider a safety margin around the ultrasound probe?

- The ultrasound probe and the beams may move during treatment
- To avoid a collision between the ultrasound probe and the patient
- To prevent the beam source from colliding with the ultrasound probe

References

[1] Badcock P C 1977 Ultrasound scanning in the radiotherapy department *Clin. Radiol.* **28** 287–93

[2] Cohen W N and Hass A C 1971 The application of B-scan ultrasound in the planning of radiation therapy treatment ports *Am. J. Roentgenol. Radium Ther. Nucl. Med.* **111** 184–8

[3] Tyagi N, Fontenla S, Zelefsky M, Chong-Ton M, Ostergren K and Shah N *et al* 2017 Clinical workflow for MR-only simulation and planning in prostate *Radiat. Oncol.* **12** 119

[4] Hoffelt S C, Marshall L M, Garzotto M, Hung A, Holland J and Beer T M 2003 A comparison of CT scan to transrectal ultrasound-measured prostate volume in untreated prostate cancer *Int. J. Radiat. Oncol. Biol. Phys.* **57** 29–32

[5] Antico M, Prinsen P, Cellini F, Fracassi A, Isola A A and Cobben D *et al* 2019 Real-time adaptive planning method for radiotherapy treatment delivery for prostate cancer patients, based on a library of plans accounting for possible anatomy configuration changes *PLoS One* **14** e0213002

[6] Leonard C, Harlow C L, Coffin C, Drose J, Norton L and Kinzie J 1993 Use of ultrasound to guide radiation boost planning following lumpectomy for carcinoma of the breast *Int. J. Radiat. Oncol. Biol. Phys.* **27** 1193–7

[7] Harrington K J, Harrison M, Bayle P, Evans K, Dunn P A and Lambert H E *et al* 1996 Surgical clips in planning the electron boost in breast cancer: a qualitative and quantitative evaluation *Int. J. Radiat. Oncol. Biol. Phys.* **34** 579–84

[8] Helyer S J, Moskovic E, Ashley S, Hastings L and Yarnold J 1999 A study testing the routine use of ultrasound measurements when selecting the electron energy for breast boost radiotherapy *Clin. Oncol. (R Coll. Radiol.).* **11** 164–8

[9] Gilligan D, Hendry J A and Yarnold J 1994 The use of ultrasound to measure breast thickness to select electron energies for breast boost radiotherapy *Radiother. Oncol.* **32** 265–7
[10] Coles C E, Cash C J C, Treece G M, Miller F N A C, Hoole A C F and Gee A H *et al* 2007 High definition three-dimensional ultrasound to localise the tumour bed: a breast radiotherapy planning study *Radiother. Oncol.* **84** 233–41
[11] Berrang T S, Truong P T, Popescu C, Drever L, Kader H A and Hilts M L *et al* 2009 3D ultrasound can contribute to planning CT to define the target for partial breast radiotherapy *Int. J. Radiat. Oncol. Biol. Phys.* **73** 375–83
[12] Wong P, Muanza T, Reynard E, Robert K, Barker J and Sultanem K 2011 Use of three-dimensional ultrasound in the detection of breast tumor bed displacement during radiotherapy *Int. J. Radiat. Oncol. Biol. Phys.* **79** 39–45
[13] Fraser D J, Wong P, Sultanem K and Verhaegen F 2010 Dosimetric evolution of the breast electron boost target using 3D ultrasound imaging *Radiother. Oncol.* **96** 185–91
[14] Heimann R and Hard D 2016 A comparison of three dimensional ultrasound, clips and CT for measuring interfractional breast lumpectomy cavity motion *J. Nucl. Med. Radiat. Ther.* **7** 1000280
[15] Rabinovitch R, Finlayson C, Pan Z, Lewin J, Humphries S and Biffl W *et al* 2000 Radiographic evaluation of surgical clips is better than ultrasound for defining the lumpectomy cavity in breast boost treatment planning: a prospective clinical study *Int. J. Radiat. Oncol. Biol. Phys.* **47** 313–17
[16] West Midlands Clinical Advisory Group 2017 *Clinical Guidelines forthe Management ofBreast Cancer* (NHS) https://www.england.nhs.uk/mids-east/wp-content/uploads/sites/7/2018/02/guidelines-for-the-management-of-breast-cancer-v1.pdf
[17] Ringash J, Whelan T, Elliott E, Minuk T, Sanders K and Lukka H *et al* 2004 Accuracy of ultrasound in localization of breast boost field *Radiother. Oncol.* **72** 61–6
[18] Serban M, Lambert C, Ruo R, Maietta C, Parker W and Evans M *et al* 2019 Computed tomography-based virtual simulation versus ultrasound-based clinical setup in electron breast boost radiotherapy: methodology for CT-based electron virtual simulation *Phys. Med.* **67** 100–6
[19] Aghili M, Barzegar Tahmtan M R, Samiee F, Haddad P, Amouzgar Hashemi F and Maddah A *et al* 2015 Ultrasound accuracy in determining the tumor depth for boost field radiotherapy in breast cancer in comparison with CT scan plus clips *Rep. Radiother. Oncol.* **2** e887
[20] Wein W, Röper B and Navab N 2007 Integrating diagnostic B-mode ultrasonography into CT-based radiation treatment planning *IEEE Trans. Med. Imag.* **26** 866–79
[21] Wein W, Röper B and Navab N 2005 Automatic registration and fusion of ultrasound with CT for radiotherapy *Med. Image Comput. Comput. Assist. Interv.* **8** 303–11
[22] Van Dyk S, Narayan K, Fisher R and Bernshaw D 2009 Conformal brachytherapy planning for cervical cancer using transabdominal ultrasound *Int. J. Radiat. Oncol.-Biol.-Phys.* **75** 64–70
[23] van Dyk S, Schneider M, Kondalsamy-Chennakesavan S, Bernshaw D and Narayan K 2015 Ultrasound use in gynecologic brachytherapy: time to focus the beam *Brachytherapy* **14** 390–400
[24] Mason S A, White I M, O'Shea T, McNair H A, Alexander S and Kalaitzaki E *et al* 2019 Combined ultrasound and cone beam CT improves target segmentation for image guided radiation therapy in uterine cervix cancer *Int. J. Radiat. Oncol. Biol. Phys.* **104** 685–93
[25] Alexander E J, Murray J R, Morgan V A, Giles S L, Riches S F and Hazell S *et al* 2019 Validation of T2- and diffusion-weighted magnetic resonance imaging for mapping intra-

prostatic tumour prior to focal boost dose-escalation using intensity-modulated radiotherapy (IMRT) *Radiother. Oncol.* **141** 181–7
[26] Wildeboer R R, van Sloun R J G, Huang P, Wijkstra H and Mischi M 2019 3-D Multi-parametric contrast-enhanced ultrasound for the prediction of prostate cancer *Ultrasound Med. Biol.* **45** 2713–24
[27] Harris E J, Miller N R, Bamber J C, Symonds-Tayler J R N and Evans P M 2010 Speckle tracking in a phantom and feature-based tracking in liver in the presence of respiratory motion using 4D ultrasound *Phys. Med. Biol.* **55** 3363–80
[28] Fuss M, Salter B J, Herman T S and Thomas C R 2004 External beam radiation therapy for hepatocellular carcinoma: potential of intensity-modulated and image-guided radiation therapy *Gastroenterology.* **127** S206–17
[29] Sanders R C, Hughes B and Hazra T A 1974 Ultrasound localization of kidneys for radiation therapy *Br. J. Radiol.* **47** 196–7
[30] Rubin J M, Feng M, Hadley S W, Fowlkes J B and Hamilton J D 2012 Potential use of ultrasound speckle tracking for motion management during radiotherapy: preliminary report *J. Ultrasound Med.* **31** 469–81
[31] De Luca V, Banerjee J, Hallack A, Kondo S, Makhinya M and Nouri D *et al* 2018 Evaluation of 2D and 3D ultrasound tracking algorithms and impact on ultrasound-guided liver radiotherapy margins *Med. Phys.* **45** 4986–5003
[32] Njeh C F 2008 Tumor delineation: the weakest link in the search for accuracy in radiotherapy *J. Med. Phys.* **33** 136–40
[33] Noble J A and Boukerroui D 2006 Ultrasound image segmentation: a survey *IEEE Trans. Med. Imag.* **25** 987–1010
[34] Meiburger K M, Acharya U R and Molinari F 2018 Automated localization and segmentation techniques for B-mode ultrasound images: a review *Comput. Biol. Med.* **92** 210–35
[35] Ghose S, Oliver A, Martí R, Lladó X, Vilanova J C and Freixenet J *et al* 2012 A survey of prostate segmentation methodologies in ultrasound, magnetic resonance and computed tomography images *Comput. Methods Prog. Biomed.* **108** 262–87
[36] Caselles V, Kimmel R and Sapiro G 1995 Geodesic active contours *Proc. of IEEE Int. Conf. on Computer Vision* (IEEE Computer Society Press) pp 694–9
[37] Li C, Xu C, Gui C and Fox M D 2010 Distance regularized level set evolution and its application to image segmentation *IEEE Trans. Image Process.* **19** 3243–54
[38] Ladak H M, Mao F, Wang Y, Downey D B, Steinman D A and Fenster A 2000 Prostate boundary segmentation from 2D ultrasound images *Med. Phys.* **27** 1777–88
[39] Vezhnevets V and Konouchine V 2005 GrowCut: interactive multi-label ND image segmentation by cellular automata. *Proc. of Graphicon*
[40] Kittler J 1983 On the accuracy of the Sobel edge detector *Image Vision Comput.* **1** 37–42
[41] Michailovich O V and Tannenbaum A 2006 Despeckling of medical ultrasound images *IEEE Trans. Ultrason. Ferroelectr. Freq. Control* **53** 64–78
[42] Cootes T F, Hill A, Taylor C J and Haslam J 1994 Use of active shape models for locating structures in medical images *Image Vis. Comput.* **12** 355–65
[43] Mason S A, White I M, Lalondrelle S, Bamber J C and Harris E J 2020 The stacked-ellipse algorithm: an ultrasound-based 3-D uterine segmentation tool for enabling adaptive radiotherapy for uterine cervix cancer *Ultrasound Med. Biol.* **46** 1040–52

[44] Siebert F-A, Kirisits C, Hellebust T P, Baltas D, Verhaegen F and Camps S *et al* 2020 GEC-ESTRO/ACROP recommendations for quality assurance of ultrasound imaging in brachytherapy *Radiother. Oncol.* **148** 51–6
[45] Betrouni N, Vermandel M, Pasquier D, Maouche S and Rousseau J 2005 Segmentation of abdominal ultrasound images of the prostate using *a priori* information and an adapted noise filter *Comput. Med. Imag. Graph.* **29** 43–51
[46] Shen D, Zhan Y and Davatzikos C 2003 Segmentation of prostate boundaries from ultrasound images using statistical shape model *IEEE Trans. Med. Imag.* **22** 539–51
[47] Ding M, Chiu B, Gyacskov I, Yuan X, Drangova M and Downey D B *et al* 2007 Fast prostate segmentation in 3D TRUS images based on continuity constraint using an autoregressive model *Med. Phys.* **34** 4109–25
[48] Cootes T F, Taylor C J, Cooper D H and Graham J 1995 Active shape models-their training and application *Comput. Vision Image Understand.* **61** 38–59
[49] Ghose S, Oliver A, Mitra J, Martí R, Lladó X and Freixenet J *et al* 2013 A supervised learning framework of statistical shape and probability priors for automatic prostate segmentation in ultrasound images *Med. Image Anal.* **17** 587–600
[50] Boda-Heggemann J, Haneder S, Ehmann M, Sihono D S K, Wertz H and Mai S *et al* 2015 Stereotactic ultrasound for target volume definition in a patient with prostate cancer and bilateral total hip replacement *Pract. Radiat. Oncol.* **5** 197–202
[51] Li M, Ballhausen H, Hegemann N-S, Ganswindt U, Manapov F and Tritschler S *et al* 2015 A comparative assessment of prostate positioning guided by three-dimensional ultrasound and cone beam CT *Radiat. Oncol.* **10** 82
[52] Lachaine M and Falco T 2013 Intrafractional prostate motion management with the clarity autoscan system *Med. Phys. Int.* **1** 72–80
[53] Ermacora D, Pesente S, Pascoli F, Raducci S, Mauro R and Rumeileh I A *et al* 2015 Automated computed tomography-ultrasound cross-modality 3-D contouring algorithm for prostate *Ultrasound Med. Biol.* **41** 2646–62
[54] Lu C, Chelikani S and Jaffray, D A 2012 Simultaneous nonrigid registration, segmentation, and tumor detection in MRI guided cervical cancer radiation therapy *IEEE Trans. Med. Imag.* **31** 1213–27
[55] Leventon M E, Grimson W E L and Faugeras O 2002 Statistical shape influence in geodesic active contours. *5th IEEE EMBS Int. Summer School on Biomedical Imaging. 2002* (IEEE) pp. V_3_1–V_3_8
[56] Fallahi A, Pooyan M, Ghanaati H, Oghabian M A, Khotanlou H and Shakiba M *et al* 2011 Uterine segmentation and volume measurement in uterine fibroid patients' MRI using fuzzy C-mean algorithm and morphological operations *Iran. J. Radiol.* **08** 150–6
[57] Militello C, Vitabile S, Rundo L, Russo G, Midiri M and Gilardi M C 2015 A fully automatic 2D segmentation method for uterine fibroid in MRgFUS treatment evaluation *Comput. Biol. Med.* **62** 277–92
[58] Langerak T, Heijkoop S, Quint S, Mens J-W, Heijmen B and Hoogeman M 2014 Towards automatic plan selection for radiotherapy of cervical cancer by fast automatic segmentation of cone beam CT scans *Medical Image Computing and Computer-Assisted Intervention—MICCAI 2014: 17th International Conf., Boston, MA, USA, September 14-18, 2014, Proc., Part I.* ed P Golland, N Hata, C Barillot, J Hornegger and R Howe (Cham: Springer International Publishing) pp 528–35

[59] Gong X-H, Lu J, Liu J, Deng Y-Y, Liu W-Z and Huang X *et al* 2015 Segmentation of uterus using laparoscopic ultrasound by an image-based active contour approach for guiding gynecological diagnosis and surgery *PLoS One* **10** e0141046
[60] Lee H J, Kim H G, Park H, Shin D and Ro Y M 2019 Region-guided adversarial learning for anatomical landmark detection in uterus ultrasound image *Medical Imaging: Image Processing* ed E D Angelini and B A Landman (Bellinham, WA: SPIE) p 115
[61] Hu N, Downey D B and Fenster A 2002 Prostate surface segmentation from 3D ultrasound images on biomedical imaging *Proc. IEEE Int. Symp. on Biomedical Imaging* pp 613–6
[62] Ghanei A, Soltanian-Zadeh H, Ratkewicz A and Yin F F 2001 A three-dimensional deformable model for segmentation of human prostate from ultrasound images *Med. Phys.* **28** 2147–53
[63] Mason S A, O'Shea T P, White I M, Lalondrelle S, Downey K and Baker M *et al* 2017 Towards ultrasound-guided adaptive radiotherapy for cervical cancer: evaluation of Elekta's semiautomated uterine segmentation method on 3D ultrasound images *Med. Phys.* **44** 3630–8
[64] Martyn M, O' Shea T, Harris E J, Bamber J C, Foley M J and Gilroy S 2016 Monte Carlo investigation of the dosimetric effect of the Autoscan ultrasound probe for guidance in radiotherapy *Medical Imaging: Ultrasonic Imaging and Tomography* ed N Duric and B Heyde (Bellingham, WA: SPIE) p 22
[65] Ipsen S, Bruder R, García-Vázquez V, Schweikard A and Ernst F 2019 Assessment of 4D ultrasound systems for image-guided radiation therapy—image quality, framerates and CT artifacts *Curr. Dir. Biomed. Eng.* **5** 245–8
[66] Schlosser J and Hristov D 2016 Radiolucent 4D ultrasound imaging: system design and application to radiotherapy guidance *IEEE Trans. Med. Imag.* **35** 2292–300
[67] Harris E J, Miller N R, Bamber J C, Symonds-Tayler J R N and Evans P M 2011 The effect of object speed and direction on the performance of 3D speckle tracking using a 3D swept-volume ultrasound probe *Phys. Med. Biol.* **56** 7127–43
[68] Edmund J M and Nyholm T 2017 A review of substitute CT generation for MRI-only radiation therapy *Radiat. Oncol.* **12** 28
[69] Preiswerk F, De Luca V, Arnold P, Celicanin Z, Petrusca L and Tanner C *et al* 2014 Model-guided respiratory organ motion prediction of the liver from 2D ultrasound *Med. Image Anal.* **18** 740–51
[70] Lee W, Chan H, Chan P, Fiorillo T, Fiveland E and Foo T *et al* 2017 A magnetic resonance compatible E4D ultrasound probe for motion management of radiation therapy *2017 IEEE Int. Ultrasonics Symp. (IUS) (Washington DC)* pp 1–4
[71] Lediju Bell M A, Şen H T, Iordachita I, Kazanzides P and Wong J 2014 *In vivo* reproducibility of robotic probe placement for a novel ultrasound-guided radiation therapy system *J. Med. Imag.* **1** 025001
[72] Şen H T, Lediju Bell M A, Zhang Y, Ding K, Wong J and Iordachita I *et al* 2015 System integration and preliminary in-vivo experiments of a robot for ultrasound guidance and monitoring during radiotherapy *Proc. Int. Conf. Adv. Robot.* 53–9
[73] Vogel L, Sihono D S K, Weiss C, Lohr F, Stieler F and Wertz H *et al* 2018 Intra-breath-hold residual motion of image-guided DIBH liver-SBRT: an estimation by ultrasound-based monitoring correlated with diaphragm position in CBCT *Radiother. Oncol.* **129** 441–8
[74] Bazalova-Carter M, Schlosser J, Chen J and Hristov D 2015 Monte Carlo modeling of ultrasound probes for image guided radiotherapy *Med. Phys.* **42** 5745–56

[75] Schlosser J, Gong R H, Bruder R, Schweikard A, Jang S and Henrie J *et al* 2016 Robotic intrafractional US guidance for liver SABR: system design, beam avoidance, and clinical imaging *Med. Phys.* **43** 5951

[76] Schlüter M, Gerlach S, Fürweger C and Schlaefer A 2019 Analysis and optimization of the robot setup for robotic-ultrasound-guided radiation therapy *Int. J. Comput. Assist. Radiol. Surg.* **14** 1379–87

[77] Gerlach S, Kuhlemann I, Jauer P, Bruder R, Ernst F and Fürweger C *et al* 2017 Robotic ultrasound-guided SBRT of the prostate: feasibility with respect to plan quality *Int. J. Comput. Assist. Radiol. Surg.* **12** 149–59

[78] Gerlach S, Kuhlemann I, Ernst F, Fürweger C and Schlaefer A 2017 Impact of robotic ultrasound image guidance on plan quality in SBRT of the prostate *Br. J. Radiol.* **90** 20160926

IOP Publishing

Modern Applications of 3D/4D Ultrasound Imaging in Radiotherapy

Emma Harris, Davide Fontanarosa, Saskia Camps and Frank Verhaegen

Chapter 6

Ultrasound for measuring interfraction organ motion

Saskia Camps and Christopher Edwards

Prior to each treatment fraction, it is important to set up the patient the same way as during the simulation stage, as this is the setup that the treatment plan was based on. Multiple solutions are available that can assist with this patient setup such as in-room laser alignment, fiducial markers, imaging of bony anatomy with CBCT and ultrasound imaging. This chapter provides information on the ultrasound based systems which have been commercialised. It covers the challenges associated with interfraction motion assessment using ultrasound and the possible use cases. For several anatomical sites, including prostate, liver and gynaecological structures, more information is provided on how the images are typically acquired, how these images can be used for motion assessment and what the associated performances are.

6.1 Introduction

As described in chapter 1 in more detail, at simulation stage, typically a computed tomography (CT) is acquired based on which a patient-specific treatment plan is prepared. After treatment plan finalisation, the treatment stage starts during which the radiation dose will be delivered to the patient in numerous daily treatment fractions [1]. The number of treatment fractions varies substantially per anatomical site and the total treatment duration can be up to eight weeks.

Prior to each treatment fraction, the patient has to be set up exactly the same way as during the simulation stage, as this is the setup based on which the treatment plan was prepared. To assist with this crucial step, several approaches are available. One frequently used approach is to align the patient with the in-room lasers available in both the CT room and the treatment room. To allow for this alignment,

doi:10.1088/978-0-7503-2552-3ch6

skin markers/tattoos are applied to the patient's skin which remain in place during the whole treatment [2].

A different approach makes use of imaging in the treatment room, which typically uses x-rays. After the patient has been aligned using the in-room lasers, a cone-beam CT (CBCT) scan (e.g. [3]) or one or multiple x-ray images are acquired to visualise the bony anatomy of the patient in the CT coordinate system. This allows matching of the bony anatomy visualised using the CT with the bony anatomy visualised using CBCT or x-rays. Subsequently, the patient setup can be fine-tuned based on the displacement of the patient anatomy estimated from the images obtained during this matching procedure.

These approaches, which can be used for patient setup prior to each treatment fraction, primarily focus on external alignment and/or on the alignment based on rigid tissues, like bones. However, even when the patient seems correctly aligned according to these approaches, soft tissue distributions might still be different. This can be caused by, for example, a different filling of the bladder (in the case of prostate and gynaecological targets), weight gain or loss, or naturally occurring organ motion (see figure 6.1 for an example).

For some types of primary cancer (e.g. prostate and liver) fiducial markers are implanted into the treatment target or the anatomical structure of interest prior to the simulation stage [4]. These markers can be used as a surrogate for the anatomical structure and/or the target and can be, for example, visualised using CBCT, planar x-ray images, (e.g. [5]) or tracked using electromagnetic tracking (e.g. [6]). The implantation of fiducial markers and imaging them with x-ray imaging allows for a better alignment of the soft tissues. However, the fiducials are only a surrogate for the tissues, so the motion of the tissues surrounding the fiducials can still not be taken into account.

As described in chapter 2, ultrasound imaging typically provides good soft tissue contrast and therefore could be of good use to assist with interfraction patient set up. It could be used after the in-room laser alignment to verify if, not only the exterior of the patient, but also the internal soft tissues are aligned correctly.

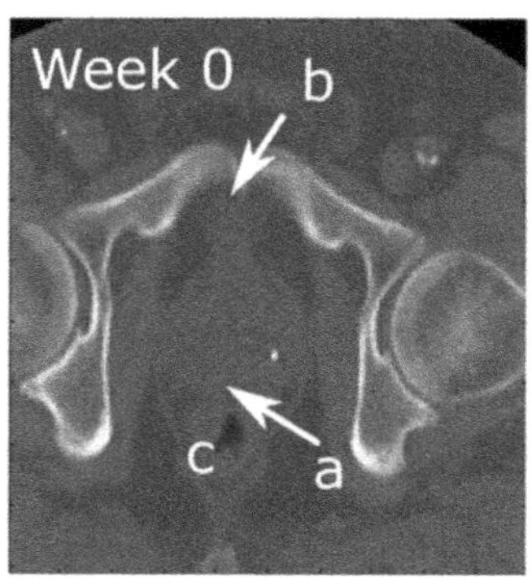

Figure 6.1. This interactive figure shows a cropped CT scan slice of a prostate cancer patient undergoing radiotherapy with (a) prostate, (b) bladder and (c) rectum. The slider can be used to visualise tissue distribution changes that occurred between the simulation CT scan (week 0) and a treatment fraction three weeks later. Animation available at https://iopscience.iop.org/book/978-0-7503-2552-3.

Ultrasound imaging allows for visualisation of the tissue boundaries in three dimensions and it allows for prolonged imaging with little risk of harm to the patient, which means that ultrasound images could be acquired multiple times during the alignment process for verification purposes.

6.2 Intermodality and intramodality imaging

Until today, there have been six medical systems commercially available that allowed for the use of ultrasound imaging for interfraction patient set up during radiotherapy workflows: I-Beam (Computerised Medical Systems Inc. Maryland Heights, MO, USA), SonArray (Varian Medical Systems, Palo Alto, CA, USA), B-mode Acquisition and Targeting (BAT) system (Best Nomos, Pittsburgh, PA, USA), the Elekta Clarity system (Elekta, Stockholm, Sweden) and the Elekta Autoscan scan (Elekta, Stockholm, Sweden). These systems can be divided into two categories: intermodality and intramodality imaging systems. The intermodality systems compare anatomical information from CT scans (simulation stage) with ultrasound images (treatment stage), while the intramodality systems compare anatomical information from ultrasound images acquired at simulation stage to ultrasound images acquired at treatment stage (see figure 6.2).

The BAT system is an intermodality system and it became available commercially about 20 years ago. This system allowed for interfraction motion monitoring of the prostate using ultrasound imaging. The BAT workflow only affects the treatment stage of the radiotherapy treatment. The first step of this workflow includes the importation of patient-specific CT structures and the treatment planning isocentre. Subsequently, the ultrasound probe which is mounted to an articulated arm is calibrated to allow for tracking of its position in space. After probe calibration,

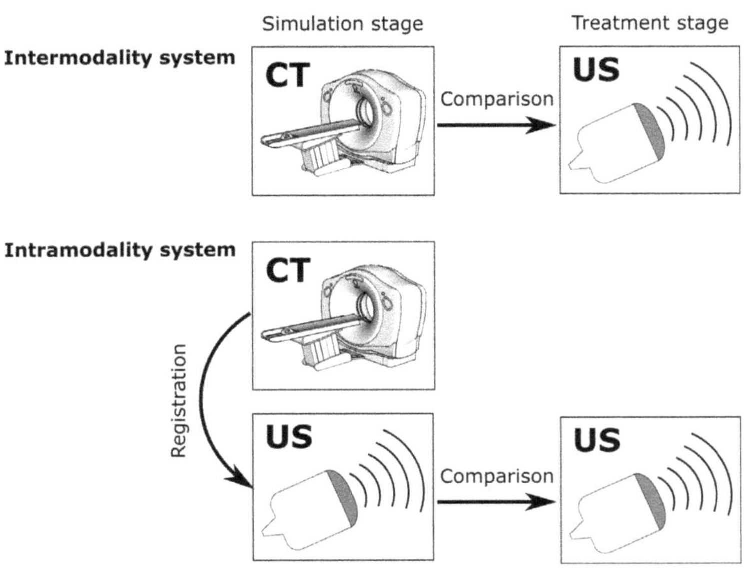

Figure 6.2. Explanation of the difference between intermodality and intramodality imaging systems.

two 2D ultrasound images with perpendicular imaging planes can be acquired of the pubic area of the patient. These ultrasound images and the CT scan are registered as they are acquired in the same coordinate systems thanks to probe calibration (see chapter 3). If the prostate visible on the ultrasound images matches the CT contour of the prostate, the patient is correctly set up. If this is not the case, the CT contour can be manually moved with respect to the ultrasound images to achieve a better match of the anatomical structures. The required treatment couch shift is then calculated by the BAT system and provided to the operator [7]. A more recent version of the BAT system (the BATCAM) no longer uses an articulated arm but instead uses optical tracking of the probe.

Several papers have been published in which, for example, the interuser variability (e.g. [8] and [9]), radiation dose coverage (e.g. [10]) and patient setup accuracy (e.g. [11] and [12]) of the BAT setup have been reported. These publications show that the patient setup accuracy improves as well as the radiation dose coverage in comparison with, for example, portal film imaging. Fontanarosa *et al* [13] provide a more complete overview of all BAT system related publications together with their results.

The SonArray system is also an intermodality system, its intended use is for prostate motion management and it has a similar workflow as the BAT system. However, instead of acquiring two ultrasound images with perpendicular imaging planes, this system allows the reconstruction of a 3D volume from several 2D ultrasound images. To enable this, the system makes use of a transabdominal ultrasound probe which is equipped with an infrared light emitting diode. While the ultrasound probe is translated or rotated on the skin of the patient, the ultrasound probe is localised, which allows the arrangement of the acquired ultrasound images in a 3D volume. As soon as the ultrasound volume is reconstructed, the contours of the planning CT are superimposed on this volume and the user can manually match the CT contours to the ultrasound volume. After the contour matching, the required treatment table shift is calculated and the table moved accordingly [14].

The SonArray system is no longer available and this might explain the very few publications available in the literature. The above referenced publication of Orton *et al* [14] presents the most extensive patient setup accuracy results and concludes that the SonArray system can be used to improve daily positioning of the patient. This seems to be in alignment with the results presented in an abstract by Tomé *et al* [15] and in a short paper by Peignaux *et al* [16].

The Elekta Clarity system is the first available intramodality imaging system. It consists of two ultrasound devices, one present in the CT room and one present in the treatment room. Thanks to optical localisation of the transabdominal ultrasound probes in both rooms, 2D ultrasound images can be reconstructed into a 3D ultrasound volume in the CT coordinate system. This allows for registration of these ultrasound volumes with the planning CT scan. At the simulation stage, the Clarity system is able to semi-automatically delineate the prostate on the acquired ultrasound volume. Then, at the treatment stage, this prostate delineation is superimposed on the newly acquired ultrasound volume. Subsequently, these contours can be manually matched by an operator to determine the required treatment table shifts to allow for correct patient setup [17].

In literature, several publications can be found that describe the use of the Elekta Clarity system. The patient setup accuracy using the Clarity system has been compared with several other setup verification tools, like fiducial markers (e.g. [18]), or CT scans (e.g. [19]). Even though the Elekta Clarity system was originally intended for prostate motion management, its use cases are broader. For example, in terms of user variability, the Clarity system has been investigated for prostate (e.g. [17]), liver (e.g. [20]) and breast (e.g. [21]). In the review paper by Fontanarosa *et al* [13] a more complete overview of the Elekta Clarity system related publications together with their results can be found.

The Elekta Autoscan system is the most recent USgRT system available on the market. Differently from the systems described above, the Autoscan makes use of a transperineal ultrasound probe instead of a transabdominal probe. This allows positioning of the probe outside of the radiation beam path, enabling continuous ultrasound imaging not only prior to a treatment fraction, but also during the radiation delivery. In addition, this transperineal probe does not require a manual sweep of the probe to construct a 3D volume, but it has a mechanical sweep built in the probe itself. This makes the presence of an operator to acquire the 3D volume unnecessary and therefore also allows for intrafraction motion monitoring. More details about the Elekta Autoscan system as well as studies that have been published in recent years can be found in chapter 7 of this book, as well as in [13, 22, 23].

6.3 Setup challenges

In the introduction of this chapter, it has been described that during a typical radiotherapy workflow a CT scan is acquired to capture the patient's anatomy. As the treatment plan is primarily based on this CT scan, all other image modalities used in the radiotherapy workflow have to be related to this scan. Therefore, in the ideal USgRT situation, one or multiple ultrasound volumes would be acquired simultaneously with this CT scan to allow for a good registration of the anatomical structures on both modalities. However, a number of challenges arise in such a scenario.

The first challenge is associated with the fact that the presence of the ultrasound probe in the beam path of the CT scanner causes (streak) artefacts on the CT scan. This could heavily compromise the quality of the CT scan, which could result in a degradation of the treatment plan quality that can be prepared based on this scan. More details on solutions that have been proposed in literature to face this challenge can be found in chapter 5 of this book.

Typically, the ultrasound probe is localised in the CT room, which then results in ultrasound images in the CT coordinate system. Several different systems are commercially available that allow localisation of objects in a room, often by making use of markers. These systems (see chapter 3) can be based on, for example, infrared (e.g. Polaris, NDI, Waterloo, Ontario, Canada) or electromagnetism (e.g. Calypso Medical Technologies, Inc., Seattle, WA, USA). The earlier mentioned Elekta Clarity and Elekta Autoscan systems both make use of the NDI system [24]. A drawback of this NDI system in the Elekta setup is that it does not allow for localisation of the ultrasound probe inside the CT bore. As the CT table moves during the scan acquisition, at some point the ultrasound probe will most probably move out of the field of view of the cameras. So even when the ultrasound probes would not cause artefacts on the CT scan, currently, there is no way to acquire them simultaneously as well as co-registered.

In addition to the challenges associated with the simultaneous acquisition of the CT scan and ultrasound volumes, also other challenges arise from the use of ultrasound imaging during simulation and treatment stages. In chapter 4 it was extensively described that a skilled operator is needed to acquire an ultrasound image of good quality. This operator needs to manually position the ultrasound probe on the skin of the patient, interpret the live images and decide if the probe setup is good enough or not. As this is an iterative process, most probably more time will be required to set up the patient correctly in comparison with, for example, a setup based on CBCT.

The operator does not only have to find a suitable acoustic window for ultrasound imaging, but also ensure that there is sufficient acoustic coupling between the ultrasound probe and the skin of the patient. In addition to the use of ultrasound gel, the application of some probe pressure could also result in a better coupling and so a better image quality. However, as described in detail in chapter 3, the application of probe pressure can result in an anatomical structure displacement in comparison with the CT. This would make it difficult if not impossible to find the correct registration between both image modalities.

6.4 Anatomical sites

6.4.1 Prostate and prostate bed

A number of anatomical sites are potentially amenable to interfraction organ assessment during radiation therapy treatment with the aid of ultrasound. The organ which has been most extensively investigated is the prostate. Imaging of the prostate with ultrasound is widely utilised and a well tolerated examination in radiology. Prostate ultrasound can be achieved using various approaches, transabdominal, transperineal and transrectal (see figure 6.3). The transabdominal approach images the prostate via the abdominal soft tissues and requires a full bladder for adequate visualisation. The quality of transabdominal images is heavily influenced by the amount of adipose tissue and the degree of bladder filling, both of which can significantly affect image quality. Transrectal ultrasound is an alternative means to image the prostate and is a more invasive technique, involving the insertion of a

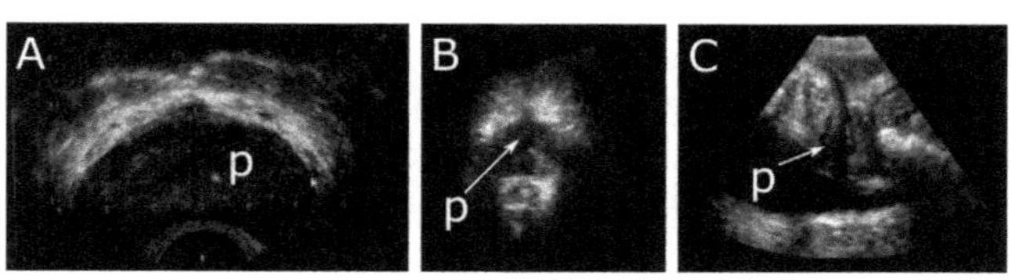

Figure 6.3. The prostate (p) imaged using transrectal (A), transabdominal (B) and transperineal ultrasound imaging.

specifically designed transducer into the rectum. A higher frequency can be used in this setting typically in the range of 8–12 MHz as the prostate is placed closer to the transducer and less susceptible to ultrasound attenuation. Improved image quality allows for a more thorough assessment of parenchymal changes and precise guidance during biopsy [25].

A third method is via transperineal ultrasound, the transducer is placed directly on the perineum and imaging of the prostate occurs via the pelvic floor. Three-dimensional matrix style transducers have also been utilised to image the prostate and provide additional volume information [26]. A transperineal approach has the advantage of being less invasive than transrectal ultrasound, does not require a full bladder and is less susceptible to ultrasound attenuation compared to trans-abdominal imaging. For most patients visualisation of the prostate via a trans-perineal approach is similar to that of transrectal ultrasound and studies have shown that volume determination on transperineal ultrasound is comparable to transrectal ultrasound [27].

Interfraction motion of the prostate is a source of treatment failure in patients undergoing prostate cancer radiotherapy [28, 29]. As a result, considerable attention has been placed on accurately localising the prostate prior to each treatment fraction independent of the surrounding bony landmarks. Both systematic and random interfraction movement of the prostate have been assessed by a large body of research using ultrasound imaging, CT, kilovoltage imaging or megavoltage CT [30]. The dominant motion of the prostate and seminal vesicles occurs in the AP (anterior posterior) with the next greatest motion occuring in the SI (superior inferior) direction. With a general trend towards the superior posterior direction being the most commonly reported. Individual examples of systematic interfraction displacement of the prostate have been reported to be as high as 10–15 mm [31]. A review of the research by McParlin and colleagues indicates that the interfraction motion of the prostate appears to have a standard deviation in the order of 1–4 mm [30]. Rectal distension is the major contributor to prostate motion and has been shown in a number of research studies [32–35]. The effect of bladder volume, however, is less clear with contradictory evidence in the literature [36], most treatment protocols employ a simple bladder filling/emptying protocol which appears sufficient to minimise the effect of bladder volume on prostate position. Even though there is not strong evidence that the degree of bladder greatly affects the clinical target volume, many centres instigate specific bladder filling protocols. For this end transabdominal ultrasound is a useful means to assess bladder filling when the patient is positioned just prior to treatment.

As described above, dedicated systems have employed transabdominal ultrasound as a means to track interfraction of the prostate, which presents some challenges. Such challenges include inaccuracies as a result of the speed of sound artefact due to the distance of the prostate from the ultrasound transducer and the variability caused by probe pressure [13]. However inaccuracies in the reference modality should also be a consideration when evaluating the utility of ultrasound as a localisation tool. The use of ultrasound remains a desirable alternative in the IGRT workflow as it is minimally invasive and does not require the use of ionising radiation. Transperineal ultrasound may become a more widespread method to monitor interfraction motion of the prostate, however, to date it is only employed as part of the Elekta Autoscan system (Elekta, Stockholm, Sweden) which is designed to monitor both interfraction and intrafraction motion via this method.

6.4.2 Gynaecology

Ultrasound plays a key role in the evaluation of the female pelvic organs and is the first line of investigation in a wide variety of clinical settings. Both transabdominal and transvaginal are well-established techniques (see figure 6.4). Transvaginal ultrasound similar to transrectal ultrasound, uses a specifically designed high frequency transducer inserted directly into the vagina allowing high resolution imaging of the cervix, uterus, endometrium, ovaries and adnexa.

Interfraction motion has been observed in gynaecological radiation therapy in the order of 2–60 mm as a result of changes in the tumour volume or variations attributed to bladder and rectal filling [37, 38]. The primary modality used to monitor the clinical target volume remains CBCT with limited reports utilising ultrasound. A recent report did however highlight the complementary role ultrasound may play when combining ultrasound and CBCT images to improve segmentation precision [39]. The study found significantly better contour agreement when ultrasound and CBCT were fused compared to using a single modality alone. Ultrasound may become a more effective means of providing high quality guidance in the future due to its real-time imaging capabilities and with the further development of three-dimensional transducers.

A common use of ultrasound in gynecological radiation therapy is during brachytherapy procedures to guide both the position of intrauterine applicators and interstitial needles. Transabdominal ultrasound is the most common technique used and has the advantage of demonstrating structures in real-time. Van Dyk *et al* [40] reported that transabdominal ultrasound is a useful tool to optimise applicator position and is used to tailor the dose distribution to individual anatomy. The use of transvaginal ultrasound is limited as there is a need to access the vagina for applicator placement, however, in certain scenarios transrectal ultrasound provides a useful alternative in complicated cases or in more advanced disease. A study by Sharma *et al* [41] describes how transrectal ultrasound provided real-time visualisation of the target volume and was able to reduce the risk of needle injury to the pelvic organs and other perioperative complications.

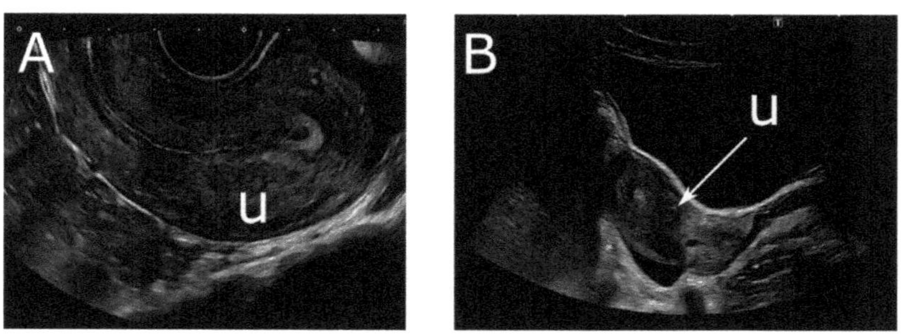

Figure 6.4. The uterus (u) imaged using tranvaginal (A) and transabdominal (B) ultrasound imaging.

6.4.3 Liver

Multiple diagnostic imaging modalities are used to image liver tumors [42]. Transabdominal ultrasound is often the first modality (see figure 6.5) to detect liver lesions and offers a fast effective technique to evaluate the liver parenchyma when there is clinical suspicion of tumor. Once detected lesions are then evaluated via cross sectional imaging modalities (CT, magnetic resonance imaging (MRI) and positron emission tomography) with the addition of contrast and/or radiopharmaceutical to provide a more definitive diagnosis. One advantage of ultrasound during the follow up of lesions is its high spatial resolution and the absence of any additional radiation dose.

This advantage together with ultrasound high temporal resolution has resulted in a body of research looking to monitor the intrafraction motion of liver lesions to mitigate the effects of respiratory changes [43]. Interfraction motion of the liver is also a significant issue, with research demonstrating that positional changes between fractions is a major source of geometric uncertainty [44]. To date however there has been limited adoption of ultrasound to assess interfraction motion. One study combined 3D ultrasound imaging for image guidance during stereotactic body radiotherapy (SBRT) for the treatment of focal lesions in a small group of patients and found the technique feasible [20]. Ultrasound monitoring has also been shown to be successful for the daily repositioning of patients undergoing SBRT using a deep inspiration breath-hold technique to treat liver metastases [45]. A standard ultrasound probe was used to acquire volumetric ultrasound data and infrared optical tracking used for positional information for planning.

6.4.4 Breast

The role of ultrasound as a diagnostic tool differs from its potential role in breast radiotherapy workflows. During the diagnostic phase ultrasound combined with

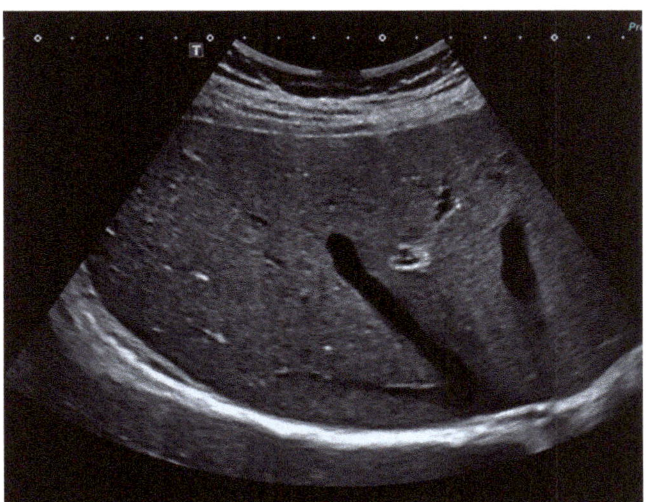

Figure 6.5. The liver imaged using transabdominal ultrasound imaging.

mammography remains one of primary means to evaluate breast lesions to determine their malignant potential [46]. A linear high frequency transducer is used typically in the order of 10–15 MHz and imaging occurs at the area of concern often as a result of a newly discovered lump. Malignant tumors are most commonly treated surgically followed by a number of radiation therapy options. These include both external beam and internal radiation (brachytherapy). With brachytherapy increasingly gaining international favour with promising results compared to external beam options [47]. Ultrasound does have a role in brachytherapy similar to gynaecology as it provides a useful modality to guide the placement and removal of interstitial applicators [48]. For patients receiving partial breast irradiation or breast boost, motion and geometric changes of the lumpectomy site between radiation fractions have been reported, and several modalities (MRI, CT and ultrasound) have been researched to monitor these changes [13]. Both 2D ultrasound and 3D ultrasound options have proven feasible, however, a number of challenges have been highlighted [49, 50]. These include the size discrepancy of the post surgical region between ultrasound and CT, the effect of probe pressure and the visibility of the cavity caused by a range of ultrasound imaging artefacts common in the postoperative setting [13]. Further studies in the future may address some of these issues.

Consolidation quiz

Q1: Why is it important to, prior to each treatment fraction, set up the patient the same way as during the simulation stage?
- ○ This was the setup based on which the treatment plan was designed
- ○ This setup was the most comfortable for the patient
- ○ This setup is the easiest to reproduce

Q2: Which of the following statements is correct?
- ○ Intermodality systems compare anatomical information from ultrasound images acquired at simulation stage with ultrasound images acquired at treatment stage
- ○ Intramodality systems compare anatomical information from CT scans (simulation stage) with ultrasound images (treatment stage)
- ○ None of the above

Q3: Which of the following challenges can be associated with ultrasoud-guided patient setup? (select all correct answers)
- ○ Probe pressure effects
- ○ Patient discomfort
- ○ Simultaneous acquisition of CT and ultrasound

Q4: Interfraction motion of a radiation therapy treatment site can be the result of….
- ○ Rectal and bladder filling
- ○ Changes in tumour volume size
- ○ All of the above

References

[1] Hoskin P 2019 *External Beam Therapy* 3rd edn (Oxford: Oxford University Press)
[2] Bentel G C 1999 *Patient Positioning and Immobilization in Radiation Oncology* (New York: McGraw-Hill)
[3] Yildirim B A, Onal C and Dolek Y 2017 Is it essential to use fiducial markers during cone-beam CT-based radiotherapy for prostate cancer patients? *Jpn. J. Radiol.* **35** 3–9
[4] Kothary N, Heit J J, Louie J D, Kuo W T, Loo B W and Koong A *et al* 2009 Safety and efficacy of percutaneous fiducial marker implantation for image-guided radiation therapy *J. Vasc. Interv. Radiol.* **20** 235–9
[5] Packard M, Gayou O, Gurram K, Weiss B, Thakkar S and Kirichenko A 2015 Use of implanted gold fiducial markers with MV-CBCT image-guided IMRT for pancreatic tumours *J. Med. Imag. Radiat. Oncol.* **59** 499–506
[6] Vanhanen A, Syrén H and Kapanen M 2018 Localization accuracy of two electromagnetic tracking systems in prostate cancer radiotherapy: a comparison with fiducial marker based kilovoltage imaging *Phys. Med.* **56** 10–8
[7] Langen K M, Pouliot J, Anezinos C, Aubin M, Gottschalk A R and Hsu I C *et al* 2003 Evaluation of ultrasound-based prostate localization for image-guided radiotherapy *Int. J. Radiat. Oncol. Biol. Phys.* **57** 635–44
[8] Serago C F, Chungbin S J, Buskirk S J, Vora S A, McLaughlin M P and Ezzell G A 2001 Initial experience with ultrasound localization for positioning prostate cancer patients for external beam radiation therapy *Int. J. Radiat. Oncol. Biol. Phys.* **51** 94
[9] Fuss M, Salter B J, Fuss C, Cavanaugh S X and Herman T S 2003 Daily stereotactic ultrasound prostate targeting *Cancer J.* **9** 511
[10] Falco T, Shenouda G, Kaufmann C, Belanger I, Procaccini C and Charrois C *et al* 2002 Ultrasound imaging for external-beam prostate treatment setup and dosimetric verification *Med. Dosim.* **27** 271–3
[11] Morr J, DiPetrillo T, Tsai J-S, Engler M and Wazer D E 2002 Implementation and utility of a daily ultrasound-based localization system with intensity-modulated radiotherapy for prostate cancer *Int. J. Radiat. Oncol. Biol. Phys.* **53** 1124–9
[12] Chandra A, Dong L, Huang E, Kuban D A, O'Neill L and Rosen I *et al* 2003 Experience of ultrasound-based daily prostate localization *Int. J. Radiat. Oncol. Biol. Phys.* **56** 436–47
[13] Fontanarosa D, van der Meer S, Bamber J, Harris E, O'Shea T and Verhaegen F 2015 Review of ultrasound image guidance in external beam radiotherapy: I. Treatment planning and inter-fraction motion management *Phys. Med. Biol.* **60** R77–114
[14] Orton N P, Jaradat H A and Tomé W A 2006 Clinical assessment of three-dimensional ultrasound prostate localization for external beam radiotherapy *Med. Phys.* **33** 4710–7
[15] Tomé W A, Meeks S L, Orton N P, Bouchet L G and Bova F J 2002 Commissioning and quality assurance of an optically guided three-dimensional ultrasound target localization system for radiotherapy *Med. Phys.* **29** 1781–8
[16] Peignaux K, Truc G, Barillot I, Ammor A, Naudy S and Créhange G *et al* 2006 Clinical assessment of the use of the Sonarray system for daily prostate localization *Radiother. Oncol.* **81** 176–8
[17] van der Meer S, Bloemen-van Gurp E, Hermans J, Voncken R, Heuvelmans D and Gubbels C *et al* 2013 Critical assessment of intramodality 3D ultrasound imaging for prostate IGRT compared to fiducial markers *Med. Phys.* **40** 071707

[18] Johnston H, Hilts M, Beckham W and Berthelet E 2008 3D ultrasound for prostate localization in radiation therapy: a comparison with implanted fiducial markers *Med. Phys.* **35** 2403–13

[19] Robinson D, Liu D, Steciw S, Field C, Daly H and Saibishkumar E P *et al* 2012 An evaluation of the Clarity 3D ultrasound system for prostate localization *J. Appl. Clin. Med. Phys.* **13** 3753

[20] Bloemen-van Gurp E, van der Meer S, Hendry J, Buijsen J, Visser P and Fontanarosa D *et al* 2013 Active breathing control in combination with ultrasound imaging: a feasibility study of image guidance in stereotactic body radiation therapy of liver lesions *Int. J. Radiat. Oncol. Biol. Phys.* **85** 1096–102

[21] Landry A, Berrang T, Gagne I, Popescu C, Mitchell T and Vey H *et al* 2014 Investigation of variability in image acquisition and contouring during 3D ultrasound guidance for partial breast irradiation *Radiat. Oncol.* **9** 35

[22] O'Shea T, Bamber J, Fontanarosa D, van der Meer S, Verhaegen F and Harris E 2016 Review of ultrasound image guidance in external beam radiotherapy part II: intra-fraction motion management and novel applications *Phys. Med. Biol.* **61** R90–137

[23] Camps S M, Fontanarosa D, de With P H N, Verhaegen F and Vanneste B G L 2018 The use of ultrasound imaging in the external beam radiotherapy workflow of prostate cancer patients *Biomed. Res. Int.* **2018** 7569590

[24] Lachaine M and Falco T 2013 Intrafractional prostate motion management with the Clarity Autoscan system *Med. Phys. Int.* **1** 72–80

[25] Tyloch J F and Wieczorek A P 2017 The standards of an ultrasound examination of the prostate gland. Part 2 *J. Ultrason.* **17** 43–58

[26] Camps S, Houben T, Edwards C, Antico M, Dunnhofer M and Martens E *et al* 2018 Quality assessment of transperineal ultrasound images of the male pelvic region using deep learning *2018 IEEE Int. Ultrasonics Symp. (IUS)* (IEEE) pp 1–4

[27] Terris M K, Hammerer P G and Nickas M E 1998 Comparison of ultrasound imaging in patients undergoing transperineal and transrectal prostate ultrasound *Urology.* **52** 1070–2

[28] de Crevoisier R, Tucker S L, Dong L, Mohan R, Cheung R and Cox J D *et al* 2005 Increased risk of biochemical and local failure in patients with distended rectum on the planning CT for prostate cancer radiotherapy *Int. J. Radiat. Oncol. Biol. Phys.* **62** 965–73

[29] Kupelian P A, Willoughby T R, Reddy C A, Klein E A and Mahadevan A 2008 Impact of image guidance on outcomes after external beam radiotherapy for localized prostate cancer *Int. J. Radiat. Oncol. Biol. Phys.* **70** 1146–50

[30] McPartlin A J, Li X A, Kershaw L E, Heide U, Kerkmeijer L and Lawton C *et al* 2016 MRI-guided prostate adaptive radiotherapy—a systematic review *Radiother. Oncol.* **119** 371–80

[31] Poli M E R, Parker W, Patrocinio H, Souhami L, Shenouda G and Campos L L *et al* 2007 An assessment of PTV margin definitions for patients undergoing conformal 3D external beam radiation therapy for prostate cancer based on an analysis of 10,327 pretreatment daily ultrasound localizations *Int. J. Radiat. Oncol. Biol. Phys.* **67** 1430–7

[32] Ghilezan M J, Jaffray D A, Siewerdsen J H, Van Herk M, Shetty A and Sharpe M B *et al* 2005 Prostate gland motion assessed with cine-magnetic resonance imaging (cine-MRI) *Int. J. Radiat. Oncol. Biol. Phys.* **62** 406–17

[33] Mah D, Freedman G, Milestone B, Hanlon A, Palacio E and Richardson T *et al* 2002 Measurement of intrafractional prostate motion using magnetic resonance imaging *Int. J. Radiat. Oncol. Biol. Phys.* **54** 568–75

[34] Padhani A R, Khoo V S, Suckling J, Husband J E, Leach M O and Dearnaley D P 1999 Evaluating the effect of rectal distension and rectal movement on prostate gland position using cine MRI *Int. J. Radiat. Oncol. Biol. Phys.* **44** 525–33

[35] Crook J M, Raymond Y, Salhani D, Yang H and Esche B 1995 Prostate motion during standard radiotherapy as assessed by fiducial markers *Radiother. Oncol.* **37** 35–42

[36] Moiseenko V, Liu M, Kristensen S, Gelowitz G and Berthelet E 2007 Effect of bladder filling on doses to prostate and organs at risk: a treatment planning study *J. Appl. Clin. Med. Phys.* **8** 55–68

[37] Chan P, Dinniwell R, Haider M A, Cho Y-B, Jaffray D and Lockwood G *et al* 2008 Inter- and intrafractional tumor and organ movement in patients with cervical cancer undergoing radiotherapy: a cinematic-MRI point-of-interest study *Int. J. Radiat. Oncol. Biol. Phys.* **70** 1507–15

[38] Jadon R, Pembroke C A, Hanna C L, Palaniappan N, Evans M and Cleves A E *et al* 2014 A systematic review of organ motion and image-guided strategies in external beam radiotherapy for cervical cancer *Clin. Oncol. (R Coll. Radiol.)* **26** 185–96

[39] Mason S A, White I M, O'Shea T, McNair H A, Alexander S and Kalaitzaki E *et al* 2019 Combined ultrasound and cone beam CT improves target segmentation for image guided radiation therapy in uterine cervix cancer *Int. J. Radiat. Oncol. Biol. Phys.* **104** 685–93

[40] van Dyk S and Bernshaw D 2008 Ultrasound-based conformal planning for gynaecological brachytherapy *J. Med. Imag. Radiat. Oncol.* **52** 77–84

[41] Sharma D N, Rath G K, Thulkar S, Kumar S, Subramani V and Julka P K 2010 Use of transrectal ultrasound for high dose rate interstitial brachytherapy for patients of carcinoma of uterine cervix *J. Gynecol. Oncol.* **21** 12–7

[42] Dulku G, Dhillon R, Goodwin M, Cheng W, Kontorinis N and Mendelson R 2017 The role of imaging in the surveillance and diagnosis of hepatocellular cancer *J. Med. Imag. Radiat. Oncol.* **61** 171–9

[43] Bertholet J, Knopf A, Eiben B, McClelland J, Grimwood A and Harris E *et al* 2019 Real-time intrafraction motion monitoring in external beam radiotherapy *Phys. Med. Biol.* **64** 15TR01

[44] Case R B, Sonke J-J, Moseley D J, Kim J, Brock K K and Dawson L A 2009 Inter- and intrafraction variability in liver position in non-breath-hold stereotactic body radiotherapy *Int. J. Radiat. Oncol. Biol. Phys.* **75** 302–8

[45] Boda-Heggemann J, Sihono D S K, Streb L, Mertens L, Vogel L and Stieler F *et al* 2019 Ultrasound-based repositioning and real-time monitoring for abdominal SBRT in DIBH *Phys Med.* **65** 46–52

[46] American College of Radiology 2013 *ACR BI-RADS Atlas* (Reston, VA: American College of Radiology)

[47] Strnad V, Ott O J, Hildebrandt G, Kauer-Dorner D, Knauerhase H and Major T *et al* 2016 5-year results of accelerated partial breast irradiation using sole interstitial multicatheter brachytherapy versus whole-breast irradiation with boost after breast-conserving surgery for low-risk invasive and *in situ* carcinoma of the female breast: a randomised, phase 3, non-inferiority trial *Lancet* **387** 229–38

[48] Trifiletti D M, Romano K D, Showalter S L, Reardon K A, Libby B and Showalter T N 2015 Accelerated partial breast irradiation with brachytherapy: patient selection and technique considerations *Breast Cancer* **7** 211–21

[49] Chadha M, Young A, Geraghty C, Masino R and Harrison L 2011 Image guidance using 3D-ultrasound (3D-US) for daily positioning of lumpectomy cavity for boost irradiation *Radiat. Oncol.* **6** 45
[50] Berrang T S, Truong P T, Popescu C, Drever L, Kader H A and Hilts M L *et al* 2009 3D ultrasound can contribute to planning CT to define the target for partial breast radiotherapy *Int. J. Radiat. Oncol. Biol. Phys.* **73** 375–83

IOP Publishing

Modern Applications of 3D/4D Ultrasound Imaging in Radiotherapy

Emma Harris, Davide Fontanarosa, Saskia Camps and Frank Verhaegen

Chapter 7

Ultrasound for measuring intrafractional organ motion

Alexander Grimwood and Svenja Ipsen

During radiotherapy delivery, the target volume and surrounding organs at risk may experience motion due to processes such as respiration, cardiovascular function, digestion and bladder filling. This intrafraction motion produces geometric uncertainties that must be accounted for both at the planning stage and during beam delivery. Planning margins account for expected patient motion relative to the static planning scans. During treatment, patient immobilisation and motion management strategies such as breath hold are used to limit intrafraction motion. State of the art radiotherapy techniques seek to use high targeting precision and intrafraction motion monitoring to deliver higher doses in fewer fractions and to adapt treatments as patients move. Ultrasound imaging is particularly suited to direct imaging of soft-tissue motion during treatment. This chapter presents the advantages and some of the challenges of using ultrasound for intrafraction motion management.

7.1 Introduction

Motion in radiotherapy can be differentiated into (1) interfractional changes observable on a day-to-day basis, such as tumour shrinkage or weight loss, and (2) intrafractional changes occurring during radiotherapy delivery, such as peristalsis or breathing motion. Translation, rotation and deformation of the target and the surrounding organs can lead to discrepancies between the static anatomy used for planning and the actual anatomy of the patient during treatment, potentially causing substantial dosimetric deviations from the original plan [1, 2]. Especially for high-dose treatments like in stereotactic body radiotherapy (SBRT), this could lead to severely overdosed healthy tissue and an underdosed tumour, compromising treatment efficacy. In this case, compensation of this motion is of highest

doi:10.1088/978-0-7503-2552-3ch7

importance. Examples of typical intrafractional motion patterns of different organs are illustrated in interactive figure 7.1.

While interfractional variations can mostly be compensated with static pretreatment imaging and plan adaptation as discussed in chapters 6 and 8, intrafractional motion requires continuous monitoring, and potentially adaptation, during treatment delivery. Even though a range of commercial and research systems can be used for intrafractional monitoring, only a brief overview of commercially available techniques used for treatment sites relevant to US monitoring will be given here. This includes external methods such as optical tracking (RPM, Varian Medical Systems Inc. Paolo Alto, CA, USA) and spirometry (ABC, Elekta AB, Stockholm Sweden), or internal methods such as kV image triangulation [3], MRI and electromagnetic fiducial transponders. External methods are mere surrogates for internal motion and, as a result, can be combined with monitoring of internal anatomy for higher accuracy, such as Exactrac (BrainLAB AG, Munich, Germany) or Synchrony (Accuray Inc. Sunnyvale, CA, USA) combining kV and optical tracking. While electromagnetic transponders (e.g., Calypso (Varian Medical Systems) or RayPilot (Micropos AB, Goteburg, Sweden)) can provide monitoring rates up to 50 Hz in patients, they require an additional implantation procedure. More recently, MRI guidance has entered the field of motion compensation with the combined MRI-linac systems MRIdian (Viewray Technologies Inc., Oakwood, OH, USA) and Unity (Elekta AB). First studies show promising results for intrafractional motion monitoring and gating [4]. However, real-time imaging with MRI is currently limited to about 2 Hz for a single 2D plane. For a comprehensive review of both commercial and research intrafractional motion compensation systems, [5] offers a detailed exploration.

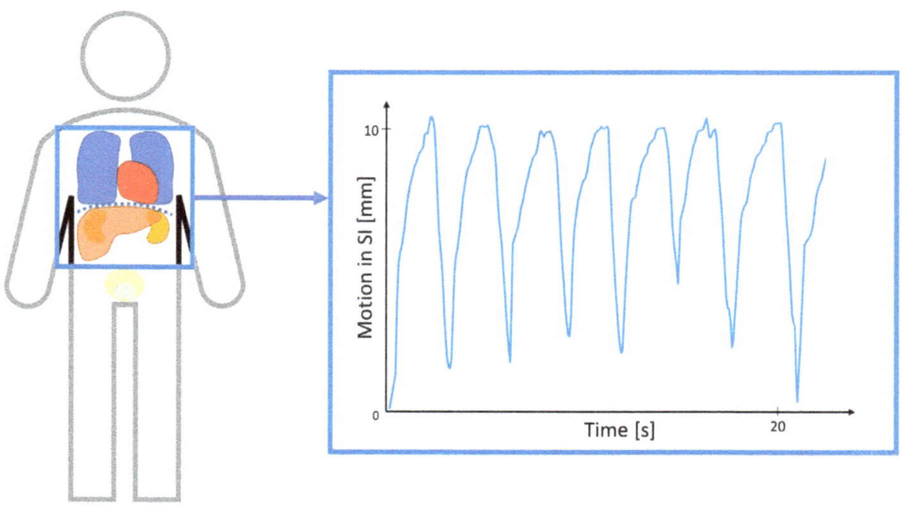

Figure 7.1. Interactive schematic of different anatomical treatment sites and corresponding typical intrafractional motion patterns. Lower abdominal and pelvic organs mainly experience slow, gradual drift, whereas periodic respiratory or cardiac motion affects the organs in the upper abdominal and thoracic area. Animation available at https://iopscience.iop.org/book/978-0-7503-2552-3.

Ultrasound imaging offers the unique advantage of being the only imaging modality that can provide volumetric image data in real-time (4D ultrasound), making it a promising candidate for intrafractional motion monitoring where target motion typically occurs in 3D space and low latency is a crucial factor. In principle, ultrasound can visualise all soft-tissue structures that are not occluded by air or bones. In a radiotherapy context, the main treatment sites suitable for ultrasound guidance are the breasts as well as inner organs in the upper and lower abdominal/pelvic area such as liver, kidneys, pancreas, prostate, uterus, cervix, bladder and rectum [6]. To date, most published studies on ultrasound guidance in radiotherapy have focussed on the prostate and the only commercially available system is using 3D ultrasound for inter- and intrafractional prostate monitoring [7].

This chapter will provide an overview of current state-of-the-art ultrasound guidance systems and monitoring approaches as well as the technical requirements and challenges this technology is facing. Section 7.2 illustrates different basic approaches for intrafractional motion monitoring in ultrasound image data, requiring accurate, robust target localisation and real-time capability. Technical and site-specific system requirements are discussed in section 7.3, as are the general limitations of ultrasound guidance. The different implementations of ultrasound guidance in phantom and patient studies are presented in section 7.4 while section 7.5 gives a glimpse into future directions and recommendations for this promising modality for real-time image guidance in radiotherapy.

7.2 Motion monitoring approaches in ultrasound

The goal of intrafractional ultrasound-guided motion monitoring is to detect a target structure in a series of ultrasound images (2D or 3D) in real time and use this information during treatment for passive monitoring or active motion compensation online. Recent years have seen notable improvements regarding ultrasound image quality, volumetric imaging and acquisition framerate, especially due to advanced imaging hardware and processing capabilities. At the same time, many approaches have been published that address the problem of reliable target localisation in ultrasound, the main challenges still often being low robustness or relatively high runtimes [8]. Several studies have shown that decreasing latency is in fact the most important factor for high-accuracy, real-time motion compensation in radiotherapy [8, 9]. However, different treatment sites often show different motion characteristics and could thus have variable demands on real-time performance and accuracy (see section 7.3.2).

In general, intrafractional motion monitoring approaches with ultrasound can be separated into two categories: (1) direct methods based only on image intensity values and (2) indirect methods based on learned correlations or motion models. To give the reader a better understanding of these basic concepts, select methods with a focus on *in vivo* application in a radiotherapy context will be presented in this section. For more details, the reader may also refer to an overview paper on intrafractional ultrasound guidance by O'Shea *et al* [6] or the results of the 'Challenge on Liver Ultrasound Tracking' (CLUST) with a variety of approaches presented in [8, 10].

7.2.1 Direct approaches

Ultrasound can visualise tissue structures and organ boundaries in real-time with good spatial resolution but the images are usually dominated by a grainy pattern referred to as speckle [11] depicted in figures 7.2 and 7.3. As described in chapter 2, speckle is caused by interference of the ultrasound waves at scattering tissue structures that are smaller than the spatial resolution limit of the ultrasound wavelength. Consequently, a speckle pattern is characteristic for a specific tissue region and generally follows its movements accordingly. It should however be noted that changes in the ultrasound imaging parameters or tissue rotation and deformation relative to the ultrasound probe can lead to decorrelation, causing differences in appearance of the local speckle pattern and even entire anatomical structures.

Direct target localisation approaches rely directly on the intensity values in the ultrasound image data and their correspondence to specific tissue structures even under motion. They can be employed locally to detect a single moving target or globally to generate entire motion fields, e.g. using template matching, features or differential methods.

Localised single-target tracking

Template matching is one of the most commonly used techniques for object localisation within an image, mainly due to its intuitive and simple implementation. It relies on the assumption that a moving structure does not significantly change its appearance when changing its position. The basic principle of template matching is illustrated in figure 7.2 and can be applied to 2D as well as 3D ultrasound data. First, a template representing the desired target is defined prior to localisation. During tracking, the location in the current frame is detected either globally or within a specified search region (region of interest (ROI)) as the point with the highest similarity to the template using similarity measures such as the sum of squared distances (SSD) or normalised cross correlation (NCC) [12].

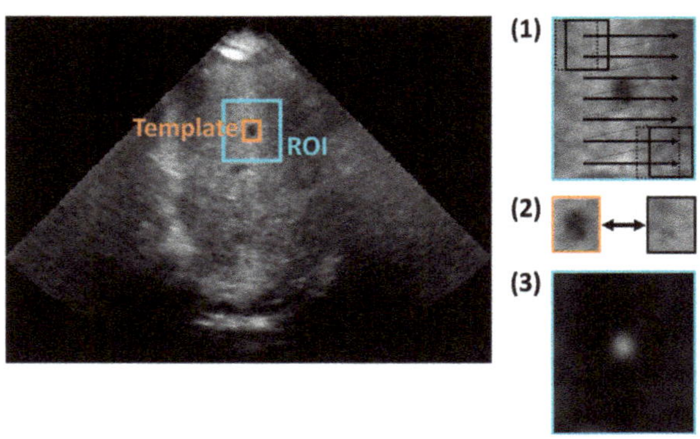

Figure 7.2. Principle of template matching in three steps. (1) The predefined template is moved iteratively over the region of interest (ROI) and (2) compared to each corresponding patch of the ROI using a suitable similarity metric. In Step (3), the point of highest similarity within the ROI is selected as the most probable target location in the current frame.

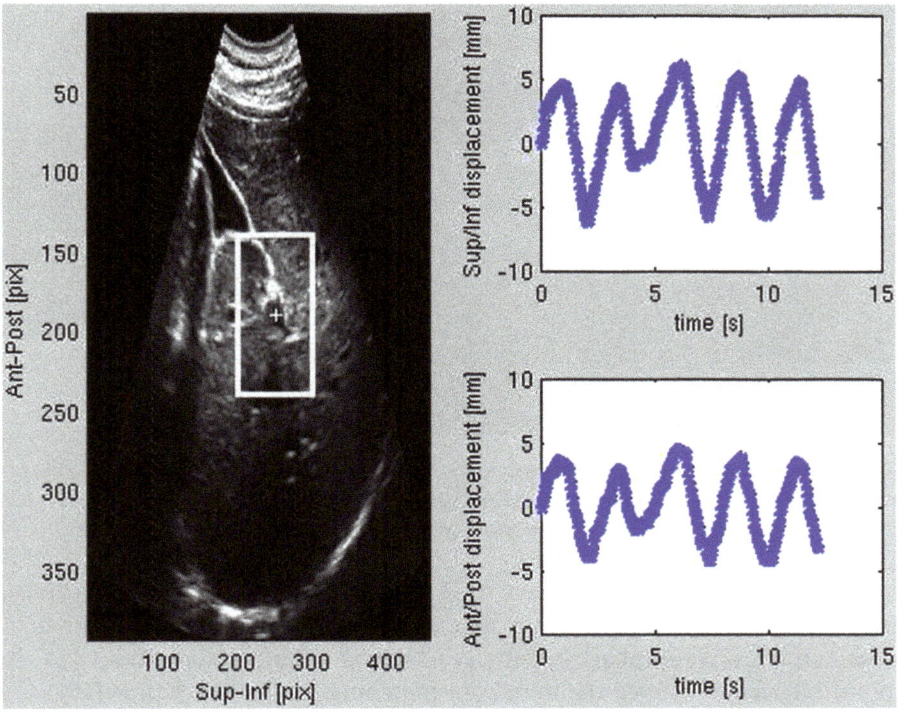

Figure 7.3. Animated schematic demonstrating the result of template matching in a 2D ultrasound sequence of the liver. A clearly resolved vessel is tracked over several breathing cycles. Animation available at https://iopscience.iop.org/book/978-0-7503-2552-3.

This concept can be used to detect resolved tissue structures, e.g. organ boundaries or vessels, as well as the speckle pattern in otherwise homogeneous tissue regions [13–15]. The latter is often referred to as speckle tracking. For accurate and robust localisation results, the template should include a unique pattern with stable appearance and visibility while the ROI should be large enough to cover the extent of interframe target motion and at the same time small enough to reduce mismatches throughout the ultrasound image. Because tumours can often not be distinguished from the surrounding healthy tissue due to similar acoustic properties, templates are often chosen at clearly resolved neighbouring structures, e.g. vessels in the liver as shown in animated figure 7.3. The target position can then be approximated based on the surrogate's motion when a fixed relationship is assumed. Template matching for target localisation is implemented in the only commercial solution currently available for ultrasound guidance in the prostate [7].

One of the main problems of using template matching for dynamic target localisation in ultrasound is the potentially changing target appearance due to decorrelation, artefacts or partial occlusion. Due to the relatively simple comparison between template and current frame on a pixel-by-pixel basis, such changes can lead to tracking errors. Especially when the search ROI is updated based on the last detected target position, these errors can accumulate over time and the target is

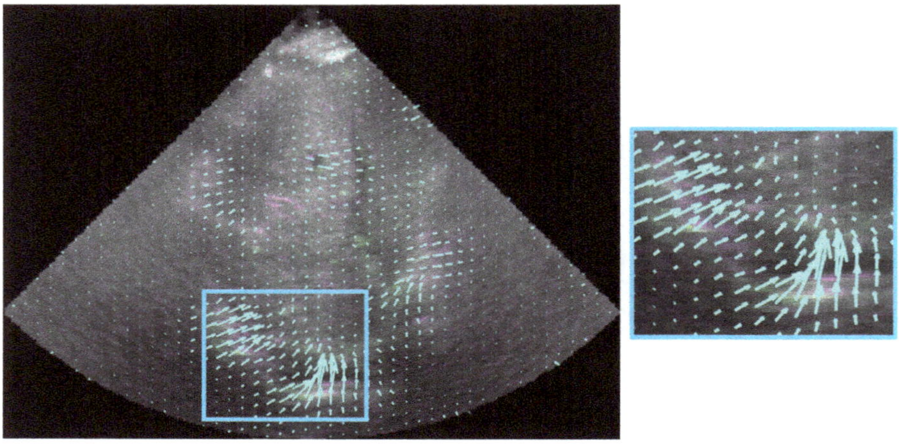

Figure 7.4. Global motion field in the liver generated over the entire field of view of the ultrasound image using optical flow. The blue arrows indicate motion from the previous frame f_{i-1} to the current frame f_i for each voxel. Both frames are plotted simultaneously using colour coding (green - f_{i-1}, purple - f_i).

ultimately lost. Different studies have tried to address the problem of low robustness by introducing regularisation mechanisms such as non-incremental tracking to avoid error accumulation [13], phase sensitivity to increase matching accuracy [14, 16] or temporal filtering to reduce the impact of matching outliers over time [17].

Another possible approach to increase matching robustness is the use of features that extend the simple pixel-based matching process. In this context, features can be considered descriptions of a localised neighbourhood around a key point based on certain key properties such as intensity value differences or gradients. Thus, features can reduce the amount of comparing operations while at the same time condense the information used for matching into the most relevant parameters. Participants of the CLUST study presented a convolutional neural network to generate lower-dimensional features that better represent the observed target motions during a training phase [8]. Another recent study used a pre-trained feature library to represent not only target motion but also deformation over the breathing cycle in 3D ultrasound data of the liver [18]. Another advantage of using multiple feature points in their library is the lower sensitivity to partial occlusion and single-feature stability.

Global tracking

In contrast to single-target techniques, global approaches try to extract multiple motion vectors, i.e. motion fields, over larger areas or even the entire ultrasound field of view (FOV) as illustrated in figure 7.4. The advantage of global approaches is that the available image data can be used more efficiently by extracting not only the current target position, but also information about organ motion surrounding the target which could be useful for improved tissue sparing or dose reconstruction. Additionally, a motion field allows the analysis of target rotation and even deformation.

One of the most obvious approaches for global tracking is block matching, an extension of template matching where the image is separated into many templates ($\leqslant$ number of voxels) and each is detected in the next frame within a localised neighbourhood. While this method can already produce a dense motion field, false or ambiguous matches will lead to sudden 'jumps' and discontinuities that are unrealistic from an anatomical point of view (tissue motion is relatively smooth and continuous). To address this problem, regularisation mechanisms must be introduced, constraining the result to reach smooth solutions. For 3D ultrasound tracking in the liver, Banerjee *et al* use a global block matching approach followed by an outlier rejection scheme for regularisation and a refinement step for localised target tracking [19]. For simplicity, the resulting motion field can then be reduced to a single rigid transform (translation + rotation) or an affine solution (rigid + scaling + shear).

Another approach to solve the global localisation problem is to exploit techniques from commonly used deformable image registration (DIR) algorithms. It has been shown that non-rigid registration can achieve high accuracy aligning ultrasound frames for motion monitoring in the liver [8]. 2D approaches such as optical flow, a technique that is widely known in the computer vision community for motion detection and 3D reconstruction tasks, have been successfully implemented for ultrasound tracking with real-time performance [8, 20]. It should be noted that DIR approaches are usually rather complex and thus computationally more demanding than simple feature or block matching techniques. In the case of 3D ultrasound, DIR is currently not real-time capable and thus not fully suitable for intrafractional monitoring purposes [21].

7.2.2 Indirect approaches

In contrast to direct, purely intensity-based techniques, indirect approaches use additional information, such as precalculated motion patterns or models, to support target localisation. In [22], the authors use a block matching algorithm combined with feature extraction and a temporal regularisation to avoid error accumulation. The latter is based on learning the typical target appearance in an initial training phase and comparing it to its current state. Similarly, Ha *et al* [23] use a pretreatment training phase to generate a motion model from dense motion fields derived offline from DIR. During tracking, only a few discrete feature locations are monitored as surrogates and global motion is approximated using the pretrained motion model, making the approach real-time capable. Instead of considering motion patterns over time, Royer *et al* [24] included a mechanical model simulating internal forces for regularisation. They combine their mechanical regularisation with a stepwise affine matching scheme with high accuracy and acceptable latency in 3D ultrasound images of the liver.

Indirect approaches can also rely on correlation models to approximate target motion based on surrogate signals. Schlosser *et al* [25] investigated respiratory gating in the liver using ultrasound guidance, showing that internal surrogates acquired close to the therapy target are superior to external surrogates on the body surface.

In [26], the authors demonstrated for the first time that correlation-based motion compensation can be achieved in real time using a correlation between continuous 3D ultrasound guidance and discrete x-ray imaging. Interestingly, this combination can also be exploited for real-time motion monitoring in the lung [27], an organ which cannot be imaged with ultrasound due to its acoustic properties.

The typical target localisation accuracy of intrafractional ultrasound tracking approaches (direct and indirect) is in the range of 1–2 mm, with *in vivo* measurements usually yielding slightly lower accuracy than controlled, phantom-based experiments. It should be noted that the definition of a ground truth as the reference position for validation is actually much more difficult for *in vivo* data where the intra- and interobserver variability can be in the range of millimetres [28]. While the accuracy of direct and indirect approaches available to date is comparable, their applicability mostly depends on the treatment site, i.e. the presence of resolved structures and possible latency restrictions.

7.3 System requirements for intrafractional ultrasound guidance

Intrafractional motion monitoring requires target localisation with low latency and high accuracy during treatment and thus poses considerable challenges for technical implementation as well as for integration into the radiotherapy workflow. However, the system requirements for an ultrasound guidance system not only depend on the modality itself but also on the method of treatment adaptation it is combined with (e.g. gating or tracking) and the treatment site it is used for. These factors could potentially influence the selection of necessary hard- and software components for the desired application and will be discussed in the following sections.

7.3.1 Site-specific requirements

A number of studies have investigated the amount of intrafractional target motion and its impact on treatment quality and dose distributions for different sites, e.g. [29, 30]. In the scope of this chapter, a broad overview of motion characteristics and their relevance for ultrasound guidance will be presented. For further details, a comprehensive overview on intrafractional organ motion ranges observable with ultrasound imaging can be found in [6].

Ultrasound-based monitoring systems should offer an FOV that covers the expected motion range of the target and a temporal resolution that allows capturing all aspects of target motion with a sufficiently high sampling rate. Lower abdominal/pelvic organs are affected by relatively slow motion typically occurring over several minutes that is mainly caused by bladder filling, gas transiting the intestines and gradual muscle relaxation, leading to a gradual drift, or rarely to erratic shifts, of the target [31]. Over the course of a single fraction, prostate motion is typically small (< 2 mm) but can exceed 18 mm in some cases [32]. Different characteristic motion patterns of the prostate have been identified [33] but are highly patient-specific.

For successful intrafractional ultrasound guidance of lower abdominal and pelvic organs, low sampling rates $\geqslant 1$ Hz and an FOV covering the target and a small margin for motion could be acceptable.

Organs in the upper abdominal and thoracic region are mainly affected by respiratory motion. The breathing cycle is generally periodic, but can have variable lengths between 3 and 6 s, with high variability between patients but even between different breaths of the same patient. Liver motion magnitudes over a single breathing cycle are usually in the range of 5–15 mm [34, 35] but can reach almost 40 mm in some patients [36]. The highest motion amplitude is typically seen in the craniocaudal direction, caused by the up-down-movement of the diaphragm. Consequently, respiratory motion is much faster than the slow drift seen in lower organs. Additionally, soft tissue organs like the liver are affected by differential motion, i.e. rotation and deformation. Rotations in the range of several degrees were observed for targets in the liver [34, 37]. Using 4D MRI, it has also been shown that liver motion magnitudes and the amount and direction of gradual drift vary substantially across the organ and can lead to systematic deviations from the initial position [38]. This type of motion is much more complex than typical pelvic motion, thus requiring higher sampling rates of $\geqslant 4$ Hz [14] and larger FOVs to cover the higher extent of possible motion for real-time target localisation. However, this could potentially be circumvented by using breath-holds as motion mitigation strategy. In this case, residual motion during the breath-hold is much smaller [39] and fast localisation is not as critical.

The most complex type of motion affects the heart with a combination of respiratory and pulsatory components. Respiratory motion of the heart lies in the range of 10 to 20 mm [29] while cardiac contraction in the ventricles can be up to 8 mm [40]. The directions of highest motion extent are craniocaudal and anterior-posterior. Due to its velocity and its added complexity, framerates $\geqslant 12$ Hz are recommended for motion monitoring in the heart [14]. The FOV is often limited by the narrow acoustic windows through the ribs but should cover the entire target and its trajectory over the course of breathing and cardiac cycles.

7.3.2 Technical requirements

Ultrasound monitoring involves direct imaging of internal tissue volumes facilitated by its excellent soft-tissue contrast and its ability to image in real time and in three dimensions without using ionising radiation. Ultrasound images are registered to the treatment isocentre by tracking the probe's position and orientation in real time within the treatment room (see chapter 3), often using optical tracking systems. This enables registration between fractions and modalities, namely simulation CT and on-treatment CBCT. Continuous visibility of the optical markers attached to the probe throughout the treatment fraction is vital for a successful registration and must be ensured for each patient and treatment site prior to delivery. For image-based monitoring, a reference volume of interest must be defined and subsequently tracked. This is typically derived from a planning structure, such as the planning target volume, previously delineated on the simulation CT scan [7]. At treatment setup, the tissues contained within reference volume (acquired at simulation CT) are localised to establish an initial position. During treatment, an image registration algorithm estimates instantaneous position relative to the reference volume. In addition to volume displacement, a measure of the monitoring quality must be provided, so that treatment can be suspended should the motion estimates fall below a predefined confidence threshold.

All monitoring systems must quantify motion at the intended target volume with adequate spatiotemporal resolution to enable adaptation of the delivered treatment (via gating or tracking, for example). To meet this requirement a system must estimate motion of the target and possibly within surrounding organs at risk. Intrafraction motion compensation requires online, real-time data transfer of monitoring data between the treatment delivery system, or radiotherapy practitioner, and the ultrasound system. The latency between motion detection and system response must be small enough to account for intrafraction motion. The method of adaptation and type of motion dictate acceptable latency times, as discussed in section 7.3.1. Response times also vary. Multi-leaf collimator (MLC) tracking is limited by the maximum collimator speed and acceleration. Similarly, couch tracking is limited by the speed and acceleration of the patient couch. For gating, the limitations are simpler—being dictated by the operator's reaction time (where manual gating is used) and the inherent beam on/beam off delay on command.

Autoscan (Elekta AB) is currently the only commercial ultrasound system designed to monitor target motion using real-time image acquisition. The system is approved for prostate and prostate bed radiotherapy. The Autoscan sample rate is ~3 Hz, which is fast enough to monitor pelvic motion with an adequate system latency of ~1 s. Autoscan is compatible with conventional linacs and uses a transperineal ultrasound probe that can be positioned outside of the treatment field to minimise disruption to standard delivery protocols.

7.3.3 Challenges and limitations

Implementing intrafractional image guidance for real-time motion monitoring comes with high requirements regarding image quality, tracking robustness and system latency. To use ultrasound imaging in this context, its technical characteristics and potential limitations must be understood. Many factors can affect the accuracy of ultrasound-based motion monitoring, including target-specific aspects such as depth and motion patterns, as well as aspects considering image acquisition, data type and tracking algorithm. Several key challenges will be discussed in this section. For further interest, a detailed analysis can be found in [6].

Many of the intrafractional ultrasound guidance approaches to date have focussed on the use of 2D imaging. The main advantages of 2D ultrasound are its widespread availability, the easy accessibility of the image data (e.g. through a frame grabber) and very high framerates. Additionally, many tracking algorithms developed by the much larger computer vision community can be adapted without much effort. However, the tracking task in radiotherapy is inherently 3D—the target volume moves, and even deforms, dynamically within the anatomy. The first 3D probes were mechanical (see chapter 2) and provided relatively low framerates (1–2 Hz) sufficient for interfractional motion compensation and slowly moving targets such as the prostate (see section 7.3.1). Fast target motion caused by respiration or pulsation requires framerates of at least 4 Hz and 12 Hz [14], respectively, and thus cannot be adequately sampled. Especially fast target motion and motion along the sweep direction of the mechanical 3D probe causes severe artefacts and high tracking errors [41]. In recent years, real-time volumetric ultrasound systems (4D ultrasound) using matrix array transducers have seen significant progress and can now provide higher framerates (5–20+ Hz) and improved image quality necessary for accurate target localisation and low-latency monitoring [42]. Another factor affecting the total latency of the system, and thus its accuracy, is the processing time of the target localisation algorithm which should be kept at a minimum, ideally lower than the image acquisition rate. Keall *et al* suggest a maximum latency of 500 ms for a real-time motion compensation system [43] as latency is the largest contributor to tracking errors overall [9]. Processing times can often be reduced by using smaller search regions or targets, employing faster hardware or implementing parallelised algorithms on graphical processing units (GPUs).

Intrafractional ultrasound guidance also suffers from the inherent limitations of ultrasound imaging due to the physical properties of image acquisition. In contrast to CT or MRI, ultrasound imaging is rotation-variant [44], i.e. target appearance depends on current orientation and deformation, complicating continuous target localisation. As described in chapter 2, severe artefacts can occur when the sound waves encounter large impedance mismatches (such as boundaries from soft tissue to bones or air-filled lungs), potentially occluding the target and thus disrupting continuous monitoring. Inconsistent speed of sound values in different tissues can lead to a distortion of the target position, potentially causing localisation errors up to several millimetres (see chapters 2 and 3).

The tracking algorithms developed for intrafractional ultrasound guidance are another limiting factor. An ideal algorithm must be able to accurately quantify the range and types of motion typically experienced within a volume of interest. For soft tissue imaging, motion can be complex and the ideal algorithm may have to account for rotations, non-rigid deformations, large periodic motion and irregular non-periodic displacements. In addition to tissue motion, large changes in the relative position of an anatomical feature with respect to the transducer will alter the appearance of the feature in the ultrasound image. Advanced DIR methods show promise, but do not yet demonstrate real-time capability. Commercial ultrasound guidance systems are able to track rigid motion in a volume of interest across six degrees of freedom, provided the target rotations are relatively small and its appearance is consistent between frames [45, 46].

Above all, one of the main disadvantages of ultrasound imaging in general is the dependence on a transducer staying in direct contact with the patient's surface. This implies that a loss of contact will lead to a loss of image data and thus tracking information, while setup reproducibility directly depends on the exact positioning of the ultrasound transducer with constant pressure. A possible approach to address these problems is the automation of the probe positioning process, as discussed in chapter 9. Furthermore, since ultrasound is used during treatment delivery, the probe could cause distortions in the precalculated dose distribution and could be damaged by the treatment beam. Thus, the presence of the probe must be considered during planning (see chapter 5).

7.4 Clinical applications

Most of the approaches on real-time target localisation described in section 7.2 have been conducted offline on previously acquired ultrasound data with a manually defined ground truth. Consequently, the results are affected by observer variability of manual landmarks in ultrasound [28] and, at the same time, explicitly exclude the errors that would usually be introduced by full system integration, such as in-room calibration and absolute tracking errors from acoustic artefacts (see chapter 3). In order to assess the performance of fully integrated ultrasound guidance, several experiments have been conducted *in vitro* and *in vivo*, using ultrasound for actual online motion compensation and for monitoring purposes.

7.4.1 *In vitro* studies

Due to their controlled conditions and predictable behaviour, *in vitro* studies are crucial when determining the accuracy, precision and latency of a motion monitoring system. The main advantage of phantom experiments is their high reliability and relative comparability of the results, especially when external reference markers are used to define the ground truth. A potential disadvantage is the lack of realism when using simplified phantoms and motion patterns.

Based on prior experiences from interfractional ultrasound guidance, the first study to assess the feasibility of intrafractional ultrasound-guided motion compensation via gating was conducted by [47]. They used a mechanical 3D US probe (Voluson730, Medison, Seoul, South Korea) and a simple water phantom moved in a sinusoidal pattern by a 1D motion platform to simulate breathing motion. A 2D template matching approach (100 ms processing time) was used for target localisation but no further quantitative results regarding accuracy or gating integration were presented. Harris *et al* [13] used a 3D programmable motion stage with a modelled respiratory trajectory to move a mechanical probe with a volumetric framerate of 1–2 Hz (Accuvix XQ, Medison, Seoul, South Korea) relative to the target. Target localisation accuracy and precision were < 1 mm and < 0.5 mm, respectively, with tracking in the elevational direction and fast target motion producing the greatest errors [41]. By relying on realistic prostate motion trajectories and external references (optical and electromagnetic markers), Abramowitz *et al* [48] confirmed an accuracy of < 1 mm using a mechanical 3D US probe (Autoscan, Elekta AB) to track a dynamically moving target. In a similar setup with an identical probe, agreement between optical and ultrasound tracking was within 1 mm in 95% of the time using simplified stepwise translational excursions to represent prostate motion [7]. Using another type of mechanical 3D probe with a volumetric framerate of 1.7 Hz (RSP6–12, GE Healthcare Inc., Chicago IL, USA), O'Shea *et al* [15] tracked stepwise static displacements as well as realistic prostate motion of a phantom. They achieved sub-millimetre accuracy comparable to the external x-ray-based reference system of a radiosurgery system (CyberKnife, Accuray Inc.), yet struggled with relatively high errors in the elevational direction that had to be eliminated using motion thresholds.

One of the first studies to implement intrafractional motion compensation based on real-time ultrasound guidance used a robotic radiosurgery system (CyberKnife, Accuray Inc.), a fast 4D US system with a volumetric framerate of 17.7. Hz, direct data access (Vivid 7 Dimension, GE Healthcare Inc.) and a correlation-based tracking approach [26] as illustrated in figure 7.5. A metal bead target was moved in a water tank with combined respiratory and pulsatory 3D motion using a robot. By replacing the optical tracking signal of superficial markers on the patient's chest with the internal target localisation from ultrasound and calculating a correlation model using the onboard Synchrony system, they could show that it is possible to compensate even for such complex motion with a geometric accuracy of 1.5 mm using x-ray images as a reference. In [49], a pseudo-3D ultrasound transducer with two perpendicular 2D planes (Mediri gMBH, Heidelberg, Germany) and online image processing at an overall framerate of 6.7 Hz was successfully used to measure 2D target motion and actively steer a proton beam. With a total system latency of about 200 ms, they achieved sub-millimetre accuracy relative to a laser sensor. Using the same ultrasound system, Schwaab *et al* [50] went one step further and implemented a full system calibration to convert ultrasound to treatment room coordinates by optically tracking the ultrasound probe (see also chapter 3). The rubber ball target was moved with a 1D sinusoidal motion trace and the real-time position derived from ultrasound was used to steer a heavy ion beam. They reported an overall accuracy of 4.8 mm when compared to time-resolved 4D positron-emission tomography (PET), with calibration as the main contributor to the tracking errors. Fast *et al* were the first to implement ultrasound-guided motion compensation on a conventional linac, using

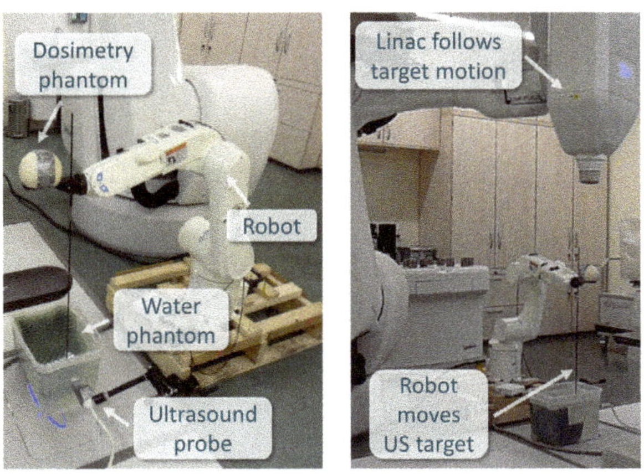

Figure 7.5. Experimental setup of real-time ultrasound-guided motion compensation using a robotic radiosurgery system as used in (Blanck *et al* [26]). A target is moved in a water phantom and localised with 4D US. Using a pre-generated correlation model, the linac position is dynamically adapted to compensate for target motion.

the Autoscan system, dynamic MLC tracking and a motion stage programmed with sinusoidal and prostate trajectories [51]. The principle of ultrasound-guided MLC tracking is illustrated in interactive figure 7.6. Due to the temporal limitations of the mechanical 3D probe, high latencies from 0.5 to 1.0 s and tracking errors below 1.8 mm were observed.

With their experimental setups, most of the previous studies were limited to monitoring or compensating quasi-static prostate motion or refrained from using 3D imaging. Faster breathing motion had not been investigated in comparable depth due to severe artefacts that would arise from interplay between slow 3D acquisition and fast target motion. This problem was addressed by Ipsen *et al* [52] who were the first to combine a fast 4D ultrasound system using a matrix array probe (3V-D, GE Healthcare Inc.) with real-time MLC tracking. At a volumetric framerate of 21.3 Hz, a metal bead target was moved in a water phantom using realistic prostate as well as more complex lung motion trajectories. They could show that ultrasound guidance led to the lowest reported latency of 172 ms for image-guided MLC tracking. Sub-millimetre accuracy was achieved for prostate tracking and even fast breathing motion could be compensated with a low tracking error 1.3 mm.

The *in vitro* studies conducted to date show that intrafractional motion monitoring and even real-time compensation can be achieved with online ultrasound guidance. It can also be concluded that sufficient temporal resolution, i.e. low system latency, at the image acquisition and processing stages is of utmost importance for this scenario to minimise the differences between ultrasound frames for accurate target localisation and to reduce the errors introduced by prediction for accurate motion compensation.

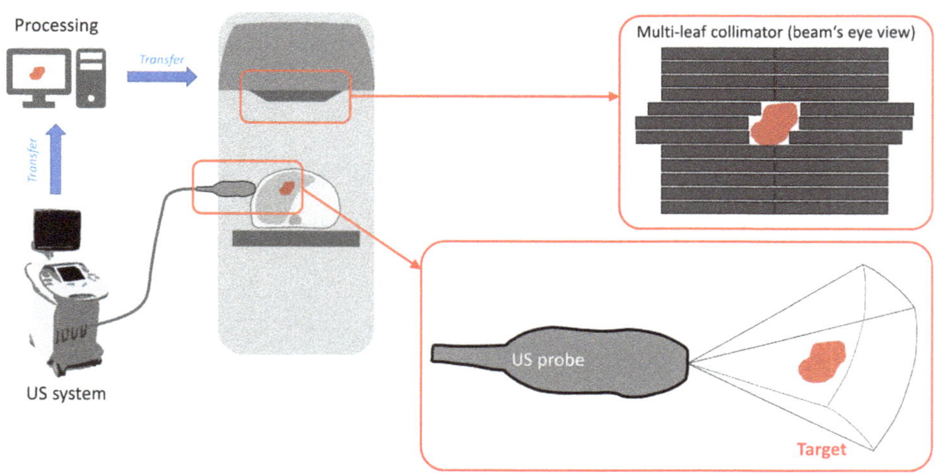

Figure 7.6. Dynamic multi-leaf collimator (MLC) aperture following a moving target. Use the slider to move the therapy target in the liver of the virtual patient. The current target location is detected with real-time ultrasound imaging and sent to the treatment system. The original MLC aperture is then adapted to the new target position by moving the separate leaves. Animation available at https://iopscience.iop.org/book/978-0-7503-2552-3.

7.4.2 *In vivo* studies

Clinically, prostate radiotherapy is the predominant application for 4D ultrasound monitoring. As a result, most *in vivo* studies focus on characterising the precision, accuracy and latency of ultrasound monitoring of the prostate and prostate bed. Direct comparisons with alternative monitoring technologies have also been made, specifically portal imaging and EM transponders. Many of these studies attempt to characterise intrafraction motion and some also identify notionally acceptable displacement thresholds. Few attempt the challenging task of examining the implications of ultrasound monitoring on dosimetry and planning strategies.

Intrafraction ultrasound monitoring has been used to successfully model prostate motion as a random walk [31, 53]. Under this assumption the prostate drifts gradually away from the isocentre during each fraction, resulting in increasing geometric uncertainty over time. Studies have also observed abrupt shifts associated with muscle clenching and rectal filling [32, 53, 54].

Prostate motion is typically small, with different studies reporting displacements below 2 mm for >92% of the total intrafraction monitoring time [32, 55]. However, intrafraction displacements >3 mm are experienced at least once by almost all patients [32, 54, 55]. This threshold is reached in approximately half of all fractions [45, 54]. Reported maximum displacements are typically close to 8 mm, but range from < 3 mm to < 18 mm over monitoring periods lasting between 100 s–600 s [32, 56]. Comparing data across centres is difficult however, because no standardised method of reporting has been devised. Obvious sources of variation include patient sample size, monitoring time and the reporting metrics used. Less clear are undeclared factors, such as user training requirements, imaging protocols and general workload.

Hypofractionated therapies where the posterior margin is 2–3 mm, or rectal sparing margins of typically 5 mm present a clear requirement for monitoring. Similarly, prostate motion is less prevalent over treatment times associated with volumetric modulated arc therapy (VMAT), but geometric uncertainties increase for longer treatments such as intensity-modulated radiotherapy (IMRT) and hypofractionation. Population-based VMAT margins have been calculated for intrafraction prostate motion using the van Herk method, resulting in small margins of 1.25 mm left-right, 1.33 mm anteroposterior and 1.10 mm craniocaudal [32]. However, the magnitude and pattern of motion in the same study was patient specific and varied between fractions. This led the authors to conclude that simple population-based models could not adequately be applied to individual patients. Motion correction strategies are still possible and are being developed by clinical centres. For example Bristol University Hospital reports pausing treatment during prostate radiotherapy if a motion threshold of 7 mm is breached and repositioning the patient couch relative to measured displacement [54].

Ultrasound monitoring has been clinically validated against other monitoring methods. An evaluation between Autoscan and Raypilot (Micropos AB) EM transponders concluded both technologies were viable monitoring solutions [45]. In the same study, both methods exhibited craniocaudal monitoring errors in the presence of rotation around the left-right axis. Autoscan proved to be more susceptible, giving a 6.9 mm error for 15° rotations compared to 3.8 mm for RayPilot. This observation underpinned a systematic divergence of motion estimates from the two monitoring techniques acquired in a single patient experiencing changes to rectal filling between planning and treatment. Agreement between Autoscan and intraprostatic markers identified in electronic portal images was within 2.5 mm for a 95% confidence threshold over 16 patients [57].

Beyond the prostate, ultrasound motion monitoring has been applied to the upper abdomen, where respiratory motion requires significant consideration. Various sites are accessible for ultrasound imaging. The feasibility of monitoring liver motion simultaneously using a customised Vivid 7 (GE Healthcare Inc.) and Calypso EM transponders (Varian Medical systems Inc.) was demonstrated in [58]. Autoscan has also been used to quantify liver motion in patients performing deep inspiration breath hold during liver radiotherapy. Here, a mean (SD) motion of 2.5 mm (0.7 mm) was reported [59]. In the same study, displacements larger than 10 mm were observed for a small proportion of measurements (0.8%). Although it is not clear if these larger shifts were confined to a single fraction or patient, they provided further justification for monitoring. To this end, the authors of the study identified a number of outstanding barriers to implementation of ultrasound monitoring for the upper abdomen. Considerations include probe positioning during treatment (section 5.4) and interobserver variation (section 4.5).

Other groups have investigated the use of ultrasound to image upper abdominal sites as surrogates for motion in the lung and pancreatic head. Good agreement was found between lung motion identified in CBCT projections and Autoscan monitoring, however, the study authors concede the three patients recruited were selected to ensure their tumours were located close to the diaphragm providing good correlation between diaphragm and treatment site [27]. Monitoring of the portal vein as a surrogate for the pancreatic head was demonstrated in patients prior to treatment delivery. The position of the portal vein relative to the pancreas was evaluated against 4DCT data acquired at simulation and found to agree with a mean absolute difference (SD) < 2.3 mm (0.8 mm) [60].

Clinical studies of intrafraction ultrasound guidance must contend with the challenge of establishing a ground truth. For *in vivo* studies, this is especially difficult. Evaluation of fully integrated ultrasound guidance methods are often performed without direct access to a measurable ground truth. Instead, performance is often compared to alternative monitoring technologies and assumptions must be made regarding the sources and magnitude of uncertainties based upon *a priori* knowledge from *in vitro* studies and previous clinical experience. The task is non-trivial and has limited the number of published studies where the relationship between ultrasound guidance and specific clinical outcomes is explicitly quantified.

7.5 Future directions and recommendations

Ultrasound intrafraction motion monitoring systems have been commercially available for over a decade and the technique is used routinely in a number of centres. Recent advances in ultrasound technology have addressed some of the modality's inherent limitations, increasing the 4D acquisition rates, expanding the field of view, improving image quality through enhanced image processing and reducing interoperator variability through automation. The translation of these technologies into the radiotherapy clinic will lead to a wider range of ultrasound monitoring applications in conjunction with the latest treatment delivery techniques.

The publication record regarding *in vitro* and volunteer studies provides a clear indication of likely future applications. A strong candidate is ultrasound monitoring of abdominal structures, especially the liver and pancreas, where early steps towards clinical translation have been reported [58, 60]. Peripheral soft-tissues, such as the breast, are also well-suited to ultrasound imaging and make good candidates for ultrasound intrafraction monitoring. Research into peripheral applications has, however, been limited, possibly because probe positioning can be difficult as contact must be maximised whilst avoiding both tissue deformation and treatment beam obstruction. Specific technical barriers to the wider implementation of ultrasound monitoring are described in section 7.3.3.

A convincing case must be made for the contribution of ultrasound monitoring towards new therapy adaptation techniques as they increasingly find their way into the clinic. Research groups need to clearly demonstrate the efficacy of integrating ultrasound monitoring with the latest treatment planning and delivery technologies, especially in relation to adaptive radiotherapy where 4D image acquisition is highly advantageous. To this end, future studies should expand upon previous research into intrafraction adaptation, such as MLC tracking, by investigating how 4D ultrasound can enhance planning strategies [51, 52]. A wider exploration of how ultrasound monitoring complements other commercial motion management technologies is also desirable. Interoperability between different monitoring solutions, treatment planning systems, and radiotherapy platforms will ensure a range of monitoring technologies can be effectively employed alongside each other to maximise patient benefit.

Recommendations regarding clinical best practice for ultrasound image guidance in radiotherapy were published in the 2011 AAPM Report Task Group Report 154 [61]. The guidance describes relevant clinical considerations, training requirements and suggested quality assurance procedures. In light of technological developments since publication, updated advice is required, especially in relation to 4D ultrasound quality assurance (QA). Specifically, the absence of QA tests (and suitable phantoms) for motion estimation algorithms needs to be addressed, with particular guidance required on quantifying accuracy and constancy for different anatomical sites. Updates are also required to address the current use of transperineal probes and to pre-empt the next generation of matrix arrays that will likely be incorporated into future guidance systems. Incorporation of intrafraction uncertainties into recommendations on end-to-end testing and the quantification of guidance errors needs to be addressed and will also help to establish what improvements in guidance accuracy and precision have been achieved by newer ultrasound monitoring systems.

Consolidation quiz

Q1: **What is the advantage of using ultrasound for intrafraction motion monitoring?**

- Every radiotherapy department has an ultrasound image guidance system
- Ultrasound is the only imaging modality that can provide volumetric soft tissue imaging in real time
- The ionising radiation dose associated with all other imaging modalities makes it impossible to rely on them for intrafraction motion monitoring

Q2: **Regularisation is a technique used in both direct and indirect monitoring. Which of these is not a regularisation method used in intrafraction monitoring?**

- Temperature regularisation
- Spatial regularisation
- Temporal regularisation

Q3: **Intrafraction motion compensation requires accurate target localisation with low latency. What is the suggested maximum latency for a real-time motion compensation system?**

- 3 s
- 10 μs
- 500 ms

Q4: **Various clinical applications of intrafraction monitoring have been studied both *in vivo* and *in vitro*. What is the most common ultrasound intrafraction monitoring application?**

- MLC tracking
- Breast SBRT
- Prostate radiotherapy

References

[1] Yu C X, Jaffray D A and Wong J W 1998 The effects of intra-fraction organ motion on the delivery of dynamic intensity modulation *Phys. Med. Biol.* **43** 91–104

[2] Colvill E, Booth J T, O'Brien R T, Eade T N, Kneebone A B and Poulsen P R *et al* 2015 Multileaf collimator tracking improves dose delivery for prostate cancer radiation therapy: results of the first clinical trial *Int. J. Radiat. Oncol. Biol. Phys.* **92** 1141–7

[3] Poulsen P R, Cho B and Keall P J 2008 A method to estimate mean position, motion magnitude, motion correlation, and trajectory of a tumor from cone-beam CT projections for image-guided radiotherapy *Int. J. Radiat. Oncol. Biol. Phys.* **72** 1587–96

[4] Fischer-Valuck B W, Henke L, Green O, Kashani R, Acharya S and Bradley J D *et al* 2017 Two-and-a-half-year clinical experience with the world's first magnetic resonance image guided radiation therapy system *Adv. Radiat. Oncol.* **2** 485–93

[5] Bertholet J, Knopf A, Eiben B, McClelland J, Grimwood A and Harris E *et al* 2019 Real-time intrafraction motion monitoring in external beam radiotherapy *Phys. Med. Biol.* **64** 15TR01

[6] O'Shea T, Bamber J, Fontanarosa D, van der Meer S, Verhaegen F and Harris E 2016 Review of ultrasound image guidance in external beam radiotherapy part II: intra-fraction motion management and novel applications *Phys. Med. Biol.* **61** R90–137

[7] Lachaine M and Falco T 2013 Intrafractional prostate motion management with the Clarity Autoscan system *Med. Phys. Int.* **1** 72–80

[8] De Luca V, Banerjee J, Hallack A, Kondo S, Makhinya M and Nouri D *et al* 2018 Evaluation of 2D and 3D ultrasound tracking algorithms and impact on ultrasound-guided liver radiotherapy margins *Med. Phys.* **45** 4986–5003

[9] Poulsen P R, Cho B, Sawant A, Ruan D and Keall P J 2010 Detailed analysis of latencies in image-based dynamic MLC tracking *Med. Phys.* **37** 4998–5005

[10] De Luca V, Benz T, Kondo S, König L, Lübke D and Rothlübbers S *et al* 2015 The 2014 liver ultrasound tracking benchmark *Phys. Med. Biol.* **60** 5571–99

[11] Burckhardt C B 1978 Speckle in ultrasound B-mode scans *IEEE Trans. Son. Ultrason.* **25** 1–6

[12] Goshtasby A A 2012 *Image Registration* (London: Springer)

[13] Harris E J, Miller N R, Bamber J C, Symonds-Tayler J R N and Evans P M 2010 Speckle tracking in a phantom and feature-based tracking in liver in the presence of respiratory motion using 4D ultrasound *Phys. Med. Biol.* **55** 3363–80

[14] Bell M A L, Byram B C, Harris E J, Evans P M and Bamber J C 2012 *In vivo* liver tracking with a high volume rate 4D ultrasound scanner and a 2D matrix array probe *Phys. Med. Biol.* **57** 1359–74

[15] O'Shea T P, Garcia L J, Rosser K E, Harris E J, Evans P M and Bamber J C 2014 4D ultrasound speckle tracking of intra-fraction prostate motion: a phantom-based comparison with x-ray fiducial tracking using CyberKnife *Phys. Med. Biol.* **59** 1701–20

[16] Byram B, Holley G, Giannantonio D and Trahey G 2010 3-D phantom and *in vivo* cardiac speckle tracking using a matrix array and raw echo data *IEEE Trans. Ultrason. Ferroelectr. Freq. Control* **57** 839–54

[17] O'Shea T P, Bamber J C and Harris E J 2016 Temporal regularization of ultrasound-based liver motion estimation for image-guided radiation therapy *Med. Phys.* **43** 455

[18] Wulff D, Kuhlemann I, Ernst F, Schweikard A and Ipsen S 2019 Robust motion tracking of deformable targets in the liver using binary feature libraries in 4D ultrasound *Curr. Dir. Biomed. Eng.* **5** 601–4

[19] Banerjee J, Klink C, Niessen W J, Moelker A and van Walsum T 2016 4D ultrasound tracking of liver and its verification for TIPS guidance *IEEE Trans. Med. Imag.* **35** 52–62

[20] Kubota Y, Matsumura A, Fukahori M, Minohara S, Yasuda S and Nagahashi H 2014 A new method for tracking organ motion on diagnostic ultrasound images *Med. Phys.* **41** 092901

[21] Vijayan S, Klein S, Hofstad E F, Lindseth F, Ystgaard B and Langø T 2014 Motion tracking in the liver: validation of a method based on 4D ultrasound using a nonrigid registration technique *Med. Phys.* **41** 082903

[22] De Luca V, Tschannen M, Székely G and Tanner C 2013 A learning-based approach for fast and robust vessel tracking in long ultrasound sequences *Med. Image Comput. Comput. Assist. Interv.* **16** 518–25

[23] Ha I Y, Wilms M, Handels H and Heinrich M P 2019 Model-based sparse-to-dense image registration for realtime respiratory motion estimation in image-guided interventions *IEEE Trans. Biomed. Eng.* **66** 302–10

[24] Royer L, Krupa A, Dardenne G, Le Bras A, Marchand E and Marchal M 2017 Real-time target tracking of soft tissues in 3D ultrasound images based on robust visual information and mechanical simulation *Med. Image Anal.* **35** 582–98

[25] Schlosser J, Salisbury K and Hristov D 2011 Image-based approach to respiratory gating for liver radiotherapy using a telerobotic ultrasound system *Int. J. Radiat. Oncol. Biol. Phys.* **81** S122

[26] Blanck O, Jauer P, Ernst F, Bruder R and Schweikard A 2013 Pilot-Phantomstudie zur ultraschallgeführten robotergestützten Radiochirurgie *44 Jahrestagung der DGMP. Cologne, Germany* 122–3

[27] Mostafaei F, Tai A, Gore E, Johnstone C, Haase W and Ehlers C *et al* 2018 Feasibility of real-time lung tumor motion monitoring using intrafractional ultrasound and kV cone beam projection images *Med. Phys.* **45** 4619–26

[28] van der Meer S, Bloemen-van Gurp E, Hermans J, Voncken R, Heuvelmans D and Gubbels C *et al* 2013 Critical assessment of intramodality 3D ultrasound imaging for prostate IGRT compared to fiducial markers *Med. Phys.* **40** 071707

[29] Korreman S S 2012 Motion in radiotherapy: photon therapy *Phys. Med. Biol.* **57** R161–91

[30] Brandner E D, Chetty I J, Giaddui T G, Xiao Y and Huq M S 2017 Motion management strategies and technical issues associated with stereotactic body radiotherapy of thoracic and upper abdominal tumors: a review from NRG oncology *Med. Phys.* **44** 2595–612

[31] Ballhausen H, Li M, Hegemann N S, Ganswindt U and Belka C 2015 Intra-fraction motion of the prostate is a random walk *Phys. Med. Biol.* **60** 549–63

[32] Sihono D S K, Ehmann M, Heitmann S, von Swietochowski S, Grimm M and Boda-Heggemann J *et al* 2018 Determination of intrafraction prostate motion during external beam radiation therapy with a transperineal 4-dimensional ultrasound real-time tracking system *Int. J. Radiat. Oncol. Biol. Phys.* **101** 136–43

[33] Ng J A, Booth J T, Poulsen P R, Fledelius W, Worm E S and Eade T *et al* 2012 Kilovoltage intrafraction monitoring for prostate intensity modulated arc therapy: first clinical results *Int. J. Radiat. Oncol. Biol. Phys.* **84** e655–61

[34] Bertholet J, Worm E S, Fledelius W, Høyer M and Poulsen P R 2016 Time-resolved intrafraction target translations and rotations during stereotactic liver radiation therapy: implications for marker-based localization accuracy *Int. J. Radiat. Oncol. Biol. Phys.* **95** 802–9

[35] Worm E S, Høyer M, Hansen R, Larsen L P, Weber B and Grau C *et al* 2018 A prospective cohort study of gated stereotactic liver radiation therapy using continuous internal electromagnetic motion monitoring *Int. J. Radiat. Oncol. Biol. Phys.* **101** 366–75

[36] Worm E S, Høyer M, Fledelius W, Hansen A T and Poulsen P R 2013 Variations in magnitude and directionality of respiratory target motion throughout full treatment courses of stereotactic body radiotherapy for tumors in the liver *Acta Oncol.* **52** 1437–44

[37] Xu Q, Hanna G, Grimm J, Kubicek G, Pahlajani N and Asbell S *et al* 2014 Quantifying rigid and nonrigid motion of liver tumors during stereotactic body radiation therapy *Int. J. Radiat. Oncol. Biol. Phys.* **90** 94–101

[38] von Siebenthal M, Székely G, Lomax A J and Cattin P C 2007 Systematic errors in respiratory gating due to intrafraction deformations of the liver *Med. Phys.* **34** 3620–9

[39] Vogel L, Sihono D S K, Weiss C, Lohr F, Stieler F and Wertz H *et al* 2018 Intra-breath-hold residual motion of image-guided DIBH liver-SBRT: an estimation by ultrasound-based monitoring correlated with diaphragm position in CBCT *Radiother. Oncol.* **129** 441–8

[40] Roujol S, Anter E, Josephson M E and Nezafat R 2013 Characterization of respiratory and cardiac motion from electro-anatomical mapping data for improved fusion of MRI to left ventricular electrograms *PLoS One* **8** e78852

[41] Harris E J, Miller N R, Bamber J C, Symonds-Tayler J R N and Evans P M 2011 The effect of object speed and direction on the performance of 3D speckle tracking using a 3D swept-volume ultrasound probe *Phys. Med. Biol.* **56** 7127–43
[42] Ipsen S, Bruder R, García-Vázquez V, Schweikard A and Ernst F 2019 Assessment of 4D ultrasound systems for image-guided radiation therapy—image quality, framerates and CT artifacts *Curr. Dir. Biomed. Eng.* **5** 245–8
[43] Keall P J, Mageras G S, Balter J M, Emery R S, Forster K M and Jiang S B *et al* 2006 The management of respiratory motion in radiation oncology report of AAPM Task Group 76 *Med. Phys.* **33** 3874–900
[44] Grau V, Becher H and Noble J A 2007 Registration of multiview real-time 3-D echocardiographic sequences *IEEE Trans. Med. Imaging* **26** 1154–65
[45] Biston M-C, Zaragori T, Delcoudert L, Fargier-Voiron M, Munoz A and Gorsse C *et al* 2019 Comparison of electromagnetic transmitter and ultrasound imaging for intrafraction monitoring of prostate radiotherapy *Radiother. Oncol.* **136** 1–8
[46] Brooks R 2017 System and method for target tracking using a quality indicator during radiation therapy *US Patent* WO/2017/001920
[47] Sawada A, Yoda K, Kokubo M, Kunieda T, Nagata Y and Hiraoka M 2004 A technique for noninvasive respiratory gated radiation treatment system based on a real time 3D ultrasound image correlation: a phantom study *Med. Phys.* **31** 245–50
[48] Abramowitz M C, Bossart E, Flook R, Wu X, Brooks R and Lachaine M *et al* 2012 Noninvasive real-time prostate tracking using a transperineal ultrasound approach *Int. J. Radiat. Oncol. Biol. Phys.* **84** S133
[49] Prall M, Kaderka R, Saito N, Graeff C, Bert C and Durante M *et al* 2014 Ion beam tracking using ultrasound motion detection *Med. Phys.* **41** 041708
[50] Schwaab J, Prall M, Sarti C, Kaderka R, Bert C and Kurz C *et al* 2014 Ultrasound tracking for intra-fractional motion compensation in radiation therapy *Phys Med.* **30** 578–82
[51] Fast M F, O'Shea T P, Nill S, Oelfke U and Harris E J 2016 First evaluation of the feasibility of MLC tracking using ultrasound motion estimation *Med. Phys.* **43** 4628
[52] Ipsen S, Bruder R, O'Brien R, Keall P J, Schweikard A and Poulsen P R 2016 Online 4D ultrasound guidance for real-time motion compensation by MLC tracking *Med. Phys.* **43** 5695
[53] Pommer T, Oh J H, Munck Af Rosenschöld P and Deasy J O 2017 Simulating intrafraction prostate motion with a random walk model *Adv. Radiat. Oncol.* **2** 429–36
[54] Richardson A K and Jacobs P 2017 Intrafraction monitoring of prostate motion during radiotherapy using the Clarity® Autoscan Transperineal Ultrasound (TPUS) system *Radiography* **23** 310–3
[55] Richter A, Exner F, Weick S, Lawrenz I, Polat B and Flentje M *et al* 2020 Evaluation of intrafraction prostate motion tracking using the Clarity Autoscan system for safety margin validation *Z. Med. Phys.* **30** 135–41
[56] Baker M and Behrens C F 2016 Determining intrafractional prostate motion using four dimensional ultrasound system *BMC Cancer.* **16** 484
[57] Grimwood A, McNair H A, O'Shea T P, Gilroy S, Thomas K and Bamber J C *et al* 2018 In vivo validation of Elekta's clarity Autoscan for ultrasound-based intrafraction motion estimation of the prostate during radiation therapy *Int. J. Radiat. Oncol. Biol. Phys.* **102** 912–21

[58] Ipsen S, Bruder R, Worm E S, Hansen R, Poulsen P R and Høyer M *et al* 2017 Simultaneous acquisition of 4D ultrasound and wireless electromagnetic tracking for in-vivo accuracy validation *Curr. Dir. Biomed. Eng.* **3** 75–8

[59] Boda-Heggemann J, Sihono D S K, Streb L, Mertens L, Vogel L and Stieler F *et al* 2019 Ultrasound-based repositioning and real-time monitoring for abdominal SBRT in DIBH *Phys Med.* **65** 46–52

[60] Omari E A, Erickson B, Ehlers C, Quiroz F, Noid G and Cooper D T *et al* 2016 Preliminary results on the feasibility of using ultrasound to monitor intrafractional motion during radiation therapy for pancreatic cancer *Med. Phys.* **43** 5252

[61] Molloy J A, Chan G, Markovic A, McNeeley S, Pfeiffer D and Salter B *et al* 2011 Quality assurance of U.S.-guided external beam radiotherapy for prostate cancer: report of AAPM Task Group 154 *Med. Phys.* **38** 857–71

Chapter 8

Applications of ultrasound to adaptive radiotherapy

Saskia Camps, Emma Harris and Sarah Mason

The field of adaptive radiotherapy is relatively new and as yet is not commonly used in the clinic. It is, however, under intense investigation by researchers who have established its superiority compared to standard image guided radiotherapy in terms of the reduction of dose to normal tissues and who now seek to establish the technologies to enable its routine use. In section 8.1 we describe the concepts of adaptive radiotherapy and the imaging requirements to support its implementation. In sections 8.2 and 8.3 we review two applications of ultrasound to adaptive radiotherapy of the prostate and cervix, respectively. In section 8.2, the use of ultrasound to create pseudo computed tomography images for the purpose of replanning is described. In section 8.3, a study of the combination of ultrasound and cone beam computed tomography (CBCT) for greater visualisation of the uterine boundary which may lead to more precise definition of the target tissue for replanning is reviewed.

8.1 Introduction

8.1.1 Adaptive radiotherapy

The previous two chapters discussed the use of ultrasound imaging to correct for interfraction and intrafraction motion. The techniques described in chapter 6 correct for interfraction motion by moving the patient, typically by adjustment of the couch position. To correct for intrafraction motion (chapter 7), the radiotherapy beam may be gated to irradiate when the target is in the planned position only, or tracked to follow the motion of the target. Shifting the couch and gating accounts for rigid motion only and does not account for any deformation (changes in both shape and size) of the target or the surrounding normal tissues. With beam tracking, when a dynamic collimator such as the multi-leaf collimator is employed, it is possible to

doi:10.1088/978-0-7503-2552-3ch8

account for deformation as well as translational motion of the target, however, tracking does not account for changes in the surrounding anatomy. Interactive figure 8.1 provides an example of how tissues can undergo deformation between treatments. In this case of the uterus, daily motion can be extreme and it is easy to see that simply shifting the couch will not account for deformation of tissue.

Adaptive radiotherapy, introduced by [1], is the practice of changing the treatment delivery plan to account for translation and deformation of the target and surrounding tissues. In general, there are two paradigms used in adaptive radiotherapy. The first, triggered replanning, responds to systematic changes in either the patient anatomy between planning and delivery; and the second responds to daily changes in the patient anatomy, using a 'plan of the day' (POTD) or by on-line replanning.

Triggered replanning can be triggered at some predefined time, i.e., mid-treatment, after the delivery of 30 Gy, weekly, etc [2–5], or by dosimetric criteria, i.e., if under or over dosing is predicted based on changes in the patient's anatomy [6, 7]; or if treatment imaging, such as CBCT has been used to recalculate dose and indicates changes in dosimetry from the treatment plan [8]. Once generated, the new plan replaces the old plan for the remainder of the patient's treatment, or until the generation of a new plan is triggered.

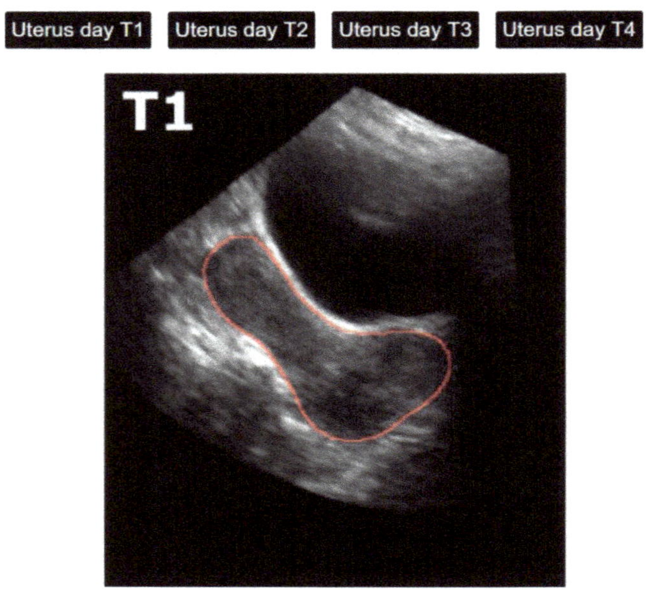

Figure 8.1. This interactive figure illustrates the large day to day deformation of the uterine motion of the uterine body. These images show central 2D slices of ultrasound volumetric images acquired on different days of treatment (T1, T2, T3 and T4). Also note how the image of the uterus has poor quality when the uterus is more upright (T2 and T4). On these days the bladder was almost empty as a result overlying tissue (the bowel) attenuated the ultrasound signal, obstructing the view of the uterus. Animation available at https://iopscience.iop.org/book/978-0-7503-2552-3.

The second approach uses a POTD, which refers to a technique where a library of treatment plans is generated prior to, or early on in, the patient's treatment to accommodate differences in daily variation in the position, size and shape of soft tissue, which for lower abdominal tissues are primarily due to different levels of bladder filling [5, 9–12]. Immediately prior to daily radiation delivery, the plan that best matches the patient's anatomy at the time of treatment is selected for use.

Both triggered and POTD approaches require in-room imaging so that clinicians and radiation therapy technologists can either determine changes in the patient anatomy which might lead to changes in dosimetry (for example, weight gain or loss or tumour regression), or visualise tissues to help select the most appropriate POTD. They also rely upon the acquisition of multiple CT scans either before treatment or during the course of treatment.

The third approach, on-line replanning, refers to rapidly generating a new treatment plan based on the internal anatomy of the patient at the time of treatment for every radiotherapy fraction. An example workflow for on-line replanning would be to (1) position the patient on the treatment couch, (2) acquire a treatment image that enables the rapid and accurate segmentation of the target structures and organs at risk (OARs), (3) generate a new treatment plan that conforms to the target whilst minimising dose to the surrounding normal tissues, and (4) deliver the radiation. Compared to other adaptive radiotherapy techniques, on-line replanning has the greatest potential for reducing normal tissue toxicity because it corrects for complex day-to-day deformation of the anatomy, i.e., differential motion between target tissues and organs at risk, and it accounts for all tissue motion, not just that caused by variation in a single variable such as target motion [13].

8.1.2 Imaging for adaptive radiotherapy

Triggered adaptive radiotherapy requires in-room imaging that should be able to inform on gross changes in the body outline or size of the tumour. For POTD selection, ideally the boundaries of the target and/or organs at risk should be visible, allowing the selection of the plan in the library that matches the daily anatomy best. Off-line evaluation of delivered dose and on-line replanning rely on in-room imaging of sufficient image quality so that images can either:

(1) be used to accurately depict the boundaries of the target and OARs such that they can be rapidly (ideally automatically) segmented and voxel gray scale values can be reliably converted to electron density for the purpose of replanning; or
(2) be used to deform the planning CT, using deformable image registration, to accurately represent the day's anatomy.

Researchers have proposed to use either in-room CT, megavoltage CBCT or megavoltage fan beam CT or kilovoltage CBCT for the purpose of adaptive radiotherapy. More recently, combined magnetic resonance imaging (MRI) scanners and linacs (MRI-linacs) have been introduced as an alternative imaging modality for adaptive radiotherapy ([14, 15]). In-room CT systems offer superior image quality but require additional space in the treatment room and can limit patient throughput [16]. Advantages of megavoltage x-ray imaging systems are that they are fully integrated with the linac and are able to more accurately characterise electron density. Unfortunately, they have poorer soft tissue contrast than kilovoltage systems due to the predominance of Compton interactions in tissue at megavoltage photon energies. Kilovoltage CBCT provides 3D images of the patient with excellent bony anatomy contrast and is commonly used for bony anatomy-based and fiducial-based assessment of setup errors ([17–20]). CBCT does provide some soft tissue contrast, though it can be difficult and not always possible to visualise the soft tissue boundaries due to scatter and reconstruction artefacts [19, 21–26]. Adaptive radiotherapy technologies that offer good soft tissue visualisation and are relatively lower cost than the highly specialised and expensive MRI-linacs, will arguably have greater benefit to the wider population of patients with cancer.

In the following two sections we briefly review how ultrasound may be used in an adaptive radiotherapy workflow to overcome the challenge of soft tissue visualisation for (1) the purpose of replanning by using ultrasound to create a pseudo CT in the context of prostate radiotherapy, and (2) as an adjunct to CBCT for visualisation of the uterus for the purpose of adaptive gynaecological radiotherapy.

8.2 Ultrasound for pseudo CT creation for adaptive prostate radiotherapy

In several chapters of this book it has been highlighted that the radiotherapy treatment plans are typically prepared based on a CT scan as this is the only image modality that provides the required electron density information. To allow for radiotherapy plan adaptation electron density information is also required which implies that, ideally, a CT scan would be acquired every time a treatment plan change is deemed necessary. However, this additional CT scan acquisition is nowadays not part of the standard clinical routine due to, among others, extra dose deposition to the patient, high costs and longer patient set up times [16].

Van der Meer *et al* [27] and Camps *et al* [28] have proposed a workflow that can provide electron density information without actually acquiring a CT scan, but using ultrasound imaging instead. The electron density information is captured in the form of a pseudo-CT scan and could potentially be used for treatment replanning.

In the proposed workflow (see figure 8.2), the simulation stage includes the acquisition of a regular simulation CT scan as well as a co-registered ultrasound volume. Subsequently, at the treatment stage, only an ultrasound volume is acquired in the CT (and radiotherapy delivery) coordinate system. By performing deformable registration of both ultrasound volumes (simulation and treatment volume) it is possible to generate a deformation field. The publications describe several approaches towards the generation of the deformation field: only rigid registration, only deformable registration or a combination of both. Also, for the registration, several similarity metrics (e.g., mutual information) have been explored. If the generated deformation field is then applied to the simulation CT scan, a pseudo-CT

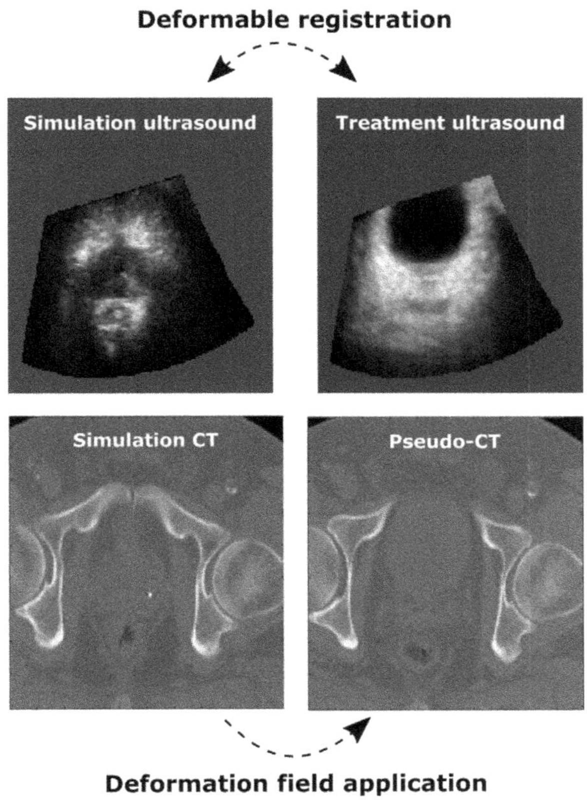

Figure 8.2. Workflow for the creation of a pseudo-CT scan of a prostate cancer patient using deformable registration of two ultrasound volumes that are acquired at simulation and treatment stage, respectively. During the deformable registration a deformation field is created which is then applied to the simulation CT scan, resulting in a pseudo-CT scan.

scan is created. It has been shown that the pseudo-CT scan better represents the patient's anatomy at the time of treatment than the simulation CT scan does.

The work by Van der Meer *et al* and Camps *et al* investigates the creation of pseudo-CT scans for prostate cancer patients based on transabdominal ultrasound volumes. This work could be expanded towards other cancer sites and could make use of other ultrasound imaging strategies, like transperineal ultrasound imaging, as well.

8.3 Ultrasound for adaptive radiotherapy for cervical cancer

The uterus is subject to large day-to-day variation in both position and shape due to changes in bladder and bowel filling (see figure 8.1). Conventional radiotherapy for cervical cancer which delivers radiation dose to the cervix, uterus and pelvic nodes requires the use of large planning target volume margins (up to 4 cm) to encompass uterine motion, which results in high doses of radiation to surrounding normal tissues. Adaptive radiotherapy is now considered optimal for the treatment of cervical cancer and the best approach to adaptation is currently being investigated [29].

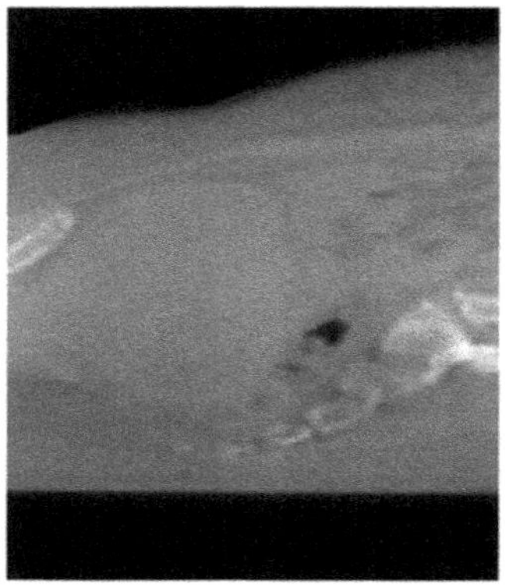

Figure 8.3. This interactive figure displays the central sagittal slices of a CBCT and a 3D ultrasound volumetric image which are co-registered using the Elekta Clarity system. Moving the slider gradually reveals the ultrasound image and the posterior boundary of the uterus becomes more visible. Animation available at https://iopscience.iop.org/book/978-0-7503-2552-3.

Ultrasound is widely used in obstetrics to perform routine diagnostic scans of the endometrium, uterus, cervix and the foetus to ensure the health of mothers and their unborn babies. This supports the suggestion that ultrasound may be a promising imaging modality to visualise the uterus as an alternative or adjunct to CBCT for image-guided radiotherapy for cervical cancer [30], and could potentially be used to enable improved soft tissue-based visualisation for adaptive radiotherapy techniques such as POTD selection or on-line replanning. Indeed, if the uterine boundary was clearly visualised on ultrasound, then the uterus could be easily segmented by observers to define the target volume for replanning or, in the the context of on-line replanning, automatically segmented. Figure 8.3 illustrates how the uterine boundary may be visualised clearly on ultrasound images but can sometimes be difficult to discern on CBCT due to poor image contrast.

A quantitative comparison of ultrasound (US) and CBCT image quality and visibility of the uterine boundary was conducted by Mason *et al* [31]. They demonstrated that on average ultrasound may be used to define the uterine boundary with precision equal to CBCT. They also showed that ultrasound can be used to complement CBCT and that combined ultrasound and CBCT (CBCT-US) enables greater boundary visualisation and observer confidence compared to ultrasound or CBCT alone, and for some cases this was due to greater visualisation of the boundary on ultrasound compared to CBCT.

Mason *et al* [31] found that the agreement of contours drawn by novice observers that had only one hour's training in the interpretation of ultrasound images of the cervix with a ground truth contour was better on CBCT-US than either ultrasound or CBCT alone. Dice Similarity Coefficient (DSC) was used to assess contour agreement, the results are illustrated in boxplots in figure 8.4(a). Interestingly, when asked to rate their certainty that their contour reflected the true uterine boundary from 1 (extremely uncertain) to 10 (extremely certain), the eight observers rated ultrasound to have the highest certainty (see figure 8.4(b)).

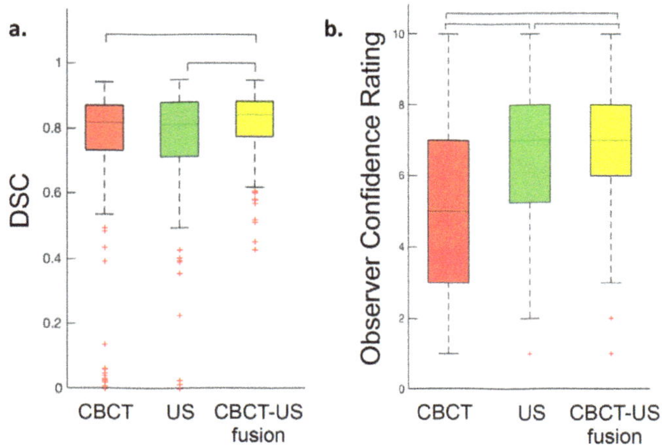

Figure 8.4. Boxplots demonstrating the DSC and Observer Confidence Rating results for each imaging method (CBCT, US, and CBCT-US-fusion) in panes a and b, respectively. Brackets indicate significant differences ($p < 0.05$) between imaging methods. Note that observers had the greatest contouring agreement and confidence on CBCT-US-fusion image.

The reason why higher observer ratings on ultrasound did not correspond to an improvement in contouring agreement on ultrasound over CBCT was unclear. It may have been due to the limited experience of the observers who had only one hour's training on ultrasound compared with CBCT, which was in routine clinical use. Inspection of the data also revealed that the observers in the 'New-to-ultrasound' cohort sometimes misinterpreted the non-homogeneous soft tissue contrast, uterine sub-structures (such as cysts or the endometrial lining) or ultrasound artefacts as the uterine boundary; errors which could potentially be overcome with more training. Examples of such ultrasound artefacts are shown in figure 8.5. It should be noted that lack of training is a perennial problem with studies comparing new techniques to established ones, and is especially pertinent to the introduction of ultrasound which typically requires a high level of user skill and experience.

The improvement in contour agreement on CBCT-US compared to the individual imaging modalities could be attributed to either (1) one of the imaging modalities displaying greater uterine boundary visibility than the other, or (2) the fusion of the two images provided complementary information. In the case of (1), the acquisition of two images essentially improved the probability of obtaining a high quality image. In the case of (2), different information was available in each image. It is recognised that there is a steep learning curve in ultrasound image interpretation which may be partially due to the fact that observers cannot rely on the body habitus or skeleton to orient themselves with the internal anatomy [32]. Potentially this is another reason for the increase in the contouring concordance and observer confidence when ultrasound is combined with CBCT above using ultrasound alone, CBCT helps the observer interpret the ultrasound image.

In the conditions in which the radiotherapy staff are adequately trained in acquiring and interpreting ultrasound images, and the ultrasound equipment is

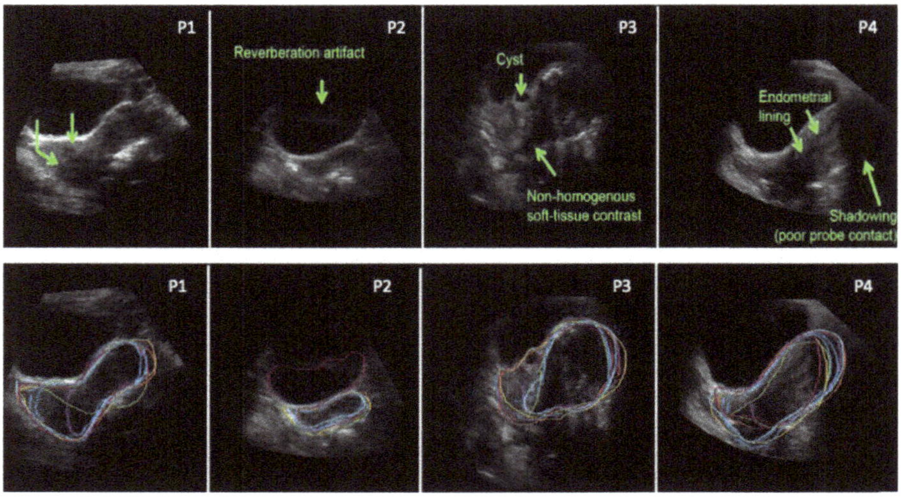

Figure 8.5. Top row: examples of ultrasound imaging features that caused contouring disagreement in four patients (P1–4); and bottom row: contouring disagreement which may result from misinterpretation of ultrasound images. Such features include non-homogeneous soft-tissue contrast in the uterus, internal structures such as cysts and the endometrial lining, and ultrasound artefacts such as shadowing and reverberations.

calibrated and set up in the treatment room, the resource investment in acquiring pre-treatment ultrasound images is small: there is no additional patient dose, ultrasound imaging equipment is relatively inexpensive and can be incorporated into pre-existing treatment room setups, and it only takes an additional few minutes (depending on how easy the uterus can be visualised) to acquire a 3D ultrasound scan. Thus, the CBCT could be augmented with ultrasound. Furthermore, the issue of using ultrasound images for replanning would not need to be addressed, the contours could be defined using CBCT-US fusion and the CBCT could be used to replan the treatment.

The fact that in some instances ultrasound gave greater observer concordance than CBCT, and that the precision of uterine segmentation was equal for both modalities alone, suggests that it may be possible that the ultrasound could replace CBCT for plan verification and POTD selection for cervical cancer patients. Ultrasound could also be implemented for image-guidance in centres without CBCT imaging systems (i.e., in low to middle income countries), or in centres that want frequent image-guidance without imparting a concomitant imaging dose to the patient.

Several challenges associated with uterine imaging using ultrasound have been noted and ultrasound image quality of the uterus has been found to be strongly influenced by: operator skill and experience, abdominal fat, bladder filling, probe pressure and acoustics obstructions, such as gas [33–36]. Furthermore, mechanically-swept 3D probes have a relatively small field of view, making it difficult to capture the entire uterus (particularly in cases where the disease is bulky), and it may be impossible to capture all of the nearby organs at risk. In these cases methods such as 3D extended aperture imaging described in section 4.5.2 could be employed to overcome the limited field of view. Further work and data from a larger cohort of patients is needed to build on the work by Mason *et al* before ultrasound can be established as an acceptable image guidance modality for adaptive radiotherapy for cervical cancer.

Consolidation quiz

Q1: In an adaptive radiotherapy workflow ultrasound will not provide:
- Accurate electron density information
- Visualisation of soft tissue boundaries
- Real-time volumetric images for dynamic replanning

Q2: Why is the acquisition of a CT scan prior to each treatment fraction not part of a standard clinical routine?
- CT equipment is commonly not available in the radiotherapy room
- The patient can experience serious discomfort during the scan acquisition
- It does not provide any clinically relevant information

Q3: In a comparison of uterine visibility on CBCT and ultrasound and ultrasound-CBCT fusion. Mason *et al* [31] did not find:
- Observers were much more confident when delineating the uterus on CBCT alone
- Observer concordance in uterine delineation was equal for CBCT and ultrasound
- Observer concordance in uterine delineation was greatest for ultrasound-CBCT fusion

References

[1] Yan D, Vicini F, Wong J and Martinez A 1997 Adaptive radiation therapy *Phys. Med. Biol.* **42** 123–32

[2] Oh S, Stewart J, Moseley J, Kelly V, Lim K and Xie J *et al* 2014 Hybrid adaptive radiotherapy with on-line MRI in cervix cancer IMRT *Radiother. Oncol.* **110** 323–8

[3] Stewart J, Lim K, Kelly V, Xie J, Brock K K and Moseley J *et al* 2010 Automated weekly replanning for intensity-modulated radiotherapy of cervix cancer *Int. J. Radiat. Oncol. Biol. Phys.* **78** 350–8

[4] van de Bunt L, van der Heide U A, Ketelaars M, de Kort G A P and Jürgenliemk-Schulz I M 2006 Conventional, conformal, and intensity-modulated radiation therapy treatment planning of external beam radiotherapy for cervical cancer: the impact of tumor regression *Int. J. Radiat. Oncol. Biol. Phys.* **64** 189–96

[5] Li T, Thongphiew D, Zhu X, Lee W R, Vujaskovic Z and Yin F-F *et al* 2011 Adaptive prostate IGRT combining online re-optimization and re-positioning: a feasibility study *Phys. Med. Biol.* **56** 1243–58

[6] Lim K, Stewart J, Kelly V, Xie J, Brock K K and Moseley J *et al* 2014 Dosimetrically triggered adaptive intensity modulated radiation therapy for cervical cancer *Int. J. Radiat. Oncol. Biol. Phys.* **90** 147–54

[7] Birkner M, Yan D, Alber M, Liang J and Nüsslin F 2003 Adapting inverse planning to patient and organ geometrical variation: algorithm and implementation *Med. Phys.* **30** 2822–31
[8] Liu C, Kim J, Kumarasiri A, Mayyas E, Brown S L and Wen N *et al* 2018 An automated dose tracking system for adaptive radiation therapy *Comput. Methods Prog. Biomed.* **154** 1–8
[9] Bondar M L, Hoogeman M S, Mens J W, Quint S, Ahmad R and Dhawtal G *et al* 2012 Individualized nonadaptive and online-adaptive intensity-modulated radiotherapy treatment strategies for cervical cancer patients based on pretreatment acquired variable bladder filling computed tomography scans *Int. J. Radiat. Oncol. Biol. Phys.* **83** 1617–23
[10] Seppenwoolde Y, Stock M, Buschmann M, Georg D, Bauer-Novotny K-Y and Pötter R *et al* 2016 Impact of organ shape variations on margin concepts for cervix cancer ART *Radiother. Oncol.* **120** 526–31
[11] Sharfo A W M, Breedveld S, Voet P W J, Heijkoop S T, Mens J-W M and Hoogeman M S *et al* 2016 Validation of fully automated VMAT plan generation for library-based plan-of-the-day cervical cancer radiotherapy *PLoS One* **11** e0169202
[12] Gill S, Pham D, Dang K, Bressel M, Kron T and Siva S *et al* 2013 Plan of the day selection for online image-guided adaptive post-prostatectomy radiotherapy *Radiother. Oncol.* **107** 165–70
[13] Sonke J-J, Aznar M and Rasch C 2019 Adaptive radiotherapy for anatomical changes *Semin. Radiat. Oncol.* **29** 245–57
[14] Fischer-Valuck B W, Henke L, Green O, Kashani R, Acharya S and Bradley J D *et al* 2017 Two-and-a-half-year clinical experience with the world's first magnetic resonance image guided radiation therapy system *Adv. Radiat. Oncol.* **2** 485–93
[15] Raaymakers B W, Jürgenliemk-Schulz I M, Bol G H, Glitzner M, Kotte A N T J and van Asselen B *et al* 2017 First patients treated with a 1.5 T MRI-Linac: clinical proof of concept of a high-precision, high-field MRI guided radiotherapy treatment *Phys. Med. Biol.* **62** L41–50
[16] Lim-Reinders S, Keller B M, Al-Ward S, Sahgal A and Kim A 2017 Online adaptive radiation therapy *Int. J. Radiat. Oncol. Biol. Phys.* **99** 994–1003
[17] Boda-Heggemann J, Köhler F M, Wertz H, Ehmann M, Hermann B and Riesenacker N *et al* 2008 Intrafraction motion of the prostate during an IMRT session: a fiducial-based 3D measurement with Cone-beam CT *Radiat. Oncol.* **3** 37
[18] Baker M, Jensen J A and Behrens C F 2014 Determining inter-fractional motion of the uterus using 3D ultrasound imaging during radiotherapy for cervical cancer ed J G Bosch and M M Doyley *Medical Imaging 2014: Ultrasonic Imaging and Tomography* (SPIE) p 90400Y
[19] Heijkoop S T, Langerak T R, Quint S, Bondar L, Mens J W M and Heijmen B J M *et al* 2014 Clinical implementation of an online adaptive plan-of-the-day protocol for nonrigid motion management in locally advanced cervical cancer IMRT *Int. J. Radiat. Oncol. Biol. Phys.* **90** 673–9
[20] Li M, Ballhausen H, Hegemann N-S, Reiner M, Tritschler S and Gratzke C *et al* 2017 Comparison of prostate positioning guided by three-dimensional transperineal ultrasound and cone beam CT *Strahlenther. Onkol.* **193** 221–8
[21] Heijkoop S T, Langerak T R, Quint S, Mens J W M, Zolnay A G and Heijmen B J M *et al* 2015 Quantification of intra-fraction changes during radiotherapy of cervical cancer assessed with pre- and post-fraction Cone Beam CT scans *Radiother. Oncol.* **117** 536–41

[22] Langerak T, Heijkoop S, Quint S, Mens J-W, Heijmen B and Hoogeman M 2014 Towards automatic plan selection for radiotherapy of cervical cancer by fast automatic segmentation of cone beam CT scans; P Golland, N Hata, C Barillot, J Hornegger and R Howe *Medical Image Computing and Computer-Assisted Intervention—MICCAI 2014: 17th Int. Conf., Boston, MA, USA, September 14–18, 2014, Proc., Part I* (Cham: Springer) p 528–35

[23] Lütgendorf-Caucig C, Fotina I, Stock M, Pötter R, Goldner G and Georg D 2011 Feasibility of CBCT-based target and normal structure delineation in prostate cancer radiotherapy: multi-observer and image multi-modality study *Radiother. Oncol.* **98** 154–61

[24] Maemoto H, Toita T, Ariga T, Heianna J, Yamashiro T and Murayama S 2017 Predictive factors of uterine movement during definitive radiotherapy for cervical cancer *J. Radiat. Res.* **58** 397–404

[25] Tyagi N, Lewis J H, Yashar C M, Vo D, Jiang S B and Mundt A J *et al* 2011 Daily online cone beam computed tomography to assess interfractional motion in patients with intact cervical cancer *Int. J. Radiat. Oncol. Biol. Phys.* **80** 273–80

[26] Wang X, Li J, Wang P, Yuan K, Yin G and Wan B 2016 Image guided radiation therapy boost in combination with high-dose-rate intracavitary brachytherapy for the treatment of cervical cancer *J. Contemp. Brachyther.* **8** 122–7

[27] van der Meer S, Camps S M, van Elmpt W J C, Podesta M, Sanches P G and Vanneste B G L *et al* 2016 Simulation of pseudo-CT images based on deformable image registration of ultrasound images: A proof of concept for transabdominal ultrasound imaging of the prostate during radiotherapy *Med. Phys.* **43** 1913

[28] Camps S, van der Meer S, Verhaegen F and Fontanarosa D 2016 Various approaches for pseudo-CT scan creation based on ultrasound to ultrasound deformable image registration between different treatment time points for radiotherapy treatment plan adaptation in prostate cancer patients *Biomed. Phys. Eng. Exp.* **2** 035018

[29] Tan L T, Tanderup K, Kirisits C, de Leeuw A, Nout R and Duke S *et al* 2019 Image-guided adaptive radiotherapy in cervical cancer *Semin. Radiat. Oncol.* **29** 284–98

[30] Fontanarosa D, van der Meer S, Bamber J, Harris E, O'Shea T and Verhaegen F 2015 Review of ultrasound image guidance in external beam radiotherapy: I. Treatment planning and inter-fraction motion management *Phys. Med. Biol.* **60** R77–114

[31] Mason S A, White I M, O'Shea T, McNair H A, Alexander S and Kalaitzaki E *et al* 2019 Combined ultrasound and cone beam CT improves target segmentation for image guided radiation therapy in uterine cervix cancer *Int. J. Radiat. Oncol. Biol. Phys.* **104** 685–93

[32] Molloy J A, Chan G, Markovic A, McNeeley S, Pfeiffer D and Salter B *et al* 2011 Quality assurance of U.S.-guided external beam radiotherapy for prostate cancer: report of AAPM Task Group 154 *Med. Phys.* **38** 857–71

[33] Fargier-Voiron M, Presles B, Pommier P, Rit S, Munoz A and Liebgott H *et al* 2014 Impact of probe pressure variability on prostate localization for ultrasound-based image-guided radiotherapy *Radiother. Oncol.* **111** 132–7

[34] Hernandez-Andrade E, Romero R, Ahn H, Hussein Y, Yeo L and Korzeniewski S J *et al* 2012 Transabdominal evaluation of uterine cervical length during pregnancy fails to identify a substantial number of women with a short cervix *J. Matern. Fetal. Neonatal Med.* **25** 1682–9

[35] Kossoff G, Griffiths K A and Dixon C E 1991 Is the quality of transvaginal images superior to transabdominal ones under matched conditions? *Ultrasound Obstet. Gynecol.* **1** 29–35

[36] Paladini D 2009 Sonography in obese and overweight pregnant women: clinical, medicolegal and technical issues *Ultrasound Obstet. Gynecol.* **33** 720–9

IOP Publishing

Modern Applications of 3D/4D Ultrasound Imaging in Radiotherapy

Emma Harris, Davide Fontanarosa, Saskia Camps and Frank Verhaegen

Chapter 9

Automation and robotics in ultrasound-guided radiotherapy

Svenja Ipsen, Floris Ernst and Alexander Schlaefer

One of the main perceived drawbacks of ultrasound guidance to date is the operator dependency and the resulting requirement for extensive training, hampering its widespread clinical use in radiotherapy motion compensation. Robotic systems and process automation could be key factors to overcome this barrier by assisting the user during setup, increasing reproducibility of ultrasound probe positioning and facilitating continuous contact pressure and motion compensation during treatment. The benefits of robotic automation for ultrasound guidance, especially regarding highly mobile target regions and active operator assistance, will be discussed in this chapter, along with technical requirements, system integration aspects and current challenges for its practical implementation.

9.1 Why automation?

The previous chapters have detailed the advantages and capabilities of ultrasound imaging and guidance in radiotherapy. Ultrasound can be used for inter- and intrafractional motion compensation by localising the target in real time prior to and during treatment. High tracking accuracy has been reported both in phantom and patient studies. However, ultrasound image acquisition conventionally relies on manual placement of the ultrasound probe on the patient, rendering it dependent on the operator. The strong dependency on the expertise of the human operator placing the probe leads to a variability in probe positions and applied probe pressures, potentially impairing image quality and ultimately tracking results. It has been shown that exceedingly high probe pressure can lead to organ displacements of several millimetres [1, 2], potentially causing mismatches between the treatment plan and the anatomy on the treatment day (for details refer to chapter 3). In the case of intrafractional motion compensation, i.e. image acquisition during treatment, manual

doi:10.1088/978-0-7503-2552-3ch9

probe handling even becomes impossible due to the radiation in the treatment room. Aside from the variability in probe positioning, ultrasound image interpretation is also much more challenging in comparison to computed tomography (CT) or magnetic resonance imaging (MRI). While the quality of ultrasound images and diagnostic results tend to improve substantially with operator experience, the users in radiotherapy are usually not trained sonographers but likely received only basic training on the system. Ultimately, reproducibility of probe positioning and target localisation accuracy cannot be guaranteed for ultrasound guidance relying solely on manual probe handling.

The goal of automation in ultrasound guided radiotherapy (USgRT) is to increase robustness and reproducibility of the individual steps in the workflow—image acquisition, target definition, motion compensation—by using robotic probe manipulation and automated image assessment. Although industrial robots have been successfully used for decades, improvements in recent years have been enormous and are now paving the way for applications in the medical field. Probably the most interesting development is the trend away from the strict separation between human and robot workspaces (i.e. the set of positions in 3D space they can reach) and towards collaborative lightweight robots optimised for operation in close contact with humans. Suitable force sensors allow the robot to both sense its environment, for example collisions, but also to quantitatively exert forces. Additional joints can lead to more flexibility, allowing the robot to reach around obstacles or avoid the treatment beam in radiotherapy. At the same time, the high positioning accuracy and reproducibility of their industrial counterparts has been retained, stressing their high potential as 'intelligent ultrasound probe manipulators' in the radiotherapy scenario.

The main advantages of the robotic ultrasound guidance system can be broken down into (1) automated probe positioning, (2) dynamic pressure control, (3) iterative optimisation of ultrasound image quality and (4) positioning flexibility during treatment. These four key tasks will be presented in section 9.2. Integration of the robot into the radiotherapy system, especially geometric alignment and collision avoidance, is featured in section 9.3. Section 9.4 provides an overview of robotic ultrasound guidance systems developed to date, while section 9.5 discusses issues of practical implementation and basic quality assurance.

9.2 Robotic ultrasound-guided radiotherapy tasks

Robots are generally used to automate industrial processes, e.g. to conduct recurring tasks with high reproducibility, and are capable of working in environments not suitable for human operators. In the ultrasound guidance context, a robot can provide assistance for the operating personnel and facilitate automation of different steps in the workflow, including operation while the radiation beam is on.

9.2.1 Technical considerations

The technical requirements for an ultrasound robot are highly task-specific and different setups regarding ultrasound and robotic hardware have been suggested to date (see section 9.4).

Ultrasound: many robotic ultrasound systems rely on 2D ultrasound imaging due to its relative simplicity, broad availability and fast framerate. However, real-time volumetric (4D) imaging offers the distinct advantage of covering the actual movements of the 3D target while at the same time requiring fewer adjustments of the ultrasound probe position to keep the target inside the field of view. At the same time, a real-time interface to the ultrasound image data is required to realise the tasks described in the following sections and integrate them into the motion compensation workflow. If ultrasound data is to be used for dynamic robot control, adequate framerates are also mandatory to ensure low latency and fast adaptation to target motion.

Robot: in an ultrasound guidance context, the most relevant parameters are workspace size and dexterity (i.e. the robot's ability to reach a certain point in the workspace from many different directions), accuracy and precision, as well as possible safety mechanisms. Workspace size and dexterity mainly depend on the robot's joint lengths and degrees of freedom and should be evaluated based on the desired task and the required amount of motion. Accuracy and precision should be assessed regarding their suitability for the desired task—especially industrial robots often provide high positioning precision (repeatability) but relatively low absolute accuracy. Finally, safety must be ensured by integrating force sensitivity, ideally along the entire kinematic chain, and by limiting velocity and acceleration of the robot movements. Computational simulations should be used to identify and avoid potential collisions.

9.2.2 Automated probe positioning

One of the biggest drawbacks of ultrasound imaging, its high operator dependency, is mainly caused by the manual probe handling process and can lead to substantial probe positioning variability. Early studies on ultrasound guidance indicated that variable probe pressure levels can cause discrepancies between planned and actual target position during scan acquisition [3]. This becomes especially problematic when the ultrasound probe is only present during setup but removed during treatment delivery. If intrafractional ultrasound guidance is used, the probe (or an artificial probe model) should ideally already be present during the acquisition of the planning CT to record the probe's position relative to the patient and to reflect any potential anatomical deformation resulting from probe pressure.

Robotic probe positioning holds the potential to overcome probe positioning variability by increasing the reproducibility of the process [4]. Depending on the desired level of automation, different positioning methods can be realised using a collaborative, i.e. force-sensitive, robot.

Robot hand guidance

The least complex but also the least automated approach for robotic probe positioning on the patient is manual control of the robot, either using remote control or a 'soft mode' where the robot can be moved by touching it and exerting forces on the different joints (also referred to as hand guidance). In particular, the latter is very close to the original process of manual probe positioning, with the distinct advantage that the robot can be used to locate the probe within the treatment room and relative to the patient, and that the forces on the ultrasound probe and thus the applied pressure can be monitored during and after positioning. However, conventional hand guidance of the robot still requires an experienced operator to interpret the ultrasound images and reposition the probe at the planned position with adequate target visibility for monitoring.

Collaborative guidance
To automatically assist the operator during probe positioning while still maintaining some measure of manual control, the robot can also be used for collaborative guidance. In work reported by Şen *et al* [5, 6], robotic hand guidance is combined with virtual constraints that signal the operator if a desirable probe position is within reach. Constraining forces can be generated by the robot to guide probe motion towards reference values from simulation, considering robot position, contact force as well as ultrasound image similarity to a reference image.

With this hybrid approach, consistent soft tissue deformation could be achieved while generally avoiding the typical drawback of a fully automated approach—getting stuck in local minima of the optimisation goals and therefore not reaching the optimal probe position—by including the human operator in the control loop.

Fully automated positioning
Aside from manual guidance, the robot could also facilitate fully automated probe positioning, as illustrated in figure 9.1. Such an operator-independent approach requires accurate in-room calibration (see section 9.3), reliable force control, as well as real-time processing of the ultrasound image data to visualise the target and detect potential imaging artefacts. Additionally, the patient position relative to the robot should be known for this approach in order to reach for a desired surface position on the patient with the probe. The patient position should be obtained with an external imaging system, such as CBCT, optical tracking or a depth-sensing camera. While CBCT is the only modality that provides true 3D information about the patient

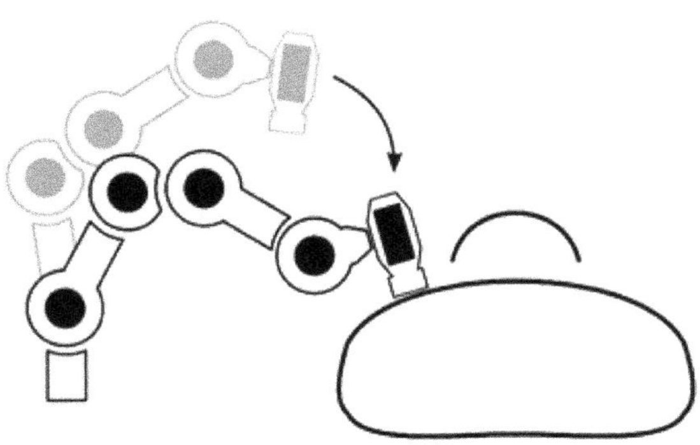

Figure 9.1. Automated probe placement on the patient using a force-sensitive robot. Alternatively, the robot could be guided manually or assist the operator during positioning.

position and internal anatomy, it can only be used to generate an initial static point of reference and is not suitable for continuous observation. In contrast, optical cameras and tracking systems can be used for real-time observation of the external patient position and can be useful for robotic ultrasound guidance [7, 8]. Depth-sensing cameras offer the additional advantage that the entire patient surface could be visualised in 3D and used for registration to the surface extracted from the planning CT for alignment.

One way to define the initial probe position on the surface of the patient is to record a suitable position manually during a planning ultrasound scan prior to treatment delivery, which will then be reproduced by the robot on each treatment day. Since this step still relies on an experienced operator defining the initial position, further automation would be desirable. Different studies have shown that it is possible to calculate optimal probe positions based on available image data such as the planning CT scan of the patient [9–13]. Based on the relationship between Hounsfield Units in the CT it is possible to identify particular tissues (e.g. muscle, fat or bone) and allocate them known acoustic properties such as absorption and reflectivity. By selecting a target within the body and calculating the acoustic properties along the resulting beam path, surface areas with high probability of good target visibility can be determined. Using this strategy, shadows caused by bones, such as the ribs, can be avoided when placing the probe. Further criteria relevant for ultrasound visibility are target depth relative to the surface, the geometry of the ultrasound probe and the ultrasound image or volume, the therapy beam directions, the dynamic behaviour of the target, up to the expected amount of speed of sound aberrations (see chapter 3). An optimisation algorithm can be used to find ideal candidates for probe positions on the patient's surface satisfying the above criteria. As shown in figure 9.2, visualisation as a 'heat map' could then also be used to assist the operator in defining a suitable initial probe position.

The ultrasound probe can then be directed towards the intended surface position, assuming the (approximate) patient position is known relative to the robot. During the positioning process, contact force must be monitored to ensure reproducible pressure as well as patient safety. Probe positioning can either be realised via position or force control, where the former aims at reproducing a predefined

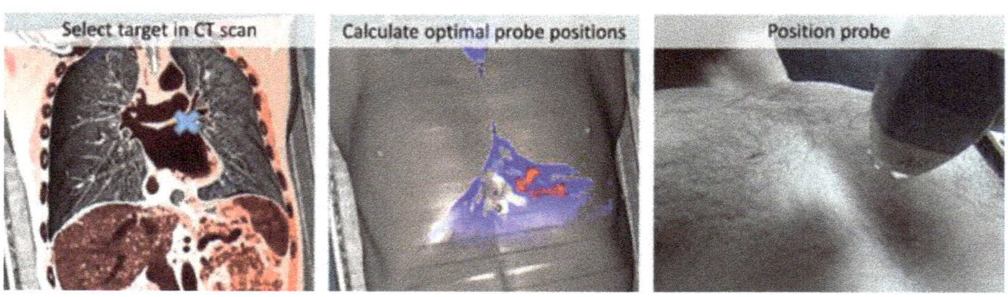

Figure 9.2. Steps to calculate optimal probe positions for robotic placement described in [9]. The target is selected in a CT scan (left). After calculating acoustic properties, surface points with high potential visibility are highlighted (centre). The probe is placed at the most suitable location, either chosen automatically or by the operator (right).

position and the latter a predefined force. For abdominal targets, position control could lead to higher reproducibility of the planned position compared to force control [4].

Once an initial surface position has been reached and contact has been established, the ultrasound image can be processed to identify the target structure defined during simulation and also to detect—and eventually compensate—imaging artefacts such as shadows caused by air or bones along the acoustic path (see section 9.2.4).

9.2.3 Dynamic adaptation

Another key advantage of robotic probe handling is the possibility to adapt the probe position dynamically as shown in figure 9.3. This could be necessary if the patient moved after the initial positioning but becomes especially important if breathing motion affects the contact surface with the probe, e.g. for abdominal targets. If left uncompensated, this type of motion can lead to undesirably high pressure levels, causing target deformation or patient discomfort, or deteriorating image quality due to a loss of probe contact [14]. Several studies have shown that force control during robotic ultrasound guidance can compensate for surface motion and thus maintain stable pressure levels for prostate, liver and pancreas [11, 15–17]. The overall goal is to move the probe in the opposite direction of the exerted force if the desired force level is exceeded, and to move it in the same direction if the current value is too low. The 'stiffness' of the robot, i.e. its reactivity to changes in measured force values, can be adapted by changing the spring constant in (x, y, z)-direction in the control parameters.

9.2.4 Optimisation of target visibility

Robotic automation can also be used to optimise target visibility in the ultrasound image without manual interference by the operator as illustrated in figure 9.4. This function, also referred to as visual servoing, relies on the ultrasound image data and uses visual input to control robot motion. Several studies have shown that visual servoing for robotic ultrasound is possible in scenarios such as diagnostic scanning or interventional navigation [18–20].

In the ultrasound guidance context, it is possible to identify imaging artefacts caused by bone or air interference by detecting the resulting 'shadowed' regions in

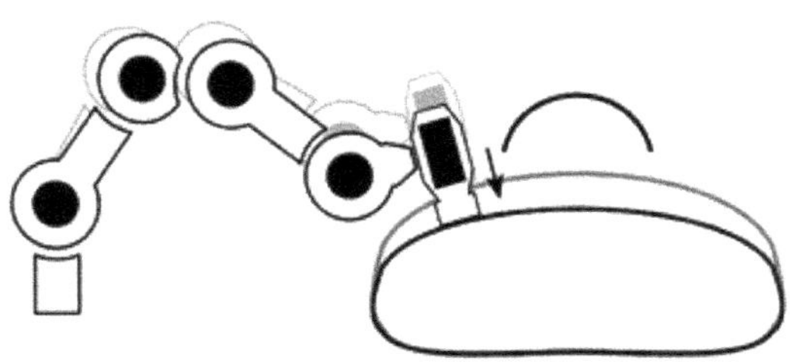

Figure 9.3. Dynamic adaptation to maintain contact with the patient's surface and to ensure constant pressure for reproducible deformation and patient safety.

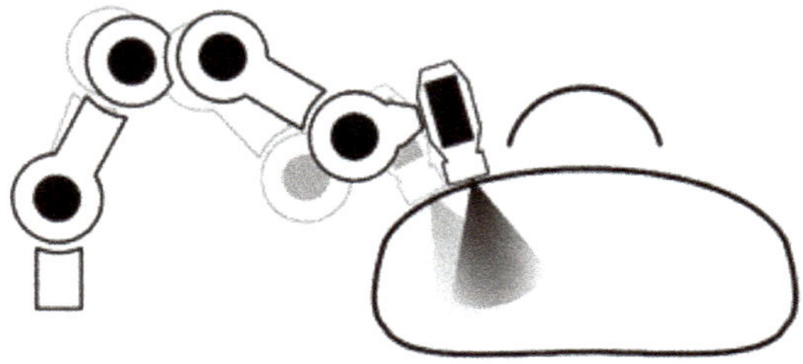

Figure 9.4. Iterative optimisation of target visibility. The robot can automatically perform minor adjustments of the probe position to bring the target within the ultrasound field of view or to avoid imaging artefacts, e.g. caused by air or bones.

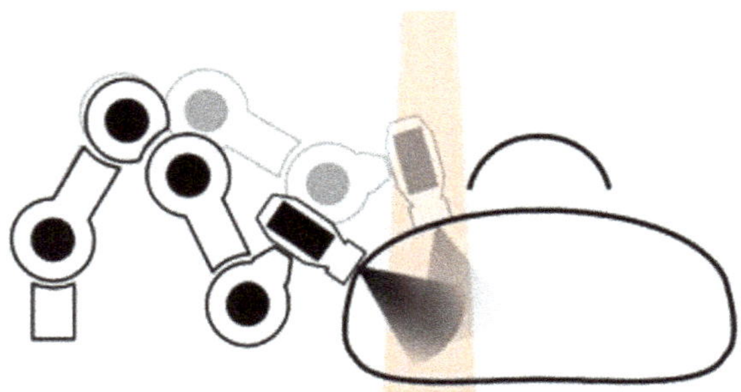

Figure 9.5. Repositioning of the probe during treatment. The robot could be controlled remotely to improve target visibility without entering the treatment room or move the probe away from an intercepting treatment beam.

the ultrasound data [15, 21]. Having located and quantified the artefact, the robot could perform small, iterative changes of the probe position, e.g. by tilting the probe away from the affected region [8], to reduce its impact on target visibility and thus tracking performance. Aside from defining these robotic movements manually, there is also high potential for solutions employing artificial intelligence to learn optimal reactions to certain types of artefacts and motion. Another example is actively following target motion if the target is approaching the boundaries of the ultrasound field of view.

9.2.5 Probe repositioning during treatment

Another key function of robotic ultrasound guidance is the ability to reposition the probe during treatment as shown in figure 9.5. Repositioning could either be performed manually via remote control by the operator in the control room or fully automatic, for example, based on the current target visibility or the direction of the treatment beam. Reconfiguring the robot or repositioning the probe during treatment (between beams) could potentially increase treatment plan quality by freeing beam angles that would otherwise have been blocked by the ultrasound probe [11, 22, 23]. Integration of robot motion into treatment planning could also open up new possibilities for dynamic treatment concepts such as RapidArc, non-coplanar or even 4pi delivery (see also chapter 5).

9.3 System integration

Integrating robotic ultrasound with beam delivery primarily requires solving two problems. First, the information gained through ultrasound imaging needs to be mapped to the patient and the system coordinate frames. Second, collisions of the robotic ultrasound with the patient and the overall system and obstruction of the treatment beams need to be avoided.

9.3.1 Calibration for robotic ultrasound guidance

Generally, the pose of an object describes the position and orientation with respect to a coordinate frame, defined for example by the planning CT, the fixed or onboard imagers, or the linac with its virtual or actual isocentre. During conventional patient setup, patient and couch are moved to realise a proper alignment of the patient with the treatment coordinate system.

Spatial relationships between different objects and structures can be expressed by transformations between the respective coordinate frames. These transformations are typically given as 4 × 4 matrices

$$T = \begin{bmatrix} r_{1,1} & r_{1,2} & r_{1,3} & t_{1,4} \\ r_{2,1} & r_{2,2} & r_{2,3} & t_{2,4} \\ r_{3,1} & r_{3,2} & r_{3,3} & t_{3,4} \\ 0 & 0 & 0 & 1 \end{bmatrix},$$

consisting of a rotation matrix with components $r_{i,j}$ and a translation vector with components $t_{i,j}$, leading to so-called homogeneous coordinates which can represent points and vectors. In the following, the notation ${}^{\mathrm{from}}T_{\mathrm{to}}$ will be used, where T is a transformation relating coordinates in the frames 'from' and 'to'.

In figure 9.6, the ultrasound transducer is positioned on the patient and the images are given in some inherent coordinate frame that defines the direction of its voxels. Using image processing techniques as described in chapters 6 and 7, the pose of the target can be determined within the ultrasound images as ${}^{\mathrm{tar}}T_{\mathrm{US}}$. If the pose of the ultrasound (US) images relative to the system ${}^{\mathrm{US}}T_{\mathrm{sys}}$ is known, the target pose

$${}^{\mathrm{tar}}T_{\mathrm{sys}} = {}^{\mathrm{tar}}T_{\mathrm{US}}\,{}^{\mathrm{US}}T_{\mathrm{sys}}$$

can be expressed in system coordinates. The transformation ${}^{\mathrm{tar}}T_{\mathrm{sys}}$ is the prerequisite for motion compensation as it facilitates aligning the treatment beam with the target. Note that from patient setup, we will typically also know the pose of the patient ${}^{\mathrm{pat}}T_{\mathrm{sys}}$ with respect to our system and thus also the expected target pose within the patient ${}^{\mathrm{tar}}T_{\mathrm{pat}}$. This also provides information on where to point the ultrasound probe to see the target. During treatment, any motion of the tumour with respect to the ultrasound images will cause a change in ${}^{\mathrm{tar}}T_{\mathrm{US}}$, as illustrated in figure 9.6(b), which can then be compensated by adjusting the beam accordingly. Likewise, if the ultrasound probe is moved relative to a stationary target, the changes in ${}^{\mathrm{tar}}T_{\mathrm{US}}$ and ${}^{\mathrm{US}}T_{\mathrm{sys}}$ cancel out as shown in figure 9.6(b).

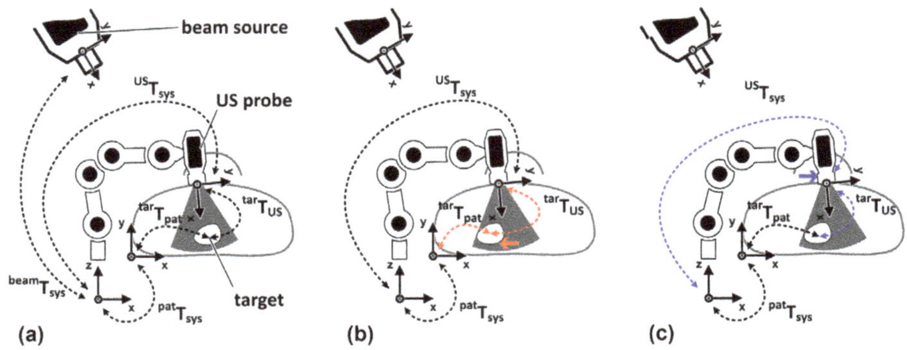

Figure 9.6. Illustration of the general setup with a beam source and a robot mounted ultrasound probe. (a) Four key coordinate frames for patient, ultrasound image, beam, and the overall system as well as the respective transformations are shown. (b) The red arrow indicates motion of the PTV, which results in a new position of the PTV with respect to the patient and the system. Dashed red arrows highlight changes in the relative pose and the new coordinates in the system frame can be obtained by ${}^{\mathrm{tar}}T_{\mathrm{sys}} = {}^{\mathrm{tar}}T_{\mathrm{US}}\,{}^{\mathrm{US}}T_{\mathrm{sys}}$. (c) The blue arrow indicates motion of the ultrasound probe, e.g., to maintain force or to slightly adjust the imaging. Here the dashed blue arrows highlight that both transformations ${}^{\mathrm{tar}}T_{\mathrm{US}}$ and ${}^{\mathrm{US}}T_{\mathrm{sys}}$ have changed compared to subfigure (a), but the resulting transformation ${}^{\mathrm{tar}}T_{\mathrm{sys}}$ would be unchanged, illustrating that the system would detect the correct target pose, even if the ultrasound robot was moved.

In order to relate the target pose as seen in the ultrasound image to the system's coordinate frame, the transformation ${}^{\mathrm{US}}T_{\mathrm{sys}}$ must be determined. As can be seen from figure 9.6(a), ${}^{\mathrm{US}}T_{\mathrm{sys}}$ can be expressed as a series of transformations

$$ {}^{\mathrm{US}}T_{\mathrm{sys}} = {}^{\mathrm{US}}T_{\mathrm{fla}}\,{}^{\mathrm{fla}}T_{\mathrm{bas}}\,{}^{\mathrm{bas}}T_{\mathrm{sys}}. $$

Clearly, an ultrasound probe rigidly mounted to the robot, i.e., at the so-called flange, will change its pose whenever the robot moves. The pose of the flange with respect to the robot's base can be expressed as a transformation ${}^{\mathrm{fla}}T_{\mathrm{bas}}$ and is determined by the joint parameters that are used for controlling the robot. The relation between joint parameters and the flange pose is known from the robot's design and the manufacturer's calibration and can be used to compute ${}^{\mathrm{fla}}T_{\mathrm{bas}}$ for any given set of joint parameters. Consequently, two transformations remain unknown: the pose of the ultrasound image coordinate frame with respect to the flange ${}^{\mathrm{US}}T_{\mathrm{fla}}$ and the pose of the robot with respect to the system ${}^{\mathrm{bas}}T_{\mathrm{sys}}$. The latter generally stays fixed, changing only when the robot's base is moved within the treatment room, e.g., due to positioning constraints based on the target region or treatment delivery.

Hand–eye-calibration

Obtaining these missing transformations is a standard procedure in robotics. It is typically approached by hand–eye or eye-in-hand calibrations, which essentially solve optimisation problems to find the best matching missing transformation matrices (see also chapter 3). The idea is best introduced considering conventional hand–eye calibration where the robot represents the 'hand' holding some object and a camera system represents the 'eye', observing the object. Figure 9.7(a) illustrates

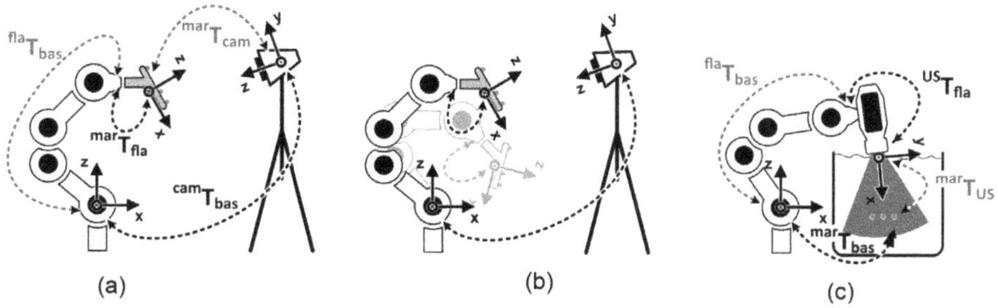

Figure 9.7. Illustration of different calibration setups involved. (a) Typical hand–eye calibration with the two known transformations ${}^{\mathrm{mar}}T_{\mathrm{cam}}$ and ${}^{\mathrm{fla}}T_{\mathrm{bas}}$ and the two unknown transformations ${}^{\mathrm{cam}}T_{\mathrm{bas}}$ and ${}^{\mathrm{mar}}T_{\mathrm{fla}}$. Generally, the features illustrated as red points define the marker geometry and need to be visible to the respective camera. Note that the camera may be an x-ray camera and the marker may contain radio-opaque patterns. (b) Calibration involves changing the known transformations while the unknown transformations remain constant and can subsequently be solved for. (c) Ultrasound calibration involves a similar setup known as eye-in-hand calibration, where the two unknown transformations ${}^{\mathrm{mar}}T_{\mathrm{bas}}$ and ${}^{\mathrm{US}}T_{\mathrm{fla}}$ are determined. Typically, only the latter is used for ultrasound tracking.

this setup where the grey object featuring some landmarks to facilitate measuring its pose with respect to the camera is referred to as marker.

The transformations relating the four coordinate frames (robot base, robot flange, camera, marker) form a cycle

$$\mathrm{I} = {}^{\mathrm{cam}}T_{\mathrm{bas}}\,{}^{\mathrm{bas}}T_{\mathrm{fla}}\,{}^{\mathrm{fla}}T_{\mathrm{mar}}\,{}^{\mathrm{mar}}T_{\mathrm{cam}}$$

so that starting at one frame and applying all four transformations will lead back to the initial pose and the total transformation becomes the identity matrix. Since the camera determines the pose of the marker and the flange pose is calculated from the known joint parameters, the transformations ${}^{\mathrm{mar}}T_{\mathrm{cam}}$ and ${}^{\mathrm{fla}}T_{\mathrm{bas}}$ are known by measurement. The remaining two transformations that relate the flange to the marker (${}^{\mathrm{fla}}T_{\mathrm{mar}}$) and the camera to the robot's base (${}^{\mathrm{cam}}T_{\mathrm{bas}}$) are generally not known but remain constant. A variety of different methods to compute the remaining two transformation matrices have been proposed. By moving the robot into different configurations and recording the resulting flange and marker poses, a system of equations can be composed and solved for ${}^{\mathrm{fla}}T_{\mathrm{mar}}$ and ${}^{\mathrm{cam}}T_{\mathrm{bas}}$. The more widely used methods by Tsai and Lenz [24] and by Daniilidis [25] preserve the properties of the transformation matrices, namely that the upper 3×3 matrix forms a valid rotation matrix. However, other approaches computing the elements of the transformation matrix independently have also been used successfully.

Ultrasound robot calibration steps

So far, the general hand–eye calibration setup has been described. When setting up the ultrasound robot, the two unknown matrices ${}^{\mathrm{bas}}T_{\mathrm{sys}}$ and ${}^{\mathrm{US}}T_{\mathrm{fla}}$ can also be determined independently. To establish the transformation ${}^{\mathrm{bas}}T_{\mathrm{sys}}$ between robot base and treatment system, a camera already calibrated to the treatment system could be used for hand–eye calibration. For example, in the case of the CyberKnife (Accuray Inc., Sunnyvale, CA, USA), the pre-installed x-ray imaging system could serve as a camera to measure the pose of a radiopaque marker mounted to the robot's flange. Hand–eye calibration would then result in the transformation from base to system as

$$^{\mathrm{bas}}T_{\mathrm{sys}} = {}^{\mathrm{bas}}T_{\mathrm{cam}}\,{}^{\mathrm{cam}}T_{\mathrm{sys}}.$$

To calculate the missing transformation $^{\mathrm{US}}T_{\mathrm{fla}}$ from ultrasound image to robot flange, the setting changes slightly to an eye-in-hand problem, where the robot moves the camera, i.e., the ultrasound transducer, instead of the marker. Figure 9.7(c) illustrates this scenario which requires some known marker geometry visible in ultrasound images for tracking. In principle, any known marker geometry could be used, but often so-called n- or z-wire phantoms are employed, as the construction is relatively simple and the wires can be easily identified in the images [26]. Similar to hand–eye calibration, the ultrasound probe can now be moved into many different poses using the robot to measure the poses of the wires and the flange and solve for the remaining transformations.

The matrices $^{\mathrm{bas}}T_{\mathrm{sys}}$ and $^{\mathrm{US}}T_{\mathrm{fla}}$ can then be used to transform ultrasound into system coordinates by calculating

$$^{\mathrm{US}}T_{\mathrm{sys}} = {}^{\mathrm{US}}T_{\mathrm{fla}}\,{}^{\mathrm{fla}}T_{\mathrm{bas}}\,{}^{\mathrm{bas}}T_{\mathrm{sys}}.$$

It should be noted that although the calibrations are fairly straightforward in principle, they can be cumbersome and error-prone in practice. Therefore, adding markers to the ultrasound robot and using an optical tracking system either calibrated to the treatment room coordinate system or seeing another precalibrated marker can facilitate a faster setup. Likewise, tracking the ultrasound probe directly has also been proposed, e.g., with the AutoScan system (Elekta AB, Stockholm, Sweden).

9.3.2 Collision avoidance

Integrating an ultrasound robot into the overall system requires a careful analysis of possible collisions. Clearly, it is of utmost importance to avoid physical collisions with the patient or other system components like linac or onboard imaging devices. A typical approach is to check whether an overlap occurs for any desired configuration of ultrasound robot and system in a virtual model. Additional sensor data like camera systems may be needed to also include the patient in collision detection. At the same time, the ultrasound robot may block beams, i.e., the virtual collision of beams with the robot needs to be considered, as attenuation and scattering may have a negative impact on the dose delivery (see chapter 4).

Different approaches have been proposed to facilitate simple system integration. The AutoScan device for prostate treatments is typically placed between the patients' legs, i.e., collisions are highly unlikely, particularly for gantry-based systems [27]. Schlosser *et al* [11] proposed a specific robot design that is placed between the legs and can thus also be used with conventional gantry-based radiation therapy systems. Moreover, they also describe simulation software that allows detecting potential collisions. Clearly, this process can be automated once the ultrasound robot has been

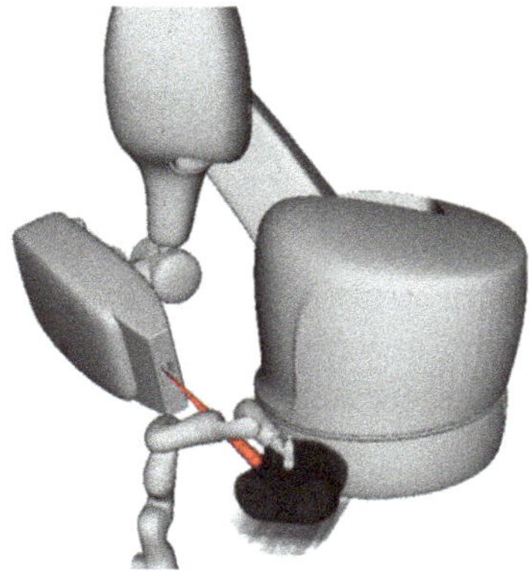

Figure 9.8. This interactive figure demonstrates how the ultrasound robot changes its configuration to allow further beams being delivered. This figure was developed with the help of Stefan Gerlach, Hamburg University of Technology. Animation available at https://iopscience.iop.org/book/978-0-7503-2552-3.

calibrated to the system. Schlüter *et al* [28] have studied approaches to automatically search for ultrasound robot position for robotic radiation therapy with the CyberKnife.

The calibrations allow determining the target pose from ultrasound images and transformation into treatment room coordinates. Depending on the type of treatment system, the actual beam delivery will be controlled accordingly, e.g., by gating the beam or by active motion compensation. Whenever the beam moves to account for target motion, checks for potential collisions with the ultrasound probe or the robot carrying it need to be performed. As such collisions during a fraction may render the treatment plan infeasible and require re-planning, it is important to minimise the likelihood of collisions by adding a safety margin during the initial collision detection at the planning stage (see chapter 5).

To further mitigate the impact of the ultrasound robot on beam delivery, kinematically redundant designs have been considered. Gerlach *et al* [23] studied how the additional flexibility of a 7-jointed robotic arm (KUKA GmbH, Augsburg, Germany) can be used to move the robot's elbow such that collisions with beams are avoided (see interactive figure 5.6). The key idea is that beams that collide with the robot in some configuration, e.g., with the elbow pointing left, may have no collision in other configurations, e.g., with the elbow pointing right. A similar approach would generally allow a tighter integration of the beam delivery system and ultrasound guidance. However, the additional motion of the ultrasound robot needs to be coordinated with the beam delivery. The same group has illustrated, for robotic radiation therapy, that the overall system motion can be optimised such that the temporal overhead is small. Interactive figure 9.8 shows how the ultrasound robot changes its configuration to allow further beams to be delivered [29].

9.4 Current robotic systems

Over the past 10–15 years, different approaches have been pursued to integrate automated robotic probe manipulation with ultrasound imaging for guidance in radiotherapy. There were two major challenges for the development of such systems: first, the requirement to accurately measure and control forces and torques with the robot when positioning the probe directly on the patient; and second, the reliance on 2D imaging for a 3D robot control and motion compensation problem can cause difficulties when trying to accurately place the probe and follow targets. Furthermore, there was—and, to a certain extent, still is—limited support or acceptance for robotic ultrasound, especially among clinicians and potential users. While these difficulties still hamper the development of robotic ultrasound systems for complex, autonomous diagnostic applications, the comparatively narrow research field of ultrasound-guided radiotherapy with its relatively static probe-holding task could be realised much faster. First systems for use in radiotherapy—like the initial ultrasound robots built in Lübeck and Stanford—already tried to address these challenges in the late 2000s.

9.4.1 First-generation systems

One of the earliest robotic ultrasound systems was developed at the University of Lübeck and is shown in figure 9.9 [30]. It was based on a conventional industrial robot (Viper s850, Omron Adept Technology Inc., Pleasanton, CA, USA) combined with an off-the-shelf force-torque sensor (ATI Industrial Automation Inc., NC, USA) mounted at the end-effector of the robot and a customised fixture to connect a volumetric (3D) ultrasound probe. Using a custom software interface [31], this was

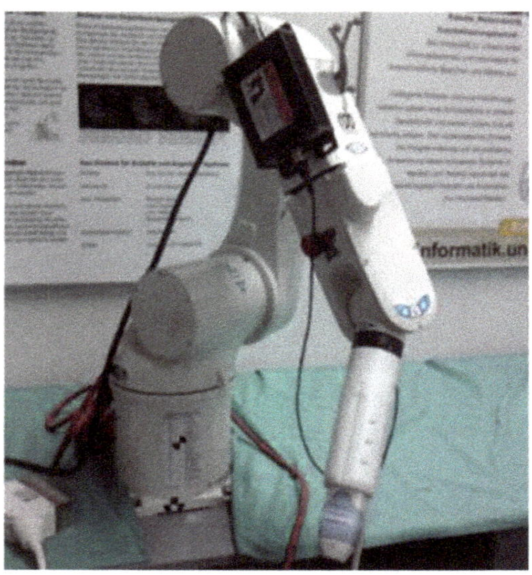

Figure 9.9. Early robotic ultrasound system from University of Lübeck featuring an industrial robot with mounted force-torque sensor and matrix array transducer described in [30].

the first system to allow real-time access to the volumetric image data acquired with a fast 2D matrix array probe (Vivid 7 Dimension ultrasound station and 3V-D probe, GE Healthcare Inc., Chicago, IL, USA). With this initial prototype, it was possible to perform the first real-time target localisation and motion compensation experiments using fast 3D US imaging in combination with force control [15]. Clear advantages of this system were the use of off-the-shelf components, making it an affordable system with well-known kinematics. Furthermore, the force-torque sensor used featured very accurate readings for contact forces and torques. On the other hand, relying on an industrial robot in a clinical scenario was and still is potentially dangerous. The robot can move extremely fast (with up to 7 m s^{-1} at the end effector) and thus can cause considerable harm when colliding with the patient. Furthermore, the robot is non-compliant, i.e. it cannot measure forces and torques anywhere but at the attached force-torque sensor. Since, at the time of development, manufacturers of 3D ultrasound systems did not provide direct access to the acquired volumetric data, the system had to rely on a modified firmware on the ultrasound station, compromising its clearance for medical purposes. Nevertheless, this is also a clear advantage: the system allowed direct access to the raw ultrasound data in spherical coordinates, making it possible to implement image processing algorithms and robot control schemes directly on the ultrasound station. Consequently, it still is one of the fastest systems with the lowest possible latency, since it is not necessary to stream volume or image data to a client machine for processing [32].

While this system was already force-sensitive and used real-time 3D imaging, other first-generation research systems relied on 2D probes and specialised kinematics. One such system, presented in 2010, was the ultrasound robot shown in figure 9.10. It was designed for motion compensation in radiotherapy by Schlosser *et al* from Stanford University [14]. Their system featured a custom-built robotic manipulator that the authors describe as 'inherently safe', mainly due to mechanical

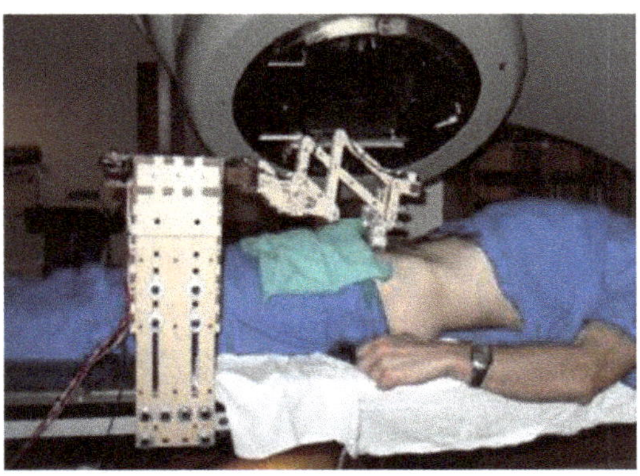

Figure 9.10. First-generation ultrasound robot from Stanford University. The system is built from radiolucent plywood and uses a 2D probe combined with force control. Figure courtesy of Jeffrey Schlosser (formerly Stanford University) and adapted from Western *et al* [37] under Creative Commons Attribution License CC BY 3.0.

constraints. The robot was built mainly from light, radiolucent materials (plywood construction) to reduce interference with treatment delivery. Further design requirements included building and positioning the robot so as to avoid linac gantry collisions and simultaneous imaging during CT simulation. Clearly, using a mostly radiolucent robot with specialised kinematics has multiple advantages. The inherent dangers of classical, often much more powerful industrial robots are avoided, the light-weight design allows for simple positioning and fixation to the treatment couch and the specialised kinematics based on moving parallelograms could be tailored to the specific application.

By design, this robot did not allow for full six degrees-of-freedom (DOF) motion compensation, due to its intended use for prostate tracking where limited motion can be expected. Active control was limited to controlling two DOFs: probe tilt and pressure against the abdomen. Another three passive DOFs used for initial positioning of the robot above the patient's prostate (transabdominal/suprapubic view, see figure 9.10) could be mechanically locked once the position was deemed adequate. Using a force-feedback system and teleoperation with a haptic device, an operator was able to steer the two motorised DOFs from outside the treatment room during beam delivery.

This system was also tested under real-world conditions imitating treatment in a volunteer study, showing that it was possible to reliably record ultrasound data over typical time periods required for beam delivery [33]. In another experiment, the robot was exposed to a treatment beam of 15 MV, where image acquisition and robot performance was not degraded [34]. In fact, this system was the first robot that was actively used for ultrasound tracking in a phantom when the treatment beam was on [35].

Another custom-built robot was developed by Şen *et al* in 2013 at Johns Hopkins University [36]. Their system, shown in figure 9.11, is unique in its high kinematic redundancy: it has five actuated and six passive DOFs, allowing for very flexible positioning. The design combines a three-DOF translational motion stage with a manually lockable arm (six DOF) and a two-DOF rotational stage. Additionally, in some experiments, the robot was mounted to a passively moveable aluminium

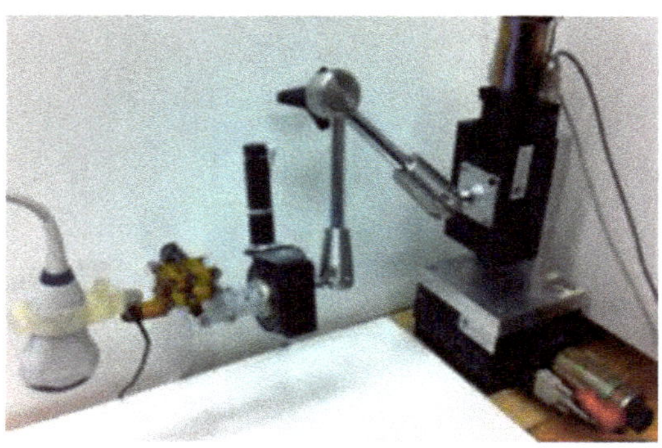

Figure 9.11. Custom ultrasound robot from Johns Hopkins University. Figure courtesy of Peter Kazanzides (Johns Hopkins University).

bridge, adding another three passive translational DOFs. A six-DOF force-torque sensor is used to measure probe contact forces and torques.

Despite the advanced robotic design, the system still relied on simple 2D ultrasound imaging or—in later studies—slow mechanical 3D probes. Nevertheless, this robot was the first to also be incorporated into treatment planning [36, 37], where an artificial probe model from plastic was positioned during the planning CT scan to mimic the deformation that would occur during treatment under ultrasound guidance. Furthermore, a collaborative control scheme has been proposed where the robot can also be used as a guidance system during treatment setup. The goal is to assist the operator, who might not be an experienced sonographer, in positioning the probe as closely as possible to the planned position [5, 6]. The authors refer to their approach as a 'human-in-the-loop image servoing co-manipulation strategy' [5]. It is based on the same technological approach as classical visual servoing, where image information is directly used for robot control, with the addition of a cooperative control framework allowing manual intervention if the automatic image processing and positioning fails. This is achieved with so-called 'soft virtual fixtures' based on a spring-damper robot control scheme. The goal of this positioning assistance is to ensure that the probe position and resulting deformation in the planning CT scan is reproduced as accurately as possible. The robotic ultrasound system from Johns Hopkins University has been successfully tested *in vivo* in a canine study [5, 6] and in three healthy volunteers [38]. They found that the use of 'soft virtual fixtures' can improve the reproducibility of patient setup and soft tissue deformation but that the manual adjustment of the passive arm was difficult to achieve for the users.

9.4.2 Second-generation systems

Based on the initial experiments described in the above section, several shortcomings could be identified in the first robotic ultrasound systems. The research groups addressed these in their second-generation systems, focussing on:

(1) adequate robotic hardware (DOFs, material, reach);
(2) incorporation of three-dimensional ultrasound imaging;
(3) use of 'compliant systems', i.e. force-sensitivity.

The robotic ultrasound system from the University of Lübeck, previously based on a rigid 6-DOF industrial robot with an external force/torque sensor, was modified to work with a state-of-the art collaborative system with integrated sensors, the LBR iiwa R800 (KUKA GmbH). Additionally, the ultilised software platform was extended to allow real-time data access from other 3D ultrasound systems (Epiq 7, Philips NV, Amsterdam, Netherlands and E95, GE Healthcare Inc.). Their second-generation system, shown in figure 9.12, was used in volunteer imaging studies for prostate (transabdominal/suprapubic view) and liver motion (intercostal view), in both cases with full compensation of respiratory motion and real-time 3D image acquisition over extended imaging sessions of 30 min [17].

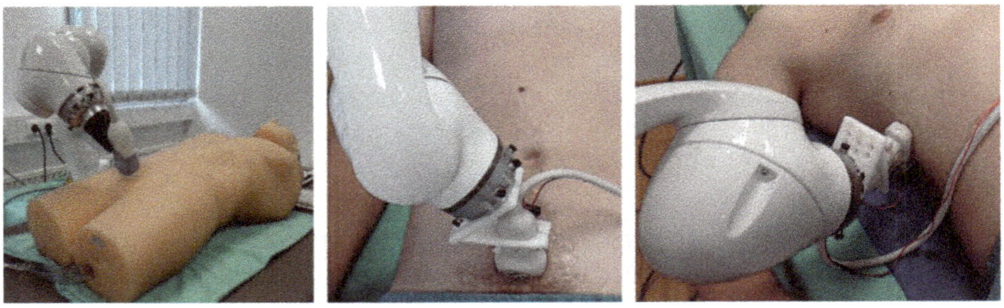

Figure 9.12. Second-generation robotic ultrasound system from Lübeck, in a phantom study (left, with 3V-D transducer, GE Healthcare Inc.), and *in vivo* acquisition for prostate (centre) and liver (right, both with X6–1 transducer, Philips NV) as described in [17].

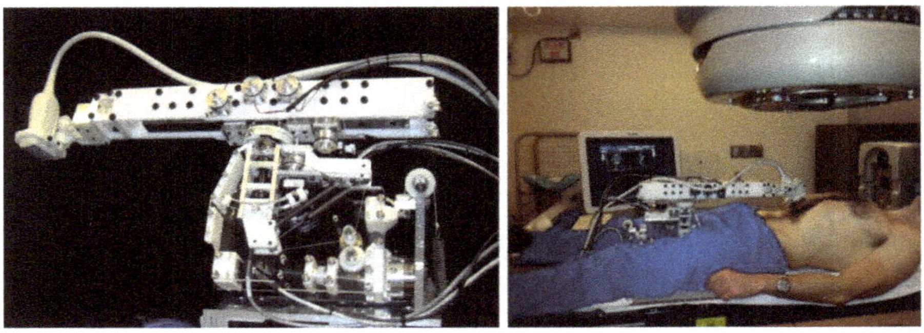

Figure 9.13. Second-generation Stanford robot, shown with X6–1 matrix probe (Philips NV). Figure courtesy of Jeffrey Schlosser (formerly Stanford University) and adapted from Western *et al* [37] under Creative Commons Attribution License CC BY 3.0.

Ipsen *et al* [39] have proposed a probe positioning extension for the platform to assist the operator during setup. To visualise the entire scene, i.e. patient CT, organ contours, ultrasound probe model and real-time ultrasound volumes, the ultrasound probe is continuously tracked either optically or robotically relative to the patient. The current superficial probe position and corresponding volume slices from CT and ultrasound can then be displayed to the operator for guidance to an optimal (potentially pre-calculated) probe position.

The second-generation system from Stanford University, shown in figure 9.13, was constructed to provide more flexibility required for abdominal targets [37]. Schlosser *et al* [11] state that their specific goal is to create a simple, human-friendly force-sensitive robot which can be used to acquire 3D/4D US data during abdominal radiotherapy. They use either an iU22 or Epiq 7 scanner with an X6–1 matrix array transducer (Philips NV) with real-time data access for ultrasound imaging. The robot was designed to eliminate most metal from the CT image acquisition and treatment areas, reducing its impact on image quality and treatment delivery. In contrast to the works at Lübeck and Johns Hopkins (see below), the Stanford group still relied on custom kinematics, mostly because this way it was possible to build a system that can be in place during CT imaging and is mostly radiolucent [40].

Furthermore, the custom robot design provides only one active degree of freedom (to control probe pressure against the patient) and a total of eight passive, electronically locking probe positioning DOFs.The robot base is positioned between the patient's legs on the treatment couch and can therefore also be placed within the CT bore for simultaneous ultrasound and CT image acquisition. Additionally, a software framework has been developed to calculate suitable ultrasound probe positions, simulate robot and gantry motion for collision avoidance and optimise treatment delivery [11].

The ultrasound robot from Stanford University has been successfully used on two liver patients during CT simulation. Using the simulation framework, ultrasound sequences were acquired via transabdominal and transcostal acoustic windows over 1–4 min at volumetric framerates of 3–4 volumes per second.

Moving away from the custom robotic platform used in their first system, Sen *et al* from Johns Hopkins University use a more standardised system in their second generation. The system, shown in figure 9.14, is based on a commercial robot (UR3/UR5, universal Robots A/S, Odense, Denmark) with integrated force/torque measurements, combined with a miniaturised wrist-mounted Nano25 force/torque sensor (ATI Industrial Automation Inc., Apex, NC, USA) and a mechanical 3D convex ultrasound probe (Ultrasonix Corp., now Analogic Corp., Richmond, BC, Canada). The system still relies on the use of virtual fixtures for guiding the operator with haptic feedback but offers the advantage of not requiring cumbersome manual adjustments of passive joints.

All three robotic ultrasound guidance systems developed to date have been shown to be flexible and useful in certain clinical tasks (prostate [4, 14, 17]; pancreas [4, 38]; liver [4, 11, 17]) and might be useful in many other imaging applications, such as cardiac imaging for treatment of arrhythmia [30, 41].

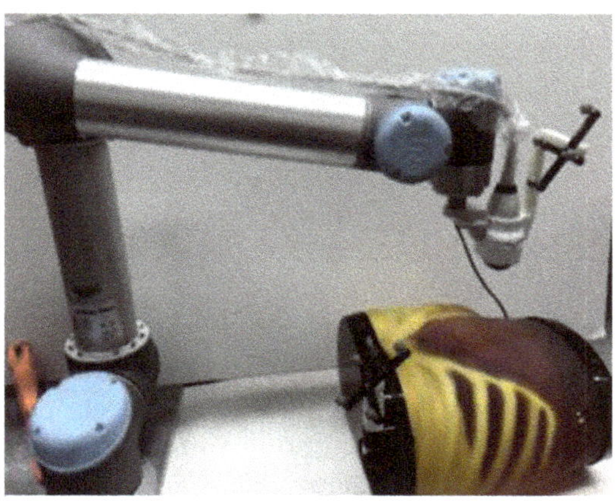

Figure 9.14. Second-generation robot from Johns Hopkins University with wrist-mounted force-torque-sensor and 3D ultrasound probe. Figure courtesy of Peter Kazanzides (Johns Hopkins University), adapted from [5] under a Creative Commons Attribution License (CC-BY).

9.5 Practical implementation and considerations

The previous sections have focussed on the general advantages, envisioned tasks and system integration of automated robotic ultrasound guidance. For practical implementation, however, several key questions still need to be addressed:

(1) Can we integrate robotic ultrasound guidance into the radiotherapy workflow?
(2) How can we ensure system accuracy?
(3) What is the expected effect on treatment quality?
(4) How can mechanical safety be realised?
(5) What are the barriers towards clinical implementation?

Considering the relative novelty of robotic systems in the radiotherapy context, potential quality assurance (QA) requirements to ensure system operation within specified parameters will be proposed and discussed in this section. These QA measures merely represent a basis for discussion and should not be considered definitive protocols at this stage.

9.5.1 Workflow integration

Successful integration of robotic ultrasound guidance into the radiotherapy workflow strongly depends on the type and placement of the robot in the treatment room. As discussed in section 9.3, the positioning of the robot base can be optimised based on the treatment site and gantry motion to minimise interference with the original treatment plan [28]. Similar to the commercial system Autoscan, which uses a static probe fixation, the robot could for example be positioned at the inferior end of the treatment table to avoid intersecting the primary beam. Another approach to further decrease the impact on the dose distribution could be a specific radiolucent robot design as proposed by Schlosser *et al* [11, 40], in contrast to using conventional industrial robots as proposed by Johns Hopkins University [5, 6] or the University of Lübeck [15, 17].

Treatment planning for robotic ultrasound guidance requires consideration of probe and robot positions expected during treatment. To ensure consistency between planned and actual patient position on the treatment day, the ultrasound probe—and resulting probe pressure—should already be present during CT simulation. This is especially important for targets located in highly deformable organs such as the liver where differences in probe position and pressure could lead to substantial discrepancies in anatomical appearance compared to the planning CT scan. To avoid probe-induced metal artefacts in the CT image data, the ultrasound probe could be replaced by a geometrically identical 'dummy' probe model as proposed by Lediju Bell *et al* [4]. Robotic placement of the probe within the CT scanner could potentially be realised with relatively small, suitably positioned robots fitting inside the CT bore. Treatment planning accounting for the dynamically adapting robot due to patient motion is discussed in more depth in chapter 5.

The main advantage of robotic ultrasound probe placement, in contrast to hand-held operation, is its high reproducibility. By recording the optimal probe position during planning (determined either fully automatically or via manual hand-guidance of the robot, see section 9.2), the exact same position can be reproduced with the same pressure on the treatment day. For *in vivo* scenarios, Lediju *et al* [4] have shown that reproducibility is superior when using position control compared to force control, i.e. reproducing the prior probe position instead of the contact pressure. They assumed the reason could be a nonlinear relationship between force and displacement in biological tissues where the same probe pressure does not necessarily place the organ in the same location. Even with position control, reproducibility was lower for highly mobile organs such as liver or pancreas compared to more constrained organs such as the prostate [4]. Since inter- and intrafractional anatomical changes will likely lead to differences in target visibility and image quality, some tolerance for deviations from the planned position will be required for online compensation. In this case, target visibility can either be assessed visually by the operator or (semi-)automatically by image processing, as described in chapter 4. Şen *et al* [5] describe it as 'a trade-off between reproducing the reference ultrasound image and bringing the probe back to the reference position and orientation' which should be weighed and resolved by the therapist. Ideally, this type of positioning tolerance should also be incorporated into a robust planning strategy for robotic ultrasound guidance. In the future, fast re-planning could potentially facilitate the use of a 'plan-of-the-day' approach where daily setup variations can be incorporated directly into an updated treatment plan, changing the focus from reproducibility towards true online adaptation.

Once the probe has been positioned on the patient in an acceptable position with good target visibility, robotic ultrasound can provide continuous, robust motion compensation by maintaining a constant contact pressure on the patient's surface. Robust treatment planning, as described in more detail in chapter 5, requires quantification of the approximate robot (and probe) motion expected during treatment. This should be done in a training session during simulation prior to treatment delivery. Probe repositioning during treatment, for example due to a planned configuration change based on the treatment plan or an unplanned spontaneous target shift outside the ultrasound field of view (FOV), could be performed from outside the treatment room both during and between beams using the remote-control capability of the robot. However, to avoid unforeseen interferences with treatment delivery, larger configuration changes should be limited to beam-off phases and might require plan adaptation if dosimetric discrepancies are expected.

9.5.2 System accuracy and quality assurance

Facilitating highly accurate target localisation is the central task of the robotic ultrasound guidance system. First and foremost, it is imperative to ensure accurate and reproducible positioning of the probe at the same coordinates in the treatment room. This can be achieved with end-to-end testing using an ultrasound QA phantom of known geometry setup in the isocentre based on the room lasers or an external optical or x-ray tracking system (with previously confirmed alignment). A discrepancy of the ultrasound probe from its intended position (external) or of a specific target location within the ultrasound image (internal) indicates an alignment error (see also chapter 3).

The main potential sources of error are discrepancies in the calibration matrices and inaccuracies of the robotic hardware, the former being far more likely and easier to correct by repeating the calibration procedure (see section 9.3). Discrepancies may arise if the probe position is changed relative to the end effector, for example if the probe has been previously detached from the robot. Geometric accuracy should be validated before every treatment to ensure correct alignment for accurate target localisation. Another potential source of uncertainty requiring regular QA is the ultrasound imaging system, as discussed in chapter 4. In addition to geometric accuracy, reliable force measurements must also be guaranteed to both ensure patient safety and reproducible probe pressure. Internal force estimations of the robot could potentially be verified using defined calibration weights and should be confirmed regularly.

Regular QA of the robotic system will be an essential part of the workflow to ensure safe and accurate operation and treatment delivery. However, since there are no commercially available robotic systems operating autonomously in direct contact with the patient to date, no comprehensive guidelines or recommendations regarding definitive QA measures exist.

9.5.3 Treatment quality

A viable concern for robotic ultrasound guidance is the presence of the ultrasound probe and the robot during treatment delivery. It has been recommended to avoid irradiation through the ultrasound probe with the primary beam to reduce dosimetric discrepancies caused by absorption and scattering [42] but also to prevent radiation-induced damage of the electronics within the probe. Several studies have addressed the concern of inferior treatment plan quality, showing that 'planning around the probe' by rejecting intersecting beams does not lead to a significant quality loss in dose distributions compared to the original plan without the probe [43]. It should also be noted that in clinical practice, the robotic ultrasound guidance system will be integrated into the planning and delivery system, allowing for optimisation of robot positions with respect to plan quality and efficiency (see also chapter 5). Another approach to further mitigate the effect on treatment delivery could be the design of radiolucent robotic components and ultrasound probe hardware [40].

Another measure for treatment quality is efficiency, in this case referring to overall treatment time. Prolonged treatment times not only increase the probability of gradual organ drift [44] but also result in a lower throughput at the linac and thus fewer patients being treated per day. Consequently, it is critical to minimise the additional time and training needed to operate the robotic ultrasound system in clinical practice. This is one of the key advantages of the robotic ultrasound system as it facilitates an automation of the workflow. Workflow automation can reduce setup time by reproducibly positioning the ultrasound probe on the patient and automatically interpreting the ultrasound image data with respect to image quality and target visibility. Assisting the operator with the difficult and cumbersome task of setting up the ultrasound equipment using a robot, either fully autonomously or via haptic feedback [5, 6], has high potential to tackle this major challenge in USgRT to date.

9.5.4 Safety

The desired operator-less manipulation of the US probe by the robot implies autonomous robotic motion with direct contact to the patient. When working in direct contact with a robot (i.e. collaborative robotics), mechanical safety is of utmost importance. The most obvious approach to achieve safe interaction between human and robot is the limitation of the maximum power, velocity, acceleration and reach of the robot, either already during the construction phase (i.e. mechanical limitations) or by implementing certain restrictions within fundamental safety layers in the control software. The major disadvantage of extensive mechanical restrictions is the loss of positioning flexibility and efficiency due to a small workspace and slow manipulation speed.

If higher flexibility is required and/or industrial robots are to be used, software-based limits should be used. Aside from globally limiting the robot's speed, in the control software it is also possible to define parts of the workspace as 'high-risk areas' with specific restrictions, e.g. by prohibiting the robot's presence entirely or only with significantly reduced speed. For example, the robotic CyberKnife system defines such a 'high-risk area' as an envelope surrounding the patient and robot motion within the envelope requires explicit confirmation by the user [45].

Especially for collaborative robotics, contact force estimation plays a critical role for safety considerations. Forces can be estimated using different techniques, e.g. by measuring torques or motor currents in the joints of the collaborative robot. Ideally, force estimation should not only be possible at the end effector but also at the other joints to facilitate collision detection along the full robot's length. Maximum force limits should then be defined to avoid collisions and thus protect the operating staff and the patients. In addition to integrated force estimations of the robot, the use of external force sensors could be considered for higher accuracy and redundancy of the measurements, either by placing several of them at critical locations along the robot or a single sensor at the end-effector with the ultrasound probe. Optical sensors, e.g. pre-installed infrared camera systems in the treatment room, can not only be used for robot calibration (see section 9.3) but also serve as a safety feature by monitoring the probe position using optical markers in addition to the robot itself. Furthermore, an emergency button for the patient should be considered to provide the option of a treatment interrupt and immediate removal of the ultrasound probe.

Ultimately, a commercial robotic ultrasound guidance system should be accompanied by a thorough risk assessment of potentially critical events such as power outages, software errors and hardware failures, and recommendations for addressing these risks to ensure operator and patient safety.

9.5.5 Acceptance

Ultimately, widespread clinical implementation of robotic ultrasound guidance will not be possible without the acceptance of potential users and patients. While the most obvious concern from the patient's point of view will likely be safety, workflow efficiency will be one of the most critical aspects for acceptance from the operator point of view. Safety, accuracy and efficiency of robotic ultrasound systems will ultimately be demonstrated in clinical studies. At the same time, robotics is a rapidly growing field becoming more and more present in the industrial context as well as in everyday life applications. Robots have also successfully entered the medical field, most notably the surgical robot DaVinci (Intuitive Inc., Sunnyvale, CA, USA) used for minimally invasive interventions and the CyberKnife system used for stereotactic radiotherapy delivery. Growing visibility of robotics and its advantages in society will likely increase trust in these systems even further.

9.6 Take home message

One of the main perceived drawbacks of ultrasound guidance to date is the operator dependency and the resulting requirement for extensive training, hampering its widespread clinical use in radiotherapy motion compensation. Robotic systems and process automation could be key factors to overcome this barrier by assisting the user during setup, increasing reproducibility of ultrasound probe positioning and facilitating continuous contact pressure and motion compensation during treatment.

To date, several robotic ultrasound guidance systems for radiotherapy have been developed and successfully tested in first *in vivo* experiments, yet none of them has reached the commercial stage. The only commercial ultrasound guidance system currently available uses a static fixture without dynamic adaptation and is currently limited to quasi-static prostate monitoring due to a slow mechanically swept ultrasound probe. The benefits of robotic automation, especially regarding highly mobile target regions and active operator assistance, make it a promising technique to increase the clinical acceptance of ultrasound-guided motion compensation and certainly warrant further investigation towards commercialisation.

Consolidation quiz

Q1: What is NOT an advantage of using robotic ultrasound guidance in radiotherapy?

- ○ Increase reproducibility of image acquisition and motion compensation
- ○ Avoidance of treatment beam angles intersecting with the robot
- ○ Reduce impact of operator dependency

Q2: What are possible applications of robotic ultrasound probe manipulation?

- ○ Adapting contact pressure dynamically and positioning remotely during treatment
- ○ Keeping a constant probe position to cause variable target deformation
- ○ Applying much higher probe pressure for better image quality

Q3: What is described by the term 'hand–eye calibration' in the context of robotic ultrasound guidance?

- ○ Geometric alignment of the robot with the treatment room and the ultrasound probe
- ○ Adjustments of the robot joints and force measurements
- ○ Detection of malfunctioning acoustic elements in the ultrasound probe

Q4: What was the focus of most second-generation robotic platforms?

- ○ Use of compliant, force-sensitive systems
- ○ Reduction of robot complexity
- ○ Reliance on two-dimensional ultrasound

Q5: What is NOT one of the major sources of error for robotic ultrasound guidance?

- ○ Misalignment due to erroneous calibration matrices (robot – isocentre / robot – ultrasound)
- ○ Positioning inaccuracy of the robot (manufacturer level)
- ○ Force measurement inaccuracies at low force levels

References

[1] Artignan X, Smitsmans M H P, Lebesque J V, Jaffray D A, van Her M and Bartelink H 2004 Online ultrasound image guidance for radiotherapy of prostate cancer: impact of image acquisition on prostate displacement *Int. J. Radiat. Oncol. Biol. Phys.* **59** 595–601

[2] van der Meer S, Bloemen-van Gurp E, Hermans J, Voncken R, Heuvelmans D and Gubbels C *et al* 2013 Critical assessment of intramodality 3D ultrasound imaging for prostate IGRT compared to fiducial markers *Med. Phys.* **40** 071707

[3] Langen K M, Pouliot J, Anezinos C, Aubin M, Gottschalk A R and Hsu I C *et al* 2003 Evaluation of ultrasound-based prostate localization for image-guided radiotherapy *Int. J. Radiat. Oncol. Biol. Phys.* **57** 635–44

[4] Lediju Bell M A, Şen H T, Iordachita I, Kazanzides P and Wong J 2014 In vivo reproducibility of robotic probe placement for a novel ultrasound-guided radiation therapy system *J. Med. Imag.* **1** 025001

[5] Şen H T, Cheng A, Ding K, Boctor E, Wong J and Iordachita I *et al* 2016 Cooperative control with ultrasound guidance for radiation therapy *Front. Robot. AI* **3** 49

[6] Şen H T, Bell M A L, Zhang Y, Ding K, Boctor E and Wong J *et al* 2017 System integration and *in vivo* testing of a robot for ultrasound guidance and monitoring during radiotherapy *IEEE Trans. Biomed. Eng.* **64** 1608–18

[7] Bin Mustafa A S, Ishii T, Matsunaga Y, Nakadate R, Ishii H and Ogawa K *et al* 2013 Human abdomen recognition using camera and force sensor in medical robot system for automatic ultrasound scan *Conf. Proc. IEEE Eng. Med. Biol. Soc.* **2013** 4855–8

[8] Mustafa A S B, Ishii T, Matsunaga Y, Nakadate R, Ishii H and Ogawa K *et al* 2013 Development of robotic system for autonomous liver screening using ultrasound scanning device *2013 IEEE Int. Conf. on Robotics and Biomimetics (ROBIO)* (Piscataway, NJ: IEEE) p 804–9

[9] Bruder R, Ernst F, Stender B, Richter L and Schweikard A 2011 SU-D-220-02: optimal transducer position for 4D ultrasound guidance in cardiac IGRT *Med. Phys.* **38** 3390

[10] Gong R, Bruder R, Schweikard A, Schlosser J and Hristov D 2015 Augmented reality system for ultrasound-guided radiation therapy *Proc. of the 29th Int. Congress and Exhibition on Computer Assisted Radiology and Surgery (CARS'15) (Barcelona, Spain)* p 39–40
[11] Schlosser J, Gong R H, Bruder R, Schweikard A, Jang S and Henrie J *et al* 2016 Robotic intrafractional US guidance for liver SABR: system design, beam avoidance, and clinical imaging *Med. Phys.* **43** 5951
[12] Camps S M, Verhaegen F, Paiva Fonesca G, de With P H N and Fontanarosa D 2017 Automatic transperineal ultrasound probe positioning based on CT scan for image guided radiotherapy ed R J Webster and B Fei *Medical Imaging 2017: Image-Guided Procedures, Robotic Interventions, and Modeling* (SPIE) p 101352X
[13] Bruder R, Bruder G and Schweikard A 2015 Method for detecting the position of a transducer. European Patent Office EP2737455B1
[14] Schlosser J, Salisbury K and Hristov D 2010 Evaluation of a telerobotic system concept for real-time soft-tissue image guidance during radiotherapy delivery *Int. J. Radiat. Oncol. Biol. Phys.* **78** S41
[15] Kuhlemann I, Bruder R, Ernst F and Schweikard A 2014 WE-G-BRF-09: force- and image-adaptive strategies for robotised placement of 4D ultrasound probes *Med. Phys.* **41** 523
[16] Şen H T, Lediju Bell M A, Zhang Y, Ding K, Wong J and Iordachita I *et al* 2015 System integration and preliminary in-vivo experiments of a robot for ultrasound guidance and monitoring during radiotherapy *Proc. Int. Conf. Adv. Robot.* **2015** 53–9
[17] Ipsen S, Kuhlemann I, Schweikard A and Ernst F 2019 Continuous long-term imaging with robotic 4D ultrasound for motion compensation in radiotherapy and beyond *Med. Phys.* **46** E287–8
[18] Abolmaesumi P, Salcudean S E, Zhu W-H, Sirouspour M R and DiMaio S P 2002 Image-guided control of a robot for medical ultrasound *IEEE Trans. Robot. Automat.* **18** 11–23
[19] Novotny P M, Stoll J A, Dupont P E and Howe R D 2007 Real-time visual servoing of a robot using three-dimensional ultrasound *Proc. 2007 IEEE Int. Conf. on Robotics and Automation* (Piscataway, NJ: IEEE) p 2655–60
[20] Zettinig O, Fuerst B, Kojcev R, Esposito M, Salehi M and Wein W *et al* 2016 Toward real-time 3D ultrasound registration-based visual servoing for interventional navigation *2016 IEEE Int. Conf. on Robotics and Automation (ICRA)* (Piscataway, NJ: IEEE) p 945–50
[21] Chatelain P, Krupa A and Navab N 2015 Optimization of ultrasound image quality via visual servoing *2015 IEEE Int. Conf. on Robotics and Automation (ICRA)* (Piscataway, NJ: IEEE) p 5997–6002
[22] Blanck O, Ipsen S, Chan M K, Bauer R, Kerl M and Hunold P *et al* 2016 Treatment planning considerations for robotic guided cardiac radiosurgery for atrial fibrillation *Cureus.* **8** e705
[23] Gerlach S, Kuhlemann I, Ernst F, Fürweger C and Schlaefer A 2017 Impact of robotic ultrasound image guidance on plan quality in SBRT of the prostate *Br. J. Radiol.* **90** 20160926
[24] Tsai R Y and Lenz R K 1989 A new technique for fully autonomous and efficient 3D robotics hand/eye calibration *IEEE Trans. Robot. Automat.* **5** 345–58
[25] Daniilidis K 1999 Hand-eye calibration using dual quaternions *Int. J. Rob. Res.* **18** 286–98
[26] Poon T C and Rohling R N 2005 Comparison of calibration methods for spatial tracking of a 3-D ultrasound probe *Ultrasound Med. Biol.* **31** 1095–108

[27] Lachaine M and Falco T 2013 Intrafractional prostate motion management with the Clarity Autoscan system *Med. Phys. Int.* **1** 72–80

[28] Schlüter M, Gerlach S, Fürweger C and Schlaefer A 2019 Analysis and optimization of the robot setup for robotic-ultrasound-guided radiation therapy *Int. J. Comput. Assist. Radiol. Surg.* **14** 1379–87

[29] Schlüter M, Fürweger C and Schlaefer A 2019 Optimizing robot motion for robotic ultrasound-guided radiation therapy *Phys. Med. Biol.* **64** 195012

[30] Bruder R, Ernst F, Schlaefer A and Schweikard A 2009 Real-time tracking of the pulmonary veins in 3D ultrasound of the beating heart *Med. Phys.* **36** 2804

[31] Martens V, Ernst F, Fränkler T, Matthäus L, Schlichting S and Schweikard A 2008 Ein Client-Server Framework für Trackingsysteme in medizinischen Assistenzsystemen Methoden. 7 Jahrestagung der Deutschen Gesellschaft für Computer- und Roboterassistierte *Chirurgie* 3–6

[32] Ipsen S, Bruder R, O'Brien R, Keall P J, Schweikard A and Poulsen P R 2016 Online 4D ultrasound guidance for real-time motion compensation by MLC tracking *Med. Phys.* **43** 5695

[33] Schlosser J, Salisbury K and Hristov D 2011 Tissue displacement monitoring for prostate and liver IGRT using a robotically-controlled ultrasound system *Med. Phys.* **38** 3812

[34] Schlosser J, Salisbury J K, Jeffrey R B and Hristov D 2010 Real-time soft-tissue imaging concurrent with external beam radiation therapy delivery *Med. Phys.* **37** 3331

[35] Schlosser J, Salisbury K and Hristov D 2012 Online image-based monitoring of soft-tissue displacements for radiation therapy of the prostate *Int. J. Radiat. Oncol. Biol. Phys.* **83** 1633–40

[36] Tutkun Şen H, Lediju Bell M A, Iordachita I, Wong J and Kazanzides P 2013 A cooperatively controlled robot for ultrasound monitoring of radiation therapy *Rep. US* **2013** 3071–6

[37] Western C, Hristov D and Schlosser J 2015 Ultrasound imaging in radiation therapy: from interfractional to intrafractional guidance *Cureus* **7** e280

[38] Su L, Iordachita I, Zhang Y, Lee J, Ng S K and Jackson J *et al* 2017 Feasibility study of ultrasound imaging for stereotactic body radiation therapy with active breathing coordinator in pancreatic cancer *J. Appl. Clin. Med. Phys.* **18** 84–96

[39] Ipsen S, Bruder R, Kuhlemann I, Jauer P, Motisi L and Cremers F *et al* 2018 A visual probe positioning tool for 4D ultrasound-guided radiotherapy *Conf. Proc. IEEE Eng. Med. Biol. Soc.* **2018** 883–6

[40] Schlosser J and Hristov D 2016 Radiolucent 4D ultrasound imaging: system design and application to radiotherapy guidance *IEEE Trans. Med. Imaging* **35** 2292–300

[41] Lydiard S, Caillet V, Ipsen S, O'Brien R, Blanck O and Poulsen P R *et al* 2018 Investigating multi-leaf collimator tracking in stereotactic arrhythmic radioablation (STAR) treatments for atrial fibrillation *Phys. Med. Biol.* **63** 195008

[42] Bazalova-Carter M, Schlosser J, Chen J and Hristov D 2015 Monte Carlo modeling of ultrasound probes for image guided radiotherapy *Med. Phys.* **42** 5745–56

[43] Boda-Heggemann J, Weiss C, Vogel L, Siebenlist K, Sihono D S K and Wertz H *et al* 2016 Ultrasound-based real-time tracking during abdominal stereotactic body radiation therapy: ultrasound probe does not influence plan quality significantly *Int. J. Radiat. Oncol. Biol. Phys.* **96** E604–5

[44] Ballhausen H, Li M, Ganswindt U and Belka C 2018 Shorter treatment times reduce the impact of intra-fractional motion: a real-time 4DUS study comparing VMAT vs. step-and-shoot IMRT for prostate cancer *Strahlenther. Onkol.* **194** 664–74

[45] Dieterich S, Cavedon C, Chuang C F, Cohen A B, Garrett J A and Lee C L *et al* 2011 Report of AAPM TG 135: quality assurance for robotic radiosurgery *Med. Phys.* **38** 2914–36

Chapter 10

Artificial intelligence applications in ultrasound-guided radiotherapy

Saskia Camps and Maria Antico

In recent years artificial intelligence has rapidly evolved and shown performance levels which are comparable to humans in many tasks, including medical image processing. This chapter provides a brief general introduction to machine learning (a subset of artificial intelligence) covering both traditional machine learning methods such as support vector machines and more novel approaches often referred to as deep learning. In addition, the differences between supervised, weakly supervised and unsupervised approaches are explained and several examples of algorithms are provided. Some machine learning based algorithms have been developed specifically for use in ultrasound-guided radiotherapy (USgRT) workflows or can be relatively easily adapted for use during these workflows. These algorithms, which can be used for, among others, automatic ultrasound image quality assessment or anatomical structure tracking, are extensively covered. Finally, some insight is provided into how artificial intelligence can be (further) implemented in the clinic.

10.1 Introduction

Ultrasound imaging provides a real-time, volumetric solution to image the patient at simulation stage as well as prior to and during treatment (i.e., USgRT). Automatic image analysis is key to make these ultrasound images usable for patient setup (chapter 6) and for radiotherapy adaptation techniques, ensuring optimal dose delivery (chapter 8). Automation of patient setup is needed to minimise the treatment duration, to reduce the operator training time and the subjectivity in the image interpretation. Time-efficient and possibly fully automated methods are required to identify the treatment target as well as the organs at risk, in order to enable the use of adaptive treatments.

doi:10.1088/978-0-7503-2552-3ch10

Image segmentation and tracking of anatomical structures for USgRT applications (e.g. pelvis, abdomen and breast) have been extensively described in chapters 5, 6 and 7. The main limitations of the algorithms described in these chapters are the low accuracy/robustness, high computational costs for target localisation and the lack of full automation in image segmentation. Most of the segmentation algorithms require the operator to manually select several initialisation points or draw an initial contour on the images. These drawbacks are associated with the inherent complexity of ultrasound images, which are caused by many factors such as speckle noise, tissue inhomogeneity, limited field of view (with possible acoustic obstruction), dependency on the probe angle and position and intra/interoperator variability.

Artificial Intelligence (AI) rapidly evolved in recent years and achieved performance levels comparable to humans in many tasks, among which is image analysis. This success can be mostly attributed to the growth of machine learning (which is a class of AI) and in particular, of deep learning, the most popular subfield of machine learning [1]. Deep learning has recently become the leading tool for automated image analysis tasks, such as classification, detection, segmentation and tracking, both in computer vision and medical imaging. These types of algorithms have been applied to ultrasound images of different anatomical regions such as breast, prostate, liver, heart, brain, foetus, kidney, spine and tongue [2], in many cases outperforming traditional image processing techniques. The main strength of deep learning is the robustness to variability in tissue appearance if a sufficient amount of varying data is provided to the algorithm for training purposes. This robustness is enabled by the automatic extraction of both low and high-level image features and high computational speed. Although machine learning and deep learning hold huge potential for automatic imaging tasks, they have not been fully explored yet for ultrasound imaging and specifically for USgRT applications.

In this chapter, the basic principles of machine learning and deep learning networks are briefly described and the current applications developed for USgRT highlighted. Three categories of machine learning can be identified: supervised, weakly-supervised and unsupervised. This subdivision is based on the technique used to train the algorithm to master the desired task (e.g. segment an anatomical structure). Reinforcement learning can be considered an additional learning category, but since it is not commonly used for ultrasound imaging, it will not be further elaborated on in this chapter. In section 10.2, supervised learning approaches are described and the most popular machine learning and deep learning architectures for automated imaging tasks introduced. Sections 10.2.1 and 10.2.2. report on the application of these algorithms to enable automation in the USgRT workflows for prostate and liver, respectively. Section 10.3 provides a description of weakly-supervised and unsupervised learning approaches and corresponding USgRT applications. Clinical implementation and limitations of AI are discussed in section 10.4.

10.2 Supervised learning approaches

Supervised learning refers to a learning approach where an algorithm is taught to perform a task (e.g. detection, classification, segmentation, etc) through a provided set of training samples and corresponding ground truth annotations or labels. These types of algorithms create a mathematical model that maps the data samples to the corresponding annotations. This is done by optimising the model variables through the minimisation of a loss function, expressing the difference between the prediction generated by the model and the expected output (i.e. the annotation provided) (figure 10.1(a)). At the end of the training, the network is tested on additional data (which the algorithm has not seen before) and the algorithm performance is assessed based on the number of correct predictions on this new dataset (figure 10.1(b)).

10.2.1 Traditional machine learning methods

Supervised machine learning algorithms aim at solving primarily classification and regression problems that involve predicting for a given object (e.g. an image) a class or a numerical label, respectively. Support vector machine (SVM) and random forest (RF) are the most famous supervised machine learning techniques for classification and regression. SVMs are used for binary classification by finding the best hyperplane separating the data in two classes, or for multi-class classification using multiple SVMs. The network architecture is composed of a first layer containing the input vectors; a hidden layer mapping the input vectors into the feature space through the kernel functions (e.g. linear, polynomial, quadratic, radial basis kernel); and an output neuron that takes the sum of the kernel outputs, each multiplied by a weight, and passes it through an activation function [3] (see figure 10.2). RF classifies data using instead an ensemble of decision trees. During training, the data samples are randomly divided between multiple decision trees [4]. To grow the trees, a subset of features is selected for each node. Then, at each node of a tree, the feature providing the best split between the data samples at that node is selected. Following this principle, each tree grows its branches until it reaches a vote for the class. The output of the RF is computed as the majority vote between the individual decision trees' outputs for a classification task and as the mean prediction of the individual decision trees' outputs for a regression task.

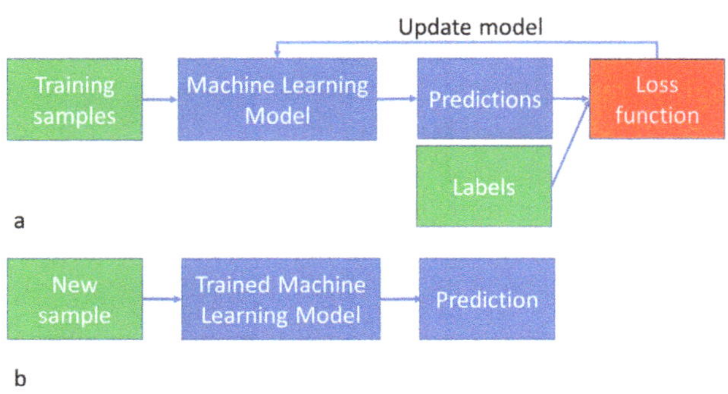

Figure 10.1. Diagram explaining supervised learning. In figures (a) and (b), the training and testing procedures are schematically represented. The green blocks in the image correspond to the data provided to the machine learning algorithm.

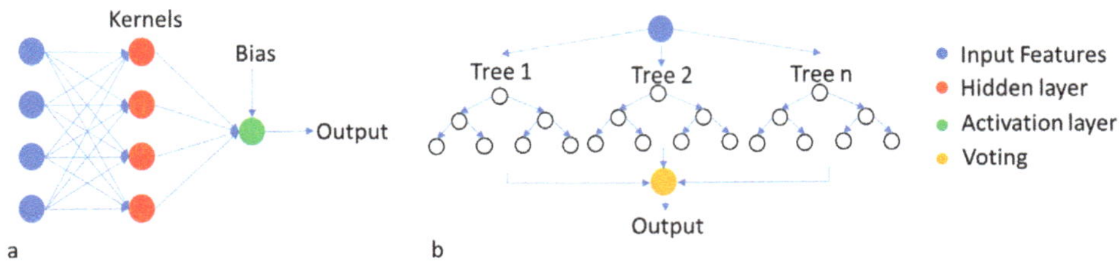

Figure 10.2. SVM (a) and RF (b) architectures.

Other popular supervised machine learning techniques include the K-Nearest Neighbors Algorithm, Naive Bayes classifier and gradient boosting algorithms, such as Adaboost [5].

For traditional machine learning approaches, the features of the training data provided to the algorithm are handcrafted. This process refers to the selection from the input images the most relevant features that characterise an image class and make it distinguishable from all the other classes. The use of these features reduces the dimensionality of the problem, but has the downside of being time-consuming to craft manually, specific to one domain/problem (and thus not reusable for other applications) and complex to design [1].

10.2.2 Deep learning methods

Different from traditional machine learning, deep learning algorithms are capable of extracting the relevant image features automatically and thus without the need for manual feature engineering. In deep learning it is also possible to use transfer learning, i.e. using a pre-trained network as starting point to re-train the network for a new task, to improve the algorithm performance and/or speed up the learning process [1].

Convolutional neural networks (CNNs) are the most popular deep learning networks that outperformed the previous state-of-the-art machine learning algorithms and imaging processing techniques used for imaging tasks such as classification and segmentation [1]. In CNNs, convolutional and pooling layers are responsible for extracting the features of the data samples. Each convolutional layer is composed of a set of filters (or features extractors), which are small arrays of numbers (or weights) representing different features (e.g. edges, curves, etc). The convolution is applied between each of the filters and the image, by translating the filter on the image by a defined stride and computing the dot product (or convolution) between the filter and the overlapped image part. For each filter, the results of the convolutions are stored in a new matrix that represents the features that were detected in the image. This feature map (see figure 10.3) will then be fed through a nonlinear activation layer (e.g. sigmoid, rectified linear unit (ReLu)) and the result will become the input of the next layer and so on. Pooling layers are generally located after each convolutional layer and are used to downsample the feature map, extracting the most important information while reducing the number of variables. As for the convolution operation, pooling consists of a filter which is

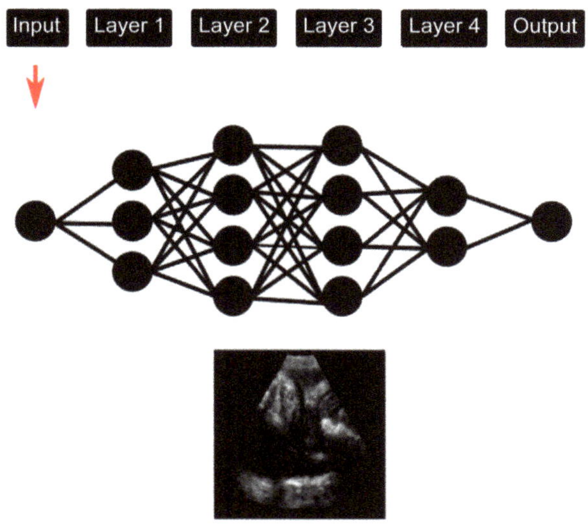

Figure 10.3. This interactive figure show an example of a neural network with an input layer, four hidden layers and an output layer. The rectangular buttons display the input image, examples of the features maps of each hidden layer and the output of the network. The further the input image propagates through the network, the more abstract the feature maps get. Animation available at https://iopscience.iop.org/book/978-0-7503-2552-3.

translated on the feature map, computing operations such as the maximum (i.e. max pool layer), or the average value of the pixels present in the window.

For classification algorithms, the CNN architecture typically ends by 'flattening' the last convolutional or pooling layer into a 1-D tensor, which is used to associate a given image with the best representative class, among the ones available, through a fully connected layer. AlexNet and DenseNet are examples of popular CNNs for classification [6]. AlexNet follows the conventional CNN structure where the input of a layer is the output of the previous layer. DenseNet is instead composed of 'dense blocks' of convolutional and pooling layers, where the input of a dense block is the concatenation of all outputs of the previous dense blocks.

While for image classification a high localisation accuracy of the image features is not required, each pixel of the image needs to be assigned to a label class to produce a semantic segmentation. For this reason, CNNs for segmentation have additional layers in comparison with CNNs for classification. They are typically composed of two symmetric parts. An encoder is used to extract coarse features of the input image exactly the same as for the classification task for the classification task (i.e. the standard CNN architecture alternating convolutional and pooling layers). A decoder is used to project the features learned in the decoder to the pixel space, recovering the original image resolution. This is achieved by up convolutions or transposed convolutions, which replace the pooling layers resizing the images in the encoder part. UNet [7] and VNet [8] are state-of-the-art CNNs for image segmentation for 2D and 3D images, respectively. In both networks, the features extracted in the encoder prior to the pooling layers are preserved by concatenating a

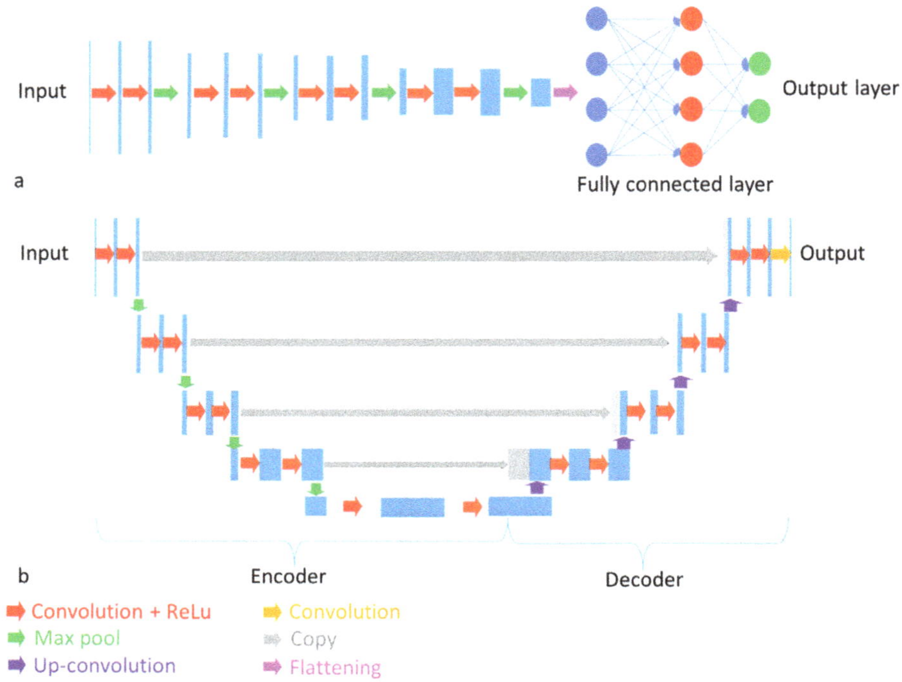

Figure 10.4. CNN for classification (a) and for segmentation (b). The blue rectangles denote the feature maps resulting from the operations indicated by the arrows. The height of each rectangle corresponds to the size of each feature map, while the width represents the number of feature maps generated. The grey rectangles in (b) correspond to the feature maps copied from the encoder network layers.

copy of these features with the convolutional layers in the decoder part (see figure 10.4(b)).

A different type of network used in deep learning is the recurrent neural network (RNN) and its variants (e.g. Long Short-Term Memory (LSTM) cell and Gated Recurrent Units) [9]. Differently from CNNs, RNNs have an internal memory (i.e. can take into account the current and previous inputs) and are used to make predictions on sequences of data. They are mostly used for speech and text recognition, and are typically used in combination with a CNN for imaging tasks such as image classification or segmentation.

In the following subsections (10.2.3 and 10.2.4), the supervised learning methods that have been implemented specifically to overcome some of the challenging aspects of prostate and liver USgRT are described. These challenges are briefly outlined and machine learning and deep learning algorithms proposed in the literature are discussed.

10.2.3 Prostate ultrasound-guided radiotherapy

Patient setup before treatment needs a trained operator to assess the quality of the ultrasound images and possibly to reposition the ultrasound probe to allow for the correct anatomical structure visualisation, as discussed in chapter 6. To support the operator and possibly automate patient setup, a few studies proposed the use of deep learning for prostate USgRT.

Camps *et al* [10] introduced a deep learning classification network for automatic image quality assessment. The algorithm was able to distinguish automatically between transperineal ultrasound images that were considered clinically usable or not usable for USgRT. Clinically usable were images with enough quality to allow for prostate identification. The algorithm implemented was a one-class regressor, combining a CNN (DenseNet) with Gaussian process regression [11]. 300 2D transperineal ultrasound images were labelled by three experts by assigning a binary score to the images based on whether it was possible or not possible to identify the prostate. Compared to the majority vote of the three experts, the algorithm achieved an accuracy of 94%, a specificity of 95% and a sensitivity of 92%.

Another approach to enable automatic patient setup has been proposed by Zhu *et al* [12]. The aim of this study was to register the simulation and the treatment transperineal ultrasound volumes. The ultrasound image content of a given anatomical area varies among ultrasound scans acquired at different times. It depends on the probe position at the moment of image acquisition and on variations in tissue distribution due to, for example, motion or deformation of the anatomical structures. A pre-trained CNN (2-channel CNN [13]) was employed to register the transperineal ultrasound volumes maximising an overall similarity score between the volumes. The registration error was smaller than 5 mm in 81% of the cases analysed, including 83 transperineal ultrasound volume pairs from 5 volunteers. The CNN performed better than manual and intensity-based registrations in terms of accuracy and reliability.

The CNNs here introduced could also be used while the patient is being treated and can be considered a step towards prostate tracking using transperineal ultrasound imaging. Existing approaches aiming at the identification of the prostate on ultrasound images have been developed only for transrectal ultrasound applications, which are not used in external beam radiotherapy. Traditional machine learning algorithms used for this task include SVM-based and RF-based algorithms [14–20]. The SVM-based methods by Akbari *et al* [14] reported a mean dice coefficient of 0.91 and 0.90, which was calculated on the 2D slices of the transrectal ultrasound volumes of 5 and 10 patients, respectively. The RF-based approach by Ghose *et al* [15] achieved a dice coefficient of 0.91 for 10 patients. In the context of deep learning instead, Yang *et al* [17] used an RNN combined with an Auto-Context scheme, while Ghavami *et al* [21] and Let *et al* [22] performed prostate segmentation on transrectal ultrasound images using a U-Net based CNN structure and a deeply supervised V-Net, respectively. The mean dice coefficient was 0.92 for the first two deep learning methods, which were tested on 7 and 44 patients and 0.91 for the third method, tested on 10 patients.

10.2.4 Liver ultrasound-guided radiotherapy

Intrafraction tissue distribution changes represent one of the main challenges in external beam radiotherapy. To compensate for anatomical structure position uncertainties, larger treatment margins are generally used which may lead to a higher dose delivered to healthy tissues. In particular, for liver cancer radiotherapy, breathing is the major cause of organ motion. The currently adopted solution is to irradiate the patient during breath-hold. This solution typically lengthens the treatment duration and does not guarantee the liver will not be subjected to drifts during and between breath-holds. Monitoring and tracking the liver using ultrasound imaging can possibly allow treatment adaptation techniques to compensate for liver motion, reducing treatment time and toxicity to the organs at risk. Two deep learning approaches have been developed to track the liver during USgRT. Both methods have been applied on the dataset of the 'The Challenge on Liver Ultrasound Tracking (CLUST) 2014 and 2015' [23].

Nouri *et al* [24] trained a CNN to learn a distance metric such that given a US image and a landmark position within the image, the CNN would locate the same landmark in the subsequent ultrasound images in the sequence. The algorithm was trained through a loss function applied to pairs of ultrasound image patches resulting in a small or a large distance whenever the pairs contained the same landmark or different landmarks, respectively. A window search was used to obtain the most likely position of the tracked landmark by finding the candidate image patch with minimum distance to the previous patches containing the same landmark. The mean tracking error for this approach was 2.83 mm. An error of less than 1.5 mm was obtained for 38 of the 62 tracked points in the test set.

Recently, Gomariz *et al* [25] used a fully-convolutional Siamese network to solve the tracking issue. While the original developed fully-convolutional Siamese network [26] was implemented to detect objects within an image, the algorithm by Gomariz *et al* has been adapted to track anatomical landmarks in a given ultrasound sequence. The network was composed of two identical CNNs (AlexNet) sharing the same network weights: the first having as input the template (i.e. an image patch containing the anatomical landmark of interest); the second was applied to a search image (i.e. the image region containing the same landmark). The outputs of the two CNNs were then compared using a cross-correlation layer, resulting in a similarity map. The maximum value within the similarity map represented the predicted landmark position. The mean tracking error was 1.34 mm.

The results obtained by Nouri *et al* [24] and Gomariz *et al* [25] were competitive with the other traditional approaches implemented for the CLUST Challenge [27] (see chapter 7), but they did not achieve the best performance in terms of accuracy and reliability. CNN methods have the advantage over the traditional methods of high computational speed (e.g. Gomariz *et al* reported 9.4 ms per 2D ultrasound image) that is fundamental to implement ultrasound guidance during treatment. However, CNNs heavily rely on the quality and amount of data provided for training that could have possibly represented a limitation for the performance achievable on this task.

10.3 Weakly supervised and unsupervised learning approaches

The deep learning approaches described in the previous section all rely on training samples which were provided to the algorithms with ground truth labels. The generation of these labels (e.g. anatomical structure contours or quality scores) is a time-consuming task, especially because deep learning algorithms tend to require a lot of data for training purposes. In addition, depending on the use case, the generation of the ground truth labels can require input from experts, whose time availability is typically even more scarce. For this reason, deep learning approaches that require only a limited number of labels (weakly supervised [28]) or no labels at all (unsupervised) have been explored.

Weakly supervised deep learning is an umbrella term for several types of deep learning strategies [28]. In the case of incomplete supervision, only a (small) subset of the data which is available for algorithm training is labelled after which the algorithm is trained with (e.g. [29, 30]) or without (e.g. [31, 32]) human intervention.

Another type of weakly supervised deep learning is the so-called inexact supervision [28]. When using this strategy, some ground truth labels are available for algorithm training; however, these labels are not as exact as the expected output. A use case for inexact supervision can be the anatomical structure localisation on ultrasound images [33] of a foetus. For every US image, there is a label available indicating which anatomical structure of the foetus is visible in the image. This label is assigned to the whole image and not to a specific anatomical structure. The deep learning algorithm is then able to classify the ultrasound images according to these labels. In addition, it can also indicate where the anatomical structure is located in the image, even though this information was never provided to the algorithm during training.

Finally, the ground truth labels provided to the algorithm might not always be the actual ground truth. In other words, those labels might contain mistakes. These mistakes can be introduced due to inexperience of the person performing the labelling or due to the difficulty of labelling. The influence of the wrong labels on the algorithm performance can be reduced by taking the label noise into account. This can be achieved by designing the neural network in such a way that it is able to better memorise clean labels than noisy labels [34].

Unsupervised learning aims at finding clusters or similarities in (image) data without ground truth labels [35]. At this moment in time, the usage of unsupervised learning for medical image processing is still in its infancy. Only a few papers have been published that make use of this approach (e.g. [36, 37]) including two that could potentially be of use during USgRT of the prostate [38, 39]. In the future, the usage of unsupervised deep learning approaches for medical image processing could be exploited further by exploring it more in depth and by potentially combining it with supervised learning approaches as well [40].

10.4 Clinical implementation

In order to make ultrasound imaging less operator dependent and to allow for its integration into standard clinical workflows, automation of ultrasound image acquisition, interpretation and utilisation are crucial to make USgRT more appealing to hospitals. Other chapters of this book have covered specific steps in USgRT workflows, like segmentation and tracking (chapter 5). In this chapter, automatic image processing has been further discussed and the use of deep learning strategies for USgRT have been reported.

Several deep learning papers have been cited that show promising and sometimes superior results in comparison with more traditional image processing approaches. All these papers have been focussing on one anatomical site (prostate, breast, pancreas, etc). However, most of the challenges associated with US imaging, such as the need for a trained operator, the need for image interpretation during the acquisition and the inaccessibility of anatomical structures shielded by bone or air, are inherent to US imaging and therefore do not depend on the anatomical structure being imaged. The advantage of deep learning is that manual crafting of features, which could be different for every anatomical structure, is obsolete, as the neural network can take care of this feature crafting. Therefore, research groups that work on different anatomical structures could join forces to create large databases that deep learning algorithms can learn from in order to tackle the generic challenges associated with ultrasound imaging first. Subsequently, transfer learning can be performed to further improve the algorithm performance for each specific anatomical structure. Alternatively, cross-domain deep learning networks, e.g. a network training with ultrasound images from different domains, can be used to address this problem. As an example, Chen *et al* [41] used a CNN to enhance detection and segmentation of anatomical structures from US images of left ventricles images acquired from different angles and foetal images.

Moreover, the growing public availability of multi-modal datasets opens new opportunities also for cross-modal transfer learning, which in some cases has been proved to be superior to the cross-domain type [42]. In the future, multi-modal datasets could also be possibly combined during training to exploit the complementary information provided by the different modalities and obtain more accurate predictions. Presently, these approaches are applied to different flavours of MRI or to the combination of MRI and CT data [43].

The deep learning strategies that are nowadays mostly used in medical imaging require learning from ground truth labels (section 10.2). These labels (segmentations, quality scores, classifications, etc) have to be provided by experts and ideally cross-validated to eliminate (part of) the operator variability. This is very time-consuming, especially concerning the fact that deep learning algorithms typically require a lot of labels to learn from. In addition, the experts have to somehow come to an agreement on the label and in particular for ultrasound imaging achieving these agreements is not always trivial.

For this reason, an eye should be kept on the advancements in weakly supervised and unsupervised deep learning strategies. In this type of deep learning, the algorithm is only provided with more high-level information to learn from. One could think of a bounding box around an anatomical structure of interest instead of a precise delineation or even just an indication of the presence of a certain anatomical structure in the image/volume. The algorithm could then learn a specific task independently and it would only need to be checked by a physician afterwards to assess its performance.

Consolidation quiz

Q1: Which of the following statements about machine learning is true?

- ○ Unsupervised learning approaches are the most commonly used for medical imaging tasks
- ○ For supervised learning approaches, the number of training images used can have a large impact on algorithm performance
- ○ None of the statements above is true

Q2: What type of CNN layer is used to transform the image features learned by the algorithm in a segmentation task to the original image resolution?

- ○ Convolutional layer
- ○ Pooling layer
- ○ Up convolutional or transposed convolutional layer

Q3: Which of the approaches can be applicable to weakly supervised deep learning? (select all correct answers)

- ○ A small subset of the available training data is labelled
- ○ A label is available for every voxel in an US image
- ○ The available data labels are different from the expected output labels

Q4: Complete the following sentence with one (or more) of the statements below: 'The deep learning algorithms tested for USgRT applications…'

- ○ always showed a better performance compared to traditional (non-machine learning) image processing techniques
- ○ showed promising results, but there is room for improvement and for further exploration of weakly-supervised and unsupervised methods
- ○ were mostly based on supervised learning methods

References

[1] Sahiner B, Pezeshk A, Hadjiiski L M, Wang X, Drukker K and Cha K H *et al* 2019 Deep learning in medical imaging and radiation therapy *Med. Phys.* **46** e1–36

[2] Liu S, Wang Y, Yang X, Lei B, Liu L and Li S X *et al* 2019 Deep learning in medical ultrasound analysis: a review *ENG.* **5** 261–75

[3] Yang X, Wu N, Cheng G, Zhou Z, Yu D S and Beitler J J *et al* 2014 Automated segmentation of the parotid gland based on atlas registration and machine learning: a longitudinal MRI study in head-and-neck radiation therapy *Int. J. Radiat. Oncol. Biol. Phys.* **90** 1225–33

[4] Breiman L 2001 Random forests *Machine Learn.* **45** 5–32

[5] Erickson B J, Korfiatis P, Akkus Z and Kline T L 2017 Machine learning for medical imaging *Radiographics.* **37** 505–15

[6] Sultana F, Sufian A and Dutta P 2018 Advancements in image classification using convolutional neural network *2018 Fourth Int. Conf. on Research in Computational Intelligence and Communication Networks (ICRCICN)* (IEEE) pp 122–9

[7] Ronneberger O, Fischer P and Brox T 2015 U-Net: convolutional networks for biomedical image segmentation *Medical Image Computing and Computer-Assisted Intervention (MICCAI)* ed N Navab, J Hornegger, W M Wells and A F Frangi (Cham: Springer) p 234–41

[8] Milletari F, Navab N and Ahmadi S-A 2016 V-Net: fully convolutional neural networks for volumetric medical image segmentation *2016 Fourth Int. Conf. on 3D Vision (3DV)* (IEEE) pp 565–71
[9] Antropova N, Huynh B, Li H and Giger M L 2019 Breast lesion classification based on dynamic contrast-enhanced magnetic resonance images sequences with long short-term memory networks *J Med Imag.* **6** 011002
[10] Camps S M, Houben T, Carneiro G, Edwards C, Antico M and Dunnhofer M *et al* 2020 Automatic quality assessment of transperineal ultrasound images of the male pelvic region, using deep learning *Ultrasound Med. Biol.* **46** 445–54
[11] Kemmler M, Rodner E, Wacker E-S and Denzler J 2013 One-class classification with Gaussian processes *Pattern Recognit.* **46** 3507–18
[12] Zhu N, Najafi M, Han B, Hancock S and Hristov D 2019 Feasibility of Image registration for ultrasound-guided prostate radiotherapy based on similarity measurement by a convolutional neural network *Technol. Cancer Res. Treat.* **18** 1533033818821964
[13] Zagoruyko S and Komodakis N 2015 Learning to compare image patches via convolutional neural networks *2015 IEEE Conf. on Computer Vision and Pattern Recognition (CVPR)* (IEEE) pp 4353–61
[14] Akbari H, Yang X, Halig L V and Fei B 2011 3D segmentation of prostate ultrasound images using wavelet transform *Proc. SPIE* **7962** 79622K
[15] Ghose S, Mitra J, Oliver A, Martí R, Lladó X and Freixenet J *et al* 2012 A supervised learning framework for automatic prostate segmentation in trans rectal ultrasound images *Advanced Concepts for Intelligent Vision Systems* ed J Blanc-Talon, W Philips, D Popescu, P Scheunders and P Zemčík (Berlin Heidelberg: Springer) 190–200
[16] Nouranian S, Ramezani M, Spadinger I, Morris W J, Salcudean S E and Abolmaesumi P 2016 Learning-based multi-label segmentation of transrectal ultrasound images for prostate brachytherapy *IEEE Trans. Med. Imaging* **35** 921–32
[17] Yang X, Schuster D, Master V, Nieh P, Fenster A and Fei B 2011 Automatic 3D segmentation of ultrasound images using atlas registration and statistical texture prior *Proc. SPIE* 7964
[18] Yang X, Rossi P J, Jani A B, Mao H, Curran W J and Liu T 2016 3D transrectal ultrasound (TRUS) prostate segmentation based on optimal feature learning framework *Proc. SPIE* 97842F
[19] Yang X and Fei B 2012 3D prostate segmentation of ultrasound images combining longitudinal image registration and machine learning *Proc. SPIE* **8316** 83162O
[20] Zaim A, Yi T and Keck R 2007 Feature-based classification of prostate ultrasound images using multiwavelet and kernel support vector machines *2007 Int. Joint Conf. on Neural Networks* (IEEE) pp 278–81
[21] Ghavami N, Hu Y, Bonmati E, Rodell R, Gibson E D and Moore C M *et al* 2018 Automatic slice segmentation of intraoperative transrectal ultrasound images using convolutional neural networks *Proc. SPIE* **10576** 1057603
[22] Lei Y, Tian S, He X, Wang T, Wang B and Patel P *et al* 2019 Ultrasound prostate segmentation based on multidirectional deeply supervised V-Net *Med. Phys.* **46** 3194–206
[23] De Luca V, Benz T, Kondo S, König L, Lübke D and Rothlübbers S *et al* 2015 The 2014 liver ultrasound tracking benchmark *Phys. Med. Biol.* **60** 5571–99
[24] Nouri D and Rothberg A 2015 Liver ultrasound tracking using a learned distance metric *Proc MICCAI Workshop: Challenge on Liver*

[25] Gomariz A, Li W, Ozkan E, Tanner C and Goksel O 2019 Siamese networks with location prior for landmark tracking in liver ultrasound sequences *2019 IEEE 16th Int. Symp. on Biomedical Imaging (ISBI 2019)* (IEEE) pp 1757–60
[26] Bertinetto L, Valmadre J, Henriques J F, Vedaldi A and Torr P H S 2016 Fully-convolutional siamese networks for object tracking *Computer vision—ECCV Workshops* ed G Hua and H Jégou (Cham: Springer) pp 850–65
[27] De Luca V, Banerjee J, Hallack A, Kondo S, Makhinya M and Nouri D *et al* 2018 Evaluation of 2D and 3D ultrasound tracking algorithms and impact on ultrasound-guided liver radiotherapy margins *Med. Phys.* **45** 4986–5003
[28] Zhou Z-H 2018 A brief introduction to weakly supervised learning *Nat. Sci. Rev.* **5** 44–53
[29] Smailagic A, Costa P, Gaudio A, Khandelwal K, Mirshekari M and Fagert J *et al* 2020 O-MedAL: online active deep learning for medical image analysis *WIREs Data Mining Knowl Discov.* **10** e1353
[30] Budd S, Robinson E C and Kainz B 2019 A survey on active learning and human-in-the-loop deep learning for medical image analysis arXiv:191002923
[31] Li M and Zhou Z-H 2007 Improve computer-aided diagnosis with machine learning techniques using undiagnosed samples *IEEE Trans. Syst. Man. Cybern. A.* **37** 1088–98
[32] Shin S Y, Lee S, Yun I D, Kim S M and Lee K M 2019 Joint weakly and semi-supervised deep learning for localization and classification of masses in breast ultrasound images *IEEE Trans. Med. Imag.* **38** 762–74
[33] Toussaint N, Khanal B, Sinclair M, Gomez A, Skelton E and Matthew J *et al* 2018 Weakly supervised localisation for fetal ultrasound images *Deep Learning in Medical Image Analysis and Multimodal Learning for Clinical Decision Support: 4th International Workshop, DLMIA 2018, and 8th International Workshop, ML-CDS 2018, Held in Conjunction with MICCAI 2018, Granada, Spain, September 20, 2018, Proc.* ed D Stoyanov, Z Taylor, G Carneiro, T Syeda-Mahmood, A Martel and L Maier-Hein *et al* (Cham: Springer) pp 192–200
[34] Cao Z, Yang G, Chen Q, Chen X and Lv F 2020 Breast tumor classification through learning from noisy labeled ultrasound images *Med. Phys.* **47** 1048–57
[35] Brattain L J, Telfer B A, Dhyani M, Grajo J R and Samir A E 2018 Machine learning for medical ultrasound: status, methods, and future opportunities *Abdom Radiol.* **43** 786–99
[36] Kallenberg M, Petersen K, Nielsen M, Ng A Y, Diao P and Igel C *et al* 2016 Unsupervised deep learning applied to breast density segmentation and mammographic risk scoring *IEEE Trans. Med. Imag.* **35** 1322–31
[37] Ng H P, Ong S H, Foong K W C, Goh P S and Nowinski W L 2006 Medical image segmentation using K-means clustering and improved watershed algorithm *2006 IEEE Southwest Symp. on Image Analysis and Interpretation* (IEEE) pp 61–5
[38] Zaim A 2005 Automatic segmentation of the prostate from ultrasound data using feature-based self organizing map *Image Analysis* ed H Kalviainen, J Parkkinen and A Kaarna (Berlin Heidelberg: Springer) 1259–65 p
[39] Richard W D and Keen C G 1996 Automated texture-based segmentation of ultrasound images of the prostate *Comput. Med. Imaging Graph.* **20** 131–40
[40] Greenspan H, van Ginneken B and Summers R M 2016 Guest editorial deep learning in medical imaging: overview and future promise of an exciting new technique *IEEE Trans. Med. Imaging* **35** 1153–9
[41] Chen H, Zheng Y, Park J-H, Heng P-A and Zhou S K 2016 Iterative multi-domain regularized deep learning for anatomical structure detection and segmentation from

ultrasound images *Medical Image Computing and Computer-Assisted Intervention—MICCAI* ed S Ourselin, L Joskowicz, M R Sabuncu, G Unal and W Wells (Cham: Springer) pp 487–95

[42] Hadad O, Bakalo R, Ben-Ari R, Hashoul S and Amit G 2017 Classification of breast lesions using cross-modal deep learning *2017 IEEE 14th Int. Symp. on Biomedical Imaging (ISBI 2017)* (IEEE) pp 109–12

[43] Cheng X, Zhang L and Zheng Y 2016 Deep similarity learning for multimodal medical images *Comp. Methods Biomechan. Biomed. Eng. Imag. Visual.* **6** 1–5

Chapter 11

Ionoacoustics

Katia Parodi and Walter Assmann

In recent years, there has been a substantial increase in the use of protons or heavy ions for the treatment of cancer. These treatments exploit the localised deposition of the majority of the kinetic energy of protons and ions at the end of their range, characterised by the Bragg peak. The localised deposition of the ions' kinetic energy results in the emission of an acoustic wave that can be detected at the surface of the body and is referred to as an ionacoustic signal. In the context of proton or ion therapy, it is important that the position of Bragg peak is known to ensure that target tissues receive a high dose and high doses to normal tissues are avoided. This chapter explores the use of ionacoustics to localise the position of the Bragg peak for the purpose of verifying the range of proton or ion beam *in vivo*. The physics underlying ionacoustics and methods to simulate the generation of the ionacoustic signal are summarised. The experiments that led to the establishment of the technique almost 50 years ago are described along with the first clinical studies. More recent work from the past decade that has exploited advances in computing and technology to optimise, through simulation, and ascertain, through experimentation, the feasibility of acoustic detection of the Bragg peak in the context of modern treatments is reviewed. Finally, opportunities for future research and clinical implementation are presented.

11.1 Introduction

The use of protons or heavier ions in external beam radiation therapy has become an interesting alternative option to photons for deep seated tumour treatment, presently counting over 90 clinical installations worldwide and a still growing number of facilities under construction or planning [1]. A major rationale for irradiation with ion beams is their characteristic depth dose distribution in tissue, represented by the Bragg curve, which shows a so-called inverted profile compared

doi:10.1088/978-0-7503-2552-3ch11

to x-rays, with a lower dose deposition before and even less after a pronounced localised dose maximum (Bragg peak) at the end of range (see figure 11.1 and interactive figure 11.2). This characteristic dose distribution entails both an advantage and a challenge: the dose maximum, if properly positioned inside the tumour, creates maximum radiation effects while minimising the damage in the concurrently irradiated healthy tissue [2]. On the other hand, a misplaced Bragg peak due to possible uncertainties in the beam penetration depth, so-called range uncertainties, can cause severe underdosage of the tumour tissue along with considerable damage in surrounding tissue, at worst in organs at risk (OAR). Therefore, information especially about the Bragg peak position with respect to the tumour boundaries is highly desirable before and even during or (less preferable) after patient treatment. To date most of the efforts aiming to verify the ion beam range *in vivo* have relied on the detection of secondary emissions induced by nuclear reactions such as positron emission tomography (PET) and different flavours of prompt gamma imaging [3]. However, also the energy deposition process itself, predominantly mediated by electromagnetic interactions of the ions with the atomic electrons, creates thermoacoustic emissions naturally enhanced at the Bragg peak. Depending on acoustic accessibility and tissue attenuation, the resulting so-called ionoacoustic signal can be detected and used for range monitoring during treatment. Although still in its infancy, this long-known phenomenon has recently regained considerable interest and could lead to an intriguing compact and cost-effective technique offering a natural combination with morphologic ultrasound imaging for

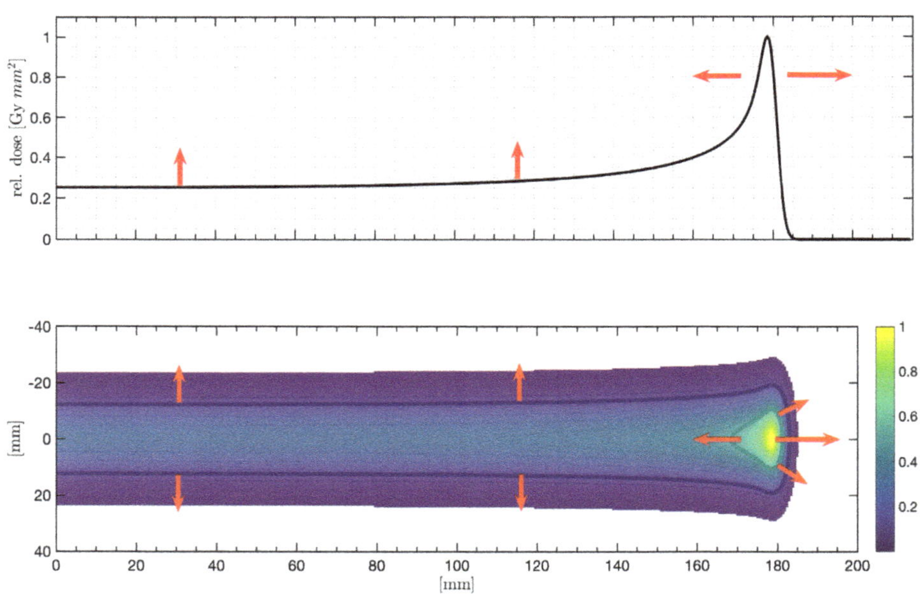

Figure 11.1. Bragg curve of 160 MeV protons in water: 2D dose distribution (below) with 1D projection along the beam penetration depth (above). Red arrows indicate the two different pressure waves (lateral and spherical, respectively).

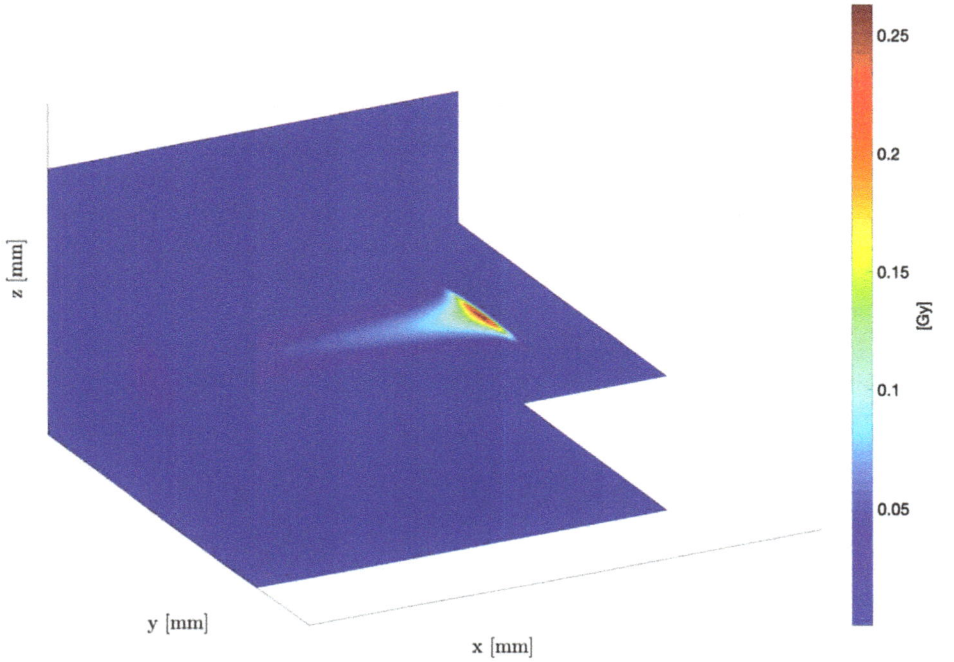

Figure 11.2. Animated 3D presentation of the proton Bragg curve of figure 11.1. Animation available at https://iopscience.iop.org/book/978-0-7503-2552-3.

quasi-simultaneous verification of the ion beam range and patient anatomy, at least in favourable anatomical locations.

11.2 Signal formation and detection

Slowing down of energetic (i.e., up to initial energies of 230 MeV) protons in matter such as water or tissue is mainly due to inelastic Coulomb interactions with target electrons (electronic energy loss) and only at their very end of range ascribed to elastic Coulomb scattering with target atoms (nuclear energy loss), while radiative losses and energy deposition in nuclear interactions can be considered negligible. There exists a large database of experimental as well as calculated stopping power values [4], which can be also simulated, e.g., by the widely used TRIM/SRIM programs [5], although more comprehensive Monte Carlo simulation codes are typically used to fully model the physics interaction processes behind dose deposition, including nuclear interactions. In the end, the energy mainly deposited through excitation/ionization of secondary (or higher generation) electrons will cause a localised heating generating thermal expansion and related thermoacoustic emissions, similar to those produced through local absorption of laser light in photo- or optoacoustics [6]. The stopping process itself takes nanoseconds at most and the resulting electrons thermalise within picoseconds [7], hence the local heating induced by a proton beam can be assumed to be instantaneous and related to the temporal beam shape. For the typical (sub)milliseconds (macro)pulse length of protons from the accelerator and individual spot delivery in pencil beam scanning [8], heat diffusion processes typically of the order of seconds in water are negligible and the energy deposition can be considered adiabatic. Moreover, for beam pulses shorter than the transit time of the sound wave across the Bragg peak width typically corresponding to a few microseconds (again for quasi-monoenergetic beams in pencil beam scanning), the energy deposition process also fulfils the condition of so-called stress confinement [9], which maximises the amplitude of the acoustic emission. An additional proton pulse microstructure e.g. due to cyclotron acceleration frequencies in the 50–100 MHz range is not of relevance for the ionoacoustic signal formation.

The generation and propagation of pressure waves in water due to transient temperature increase $T(r,t)$ can be described by the general thermoacoustic equation (11.1)

$$\left(\nabla^2 - \frac{1}{v_s^2}\right)\frac{\partial^2 p(\vec{r}, t)}{\partial t^2} = -\frac{\beta}{\kappa v_s^2}\frac{\partial^2 T(\vec{r}, t)}{\partial t^2} \quad (11.1)$$

with the induced pressure $p(r,t)$, the speed of sound in water v_s, the thermal coefficient of volumetric expansion β, and the isothermal compressibility κ. Under the above-mentioned conditions of thermal and stress confinement, the heat equation can be reduced to $\rho C_V \frac{\partial}{\partial t} T(\vec{r}, t) = H(\vec{r}, t)$, with the mass density ρ and specific heat capacity at constant volume C_V. Furthermore, the heating function $H(\vec{r}, t)$ can be separated into its temporal and spatial components to $H(\vec{r},',, , t,') = Q(\vec{r},')H'(t,')$. With this simplification, equation (11.1) can be solved analytically for pressure $p(r,t)$ resulting in expression

$$p(\vec{r}, t) = \frac{\beta}{4\pi v_s \kappa \rho C_V}\frac{\partial}{\partial t}\int_{A(t)} \frac{Q(\vec{r},')}{R} dA' \quad (11.2)$$

where the source term $Q(\vec{r},')$ is the energy deposition density (J m^{-3}) represented by the Bragg curve, integrated for $R = |\,\vec{r}, - ,\vec{r},'|$ and $A(t)$ is the surface, on which $R = v_s t$ and is thus a function of time.

Hence, the acoustic wave amplitude depends on both the deposited energy and temporal shape of the excitation pulse. In simulation studies, Albul *et al* [10] distinguished one signal originating before the Bragg peak, resulting in a cylindrical wave emitted laterally, and another one originating at the Bragg peak, approximately corresponding to a spherical wave (see arrows in figure 11.1). The latter signal was postulated by Jones *et al* [11] to be of higher interest for range verification based on time-of-flight (TOF) techniques, best placing single detectors in (near) axial configuration distal to the Bragg peak.

The ionoacoustic signal amplitude and the signal-to-noise ratio determine the required detector sensitivity, but the expected frequency spectrum also has to be considered for the right detector choice, which depends on the energy- and facility-dependent Bragg curve and the temporal profile of the beam pulse. Both, amplitude and frequency spectrum, can be deduced from the dose distribution of protons in

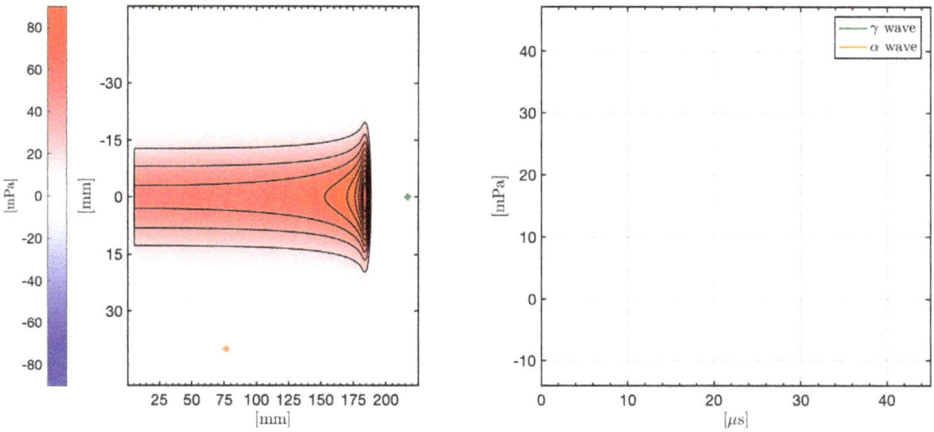

Figure 11.3. Animation of a k-Wave simulation of the ionoacoustic pressure wave development created by 160 MeV protons in water (corresponding Bragg curve in figures 11.1 and 11.2). Axial g wave (green) seen by a transducer in axial position (green cross) and lateral a wave (brown) seen in lateral position (brown cross). Animation available at https://iopscience.iop.org/book/978-0-7503-2552-3.

tissue, calculated e.g. with a general purpose Monte Carlo code like Geant4 [12], along with the medium properties (for conversion of dose into initial pressure and for speed of sound estimation) and beam temporal profile, to be input in an acoustic propagation engine like the k-Wave simulation platform [13] to determine in a second step the acoustic signal at the detector position (see interactive figure 11.3). One important finding of such simulations is the very low pressure to be expected at typical clinical proton pulse intensities in the range of tens of mPa, which is orders of magnitude lower than typical pressures for ultrasound imaging of up to 10 kPa or more, and certainly one major challenge for clinical application of ionoacoustics. In stress confinement, the mean signal frequency can be approximately estimated from the calculated Bragg peak width divided by the speed of sound and ranges from a few MHz for proton test energies around 20 MeV down to tens of kHz for clinical energies above 140 MeV, also in agreement with results of more refined k-Wave simulations.

One unique feature of the ionoacoustic method, which distinguishes it from all other investigated range monitoring techniques [3], is the possibility to correlate the ionoacoustic signal with ultrasound images of the irradiated region, especially when using the same ultrasound transducer. However, in view of the expected very low ionoacoustic signal frequency in proton therapy (10–50 kHz) compared to ultrasound imaging (2–10 MHz), the choice of appropriate detectors eventually combined with concurrent ultrasound imaging poses the other major challenge and, thus, is the subject of ongoing investigations. As seen in the following sections, two types of commercially available US detectors have been used so far for ionoacoustics: PZT (lead zirconate titanate) based single or multi-element immersion transducers and PVDF (Polyvinylidene fluoride) foils in hydrophones. PZT transducers can be ordered with mean frequencies from 0.5 to 25 MHz and 70% bandwidth typically, whereas special PVDF detectors are available with an almost constant sensitivity from 50 kHz to 5 MHz. Signals from a PZT transducer are usually sent to an external low noise preamplifier, whereas hydrophones often use integrated frontend amplification to improve signal-to-noise ratio.

11.3 Pioneering investigations on ionoaoustics and first clinical testing

Back in the 1970s Sulak *et al* [14] reported first extensive experimental characterisation of acoustic signals generated by ions in water, using different hydrophones placed at variable distances from collimated (1–10 cm diameter) proton beams of 158 MeV and 200 MeV delivered to large water tanks at the Brookhaven linear accelerator and Harvard cyclotron. Although this seminal work and successive activities of different groups were primarily focussed on understanding the ion-induced thermoacoustic emissions for application to beam monitoring or cosmic neutrino detection, the potential of the method for localisation of the Bragg peak during radiation therapy was already recognised in the 1990s. At this time, a group at the Proton Medical Research Center Tsukuba in Japan started a campaign to explore the potential of the ionoacoustic technique for radiation therapy [15]. In particular, the ionoacoustic signature could be detected with a hydrophone placed on the patient skin during hepatic treatment with passively scattered proton delivery, using a pulsed proton beam of 50 ns duration at 50 ms separation and a dose rate of 0.25 cGy/pulse [16]. In order to obtain sufficient signal-to-noise ratio, the acoustic signal was amplified 10 000 times and accumulated for 100 up to 700 proton pulses, and physiological noise (e.g., from respiration or blood circulation) was found negligible for the frequencies of interest above 10 kHz. The authors already described visionary applications of 2D arrays for 3D dose reconstruction, which they also studied in simulations [17], as well as combination with anatomical ultrasound imaging. However, the employed passively scattered beam delivery, implying quasi-simultaneous concentration of energy deposition over large volumes, complicated this line of research, which was finally given up. After astonishingly low awareness of this promising clinical experience among the international ion therapy community, different groups in Europe and USA recently regained interest in the technique, apparently almost at the same time and initially independently from each other (see references in [3]). Such renewed interest can be attributed to the recent developments in proton therapy, where ionoacoustic emissions are naturally favoured by the concentration of energy deposition in space (via sequential application of beam spots in pencil beam scanning) and time (via the development of intrinsically pulsed compact machines such as synchrocyclotrons). Interestingly, the thermoacoustic effect found at that time also new interest in high energy x-ray imaging and radiotherapy, where Xiang *et al* proposed x-ray acoustic computed tomography (CT) [18] and other groups explored photon induced acoustics for photon beam dosimetry [19].

11.4 Renaissance of ionoacoustics and ongoing developments

In 2013 Stantz *et al* reported first simulation studies supporting the feasibility of radio-acoustic computed tomography for dosimetry of pulsed proton pencil beams stopped in water using a cylindric scanner design with a 128-element transducer array [20]. Shortly afterwards, Jones *et al* published computational studies addressing the acoustic signal formation in dependence of several spatial and temporal beam properties (e.g., temporal pulse duration, lateral beam size, Bragg peak width), as well as its optimal detection by considering several spatial detector arrangements and different metrics for analysis of TOF measurements [11]. This theoretical work provided the basis for a first experimental demonstration of ionoacoustics at the IBA clinical isochronous cyclotron in Philadelphia, artificially modulated to create proton pulses with (still suboptimal) rise times of 18 μs and a maximum measured instantaneous proton current of 790 nA stopped in water [21]. Over the same years, Assmann *et al* thoroughly characterised the Bragg peak position resolution in water under idealised conditions of narrow (2 mm diameter) proton beams of very low energy (20 MeV) delivered by a Tandem accelerator, exploring the impact of different pulsing structure (from 8 ns to 4.3 μs with a rise time of 3 ns) and intensity (1 nA–10 μA beam current) at 1–10 kHz repetition frequencies. To this end, the ionoacoustic signal was detected in the most favourable axial position distal to the Bragg peak, using PZT transducers of different central frequency in the MHz range [22]. Extension to ionoacoustic tomography with first-time co-registration to optoacoustic and ultrasonic imaging was reported by the same collaboration for an *ex vivo* mouse experiment under similar irradiation conditions in Kellnberger *et al* [23]. Ionoacoustic and optoacoustic imaging was performed with an ultrasonic 64-element curved array of 5 MHz central frequency and 532 nm laser illumination for optoacoustics, whereas a co-localised linear ultrasound array was used for additional ultrasound imaging (see figure 11.4). Shortly afterwards, Patch *et al* reported the first intrinsically co-registered ionoacoustic and ultrasonic acquisitions, performed with the same US transducer array for a high dose rate irradiaton (~2 Gy/pulse at the Bragg peak) of a water tank and a gelatine phantom with a cavity, either left empty or filled with olive oil [24]. In this case, a 4 mm diameter low-energy 50 MeV proton beam of high current (2 μA) was pulsed to 1.5 μs by a fast chopper at a repetition frequency of 100 Hz. However, a signal integration of 1024 pulses was performed by the clinical cardiac array, corresponding to over 2000 Gy of total dose delivery, which underlined the low signal-to-noise challenge.

Following the promising simulated extrapolations to higher beam energies, Lehrack *et al* [25] reported the first ionoacoustic measurements at a clinical synchrocyclotron, using high energy proton beams (from 145 MeV to 227 MeV) intrinsically pulsed to a macrostructure of 2.5–3.7 μs carrying 0.1–2 pC/pulse at 1 kHz repetition. By measuring the ionoacoustic emission with a broadband hydrophone distally placed at a known position in a water phantom, axial to the beam direction, absolute range measurements could be obtained, which showed again submillimeter agreement (both in terms of accuracy and precision) with Geant4 simulations and with reference data of the on-site calibrated detector system for Bragg peak doses of more than 4 Gy. This study also showed the degradation of the ionoacoustic measuring precision, when reducing the applied dose, however still suggesting the potential of millimetre range verification for doses above 2 Gy, as typically carried by the most energetic pencil beams in clinical treatment.

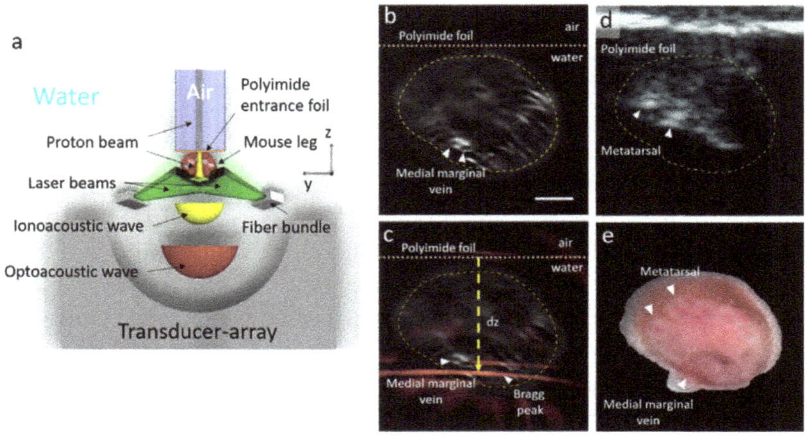

Figure 11.4. Triple-modality imaging of a mouse leg using optoacoustics, ionoacoustics, and ultrasonography. (a) Schematic of the opto- and ionoacoustic experiment. For ultrasonography, we replaced the curved array with a linear ultrasound array (picture not shown). (b) Optoacoustic reconstruction of a mouse leg positioned in the proton beam line using the curved array (arrows mark the medial marginal vein; the polyimide foil in dashed lines define the interface air—water; scale bar equals 2 mm). (c) Dual-modality opto-ionoacoustic image, showing the overlay of the Bragg peak in red color onto the optoacoustic image in grayscale. The distance $dz = 4.7 \pm 0.2$ mm defines the proton range from the polyimide foil to the Bragg peak. (d) Ultrasonography of the mouse leg obtained with a linear ultrasound array, showing metatarsal bones as positive contrast; blood vessels cannot be resolved with a conventional ultrasound imaging system. (e) Cryoslice of the mouse leg, showing the metatarsal which can be seen with conventional ultrasound and the medial marginal vein, which can be resolved with optoacoustics based on the optical absorption of blood.

Important to note, and similar to what is observed also in PET and prompt gamma imaging, resolvability of the Bragg peak position (i.e., edge detection) with TOF-techniques was not found to be affected by the imaging spatial resolution, which is related to the signal frequency in conventional ultrasound imaging. Ionoacoustic range determination relying on TOF measurements basically depends on the (almost frequency independent) time resolution of the detector system and, hence, the lower frequency spectrum in the kHz region does not prevent the prospect of obtaining (sub)millimetre-accurate range monitoring [25]. On the contrary, low frequencies can also help to reduce signal attenuation. In fact, as already mentioned, the strength of the measured signal, which depends on the initial acoustic emission (related to the spatial and temporal characteristics of the energy deposition), on the signal attenuation in tissue and on the sensitivity and bandwidth of the transducer, is one major factor influencing the achievable resolution of ionoacoustics for range monitoring.

11.5 Future clinical implementation

Generation of a measurable ionoacoustic signal under clinical conditions critically depends on the time structure and local intensity of the beam. Whereas new-generation compact synchrocyclotrons already exhibit suitable properties for ionoacoustic monitoring during treatment delivery, conventional isochronous cyclotrons require additional beam modulation into pulses matched to optimise thermoacoustic emissions.

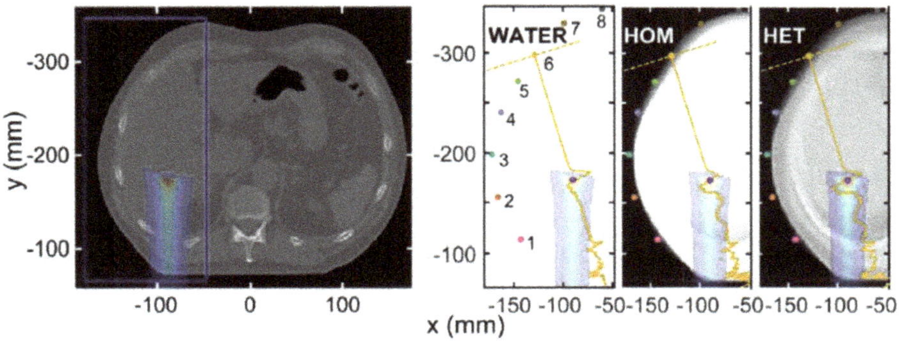

Figure 11.5. Axial CT image with superimposed proton pencil beam dose delivery to the liver (left), with a blue box indicating the dose deposition and simulation volume boundary. The average HU of each simulation volume for the three cases is given by the grey scale level shown in the right images, along with the average *x*, *y* position of each detector set. The yellow line indicates a characteristic acoustic trace superimposed on the image, showing the effect of the simulation in a pure box of water ('WATER'), a homogeneous anatomy reflecting the patient body contour ('HOM') and a realistic heterogeneous representation of the patient anatomy deduced from the patient CT ('HET'). Reproduced from [26] with permission. Copyright IOP Publishing. Reproduced with permission. All rights reserved.

Depending on the respective injection technique and used ion source, several methods are possible, such as pulsing of the deflector voltage or the ion source current, which was demonstrated by Jones *et al* [21]. In this latter case, clinical workflows have been proposed entailing a pre-treatment range verification with the artificially created proton pulses of reduced temporal length and high current ('diagnostic shots'), followed by conventional dose delivery for treatment [21, 25]. Although further speculations on future clinical workflows of ionoacoustics can still be considered too premature, the commonly perceived strategy already envisioned in the pioneering works of the 1990s should combine multiple transducers placed in contact to the patient, ideally with robotic or auto-adhesive means. Especially in the modern era of pencil beam scanning delivery, the usage of multiple detectors is foreseen to enhance the performance of the method by providing increased sensitivity and enabling proper multilateration or image reconstruction techniques to localise individual Bragg peaks or even reconstruct the delivered dose (at least for those spots depositing sufficiently high dose) [26, 27]. Corresponding simulation studies in realistic patient geometries support the possibility to overcome issues from signal distortion and attenuation in tissue heterogeneities. The example shown in figure 11.5 (from [11]) illustrates the influence of inner tissue heterogeneities and body contour in comparison to a box of water on the acoustic traces detected by transducers placed on the patient skin for pencil beam irradiation of a liver tumour. First experimental studies of Patch *et al* [28] acquiring data with a 96-channel ultrasound array and a programmable ultrasound system demonstrated the robustness of ionoacoustic range verification to acoustic heterogeneities and discrepancies between assumed and true propagation speed, i.e., speed of sound errors, thus giving confidence that those problems can be solved. Furthermore, the method could greatly benefit from additional prior tissue knowledge, derived from pre-treatment x-ray CT images (similar to proposed aberration corrections in ultrasound image guidance [29]) together with co-registered ultrasound images. The latter could be enhanced in contrast either by ultrasound specific contrast agents or additional signal evaluation techniques such as elastography [30].

Aiming at (sub)millimetre accuracy of the method, the Bragg peak position must be correlated as exactly as possible with the tumour location during treatment. To this purpose, different imaging modalities can be combined with ultrasound imaging before treatment to enhance the detectability of the tumour tissue, which often shows poor contrast in ultrasound imaging. Examples are automatic CT to ultrasound registration for diagnostic imaging, magnetic resonance imaging (MRI) combined with prostate ultrasound imaging [31] or clinical optoacoustic imaging combined with ultrasound for co-registered anatomical mapping of breast tumors [32]. Those multimodal approaches of pre-treatment imaging could help increasing the ionoacoustic position accuracy inside co-registered ultrasound images during patient treatment. Usage of commonly used fiducial markers could also be envisaged, which should be detectable in pre-treatment CT or MRI as well as during ultrasound image guidance, and on the other hand, should create minimal imaging artefacts or treatment dose perturbations [33]. Solid and liquid markers have been studied and compared for those properties and one liquid marker (BioXmark, Nanovi, Denmark) was found to best meet all requirements, in addition to exclusively offering ultrasound visibility [34, 35]. Hence, this marker, which solidifies after injection in tissue and degrades only after months, could offer an interesting prospect for ionoacoustic co-registration in image guidance.

Translation of photon therapy motion monitoring concepts to particle therapy was discussed by Bertholet *et al* [36], pointing at still rare clinical applications of ultrasound imaging for particles, except for phantom-based tracking and the above-mentioned co-registration studies [28, 37]. An obvious example of future ionoacoustic motion monitoring could be prostate cancer, where proton therapy cannot exploit its strengths due to OARs within the currently large safety margins partly caused by unpredictable prostate movements [38]. For photon therapy, a clinically approved ultrasound tracking system has been developed (Clarity, Elekta, Sweden) and applied to collect a large dataset of prostate intra-fractional motion [39]. A similar system could be used to improve time-resolved ionoacoustic range monitoring with co-registered ultrasound guidance, similar to the successful application of 4D ultrasound to beam tracking motion mitigation techniques in moving phantom experiments with scanned carbon ion beams in [37].

Although the mentioned separation of the frequency spectra employed in US imaging (~MHz) and those produced under realistic clinical conditions at intrinsically or artificially pulsed sources (~kHz) currently prevents the usage of the same detector, future solutions might enable integration of different transducer technologies in a single system (hybrid detector) for more straightforward image co-registration. With extremely fast data processing, it might become possible to visualise both the Bragg peak position and tissue anatomy in quasi real-time, thus promising very appealing means for checking the correctness of the beam delivery on a spot-by-spot basis. Although clinical applicability and performance will ultimately depend on sonic accessibility, signal strength and related localisation accuracy in presence of tissue heterogeneities, ionoacoustics might prove highly beneficial for those more critical tumour indications, which are currently challenged by intra-fractional organ motion, such as prostate, breast, liver and pancreas [30].

11.6 Conclusion and outlook

Ionoacoustics promises a cost-effective and accurate range verification modality, ideally suited for combination with 3D/4D ultrasound imaging for certain favorable tumour entities in proton therapy. However, despite the promising recent results reported by several groups in experiments and simulation studies on various water phantoms, the major challenges of ionoacoustic range verification resides in: (i) the measurable signal strength for individual pencil beams at typical therapeutic doses, (ii) the large frequency range to be detected, (iii) the knowledge of the patient-specific acoustic tissue properties and (iv) (sub)millimetre accuracy in presence of strong acoustic heterogeneities in the patient body. Concerning the weak acoustic signal, current trends of modern compact synchrocyclotrons, delivering pulsed beams of high local intensity, intrinsically favour the strength of ionoacoustic emissions. This trend would be enhanced by FLASH, a technological advance in radiation therapy ascending on the horizon, which requires even higher pulse intensities, already demonstrated at a synchrocyclotron [40, 41]. Along with further possibilities of signal enhancement at production, major developments are expected on the detection site, to enable utmost sensitivity in the relatively low frequency range (10–100 kHz) of ionoacoustic emissions, ideally integrating solutions for additional ultrasound imaging. And while most of the measurements and simulations reported so far were almost limited to homogenous targets, it is well known that tissue heterogeneities will increase the attenuation of the signal and distort its shape. Nevertheless, preliminary simulation studies in realistic patient geometries support the possibility to maintain millimeter range accuracy in favorable anatomical locations, when using multiple detectors or detector arrays along with multilateration or proper image reconstruction techniques. Still, more work will be required, also to extrapolate the needed information on the tissue acoustic properties from proper pre-treatment imaging or co-registered ultrasound images. Along with the encouraging findings of the early clinical testing in the 1990s, despite the complications of the at that time employed passively scattered beam delivery, the current state of knowledge encourages the ongoing or planned further developments, eventually aiming at realising a precise and cost-effective modality for real-time *in vivo* range/dose (and possibly also anatomy) verification for suitable clinical locations based on ionoacoustics (and ultrasound).

Acknowledgement

The authors would like to thank Dr Hans-Peter Wieser from LMU for support with figure 11.1 and the interactive material and Dr Stephan Kellnberger from IBMI/HZM for help with figure 11.5, and acknowledge Drs Julie Lascaud and Sebastian Lehrack from LMU along with Dr Stephen Avery from University of Pennsylvania for several fruitful discussions on ionoacoustics.

Consolidation quiz

Q1: How are thermoacoustic emissions produced during pulsed proton therapy delivery?

- ○ Upon tissue irradiation, a localised (in space and time) energy deposition, especially pronounced at the Bragg peak, can lead to thermal expansion and related acoustic emissions, with properties depending on the initial beam characteristics (especially energy deposition pattern and time profile)
- ○ Upon tissue irradiation acoustic waves result from photoacoustic emissions induced by the prompt gamma produced along the beam penetration depth, until the energy drops below threshold for nuclear interaction
- ○ Thermoacoustic emissions can only be produced by continuous beams of ionising irradiation

Q2: What defines the mean frequency of the ionoacoustic signal originating from the Bragg peak?

- ○ The ionoacoustic signal frequency depends only on the temporal ion pulse shape
- ○ The mean signal frequency is independent of the generation mechanism and only determined by the ultrasound detector properties
- ○ The ionoacoustic signal mean frequency is mainly defined by the Bragg peak space distribution and partly by the temporal ion pulse shape

Q3: Which kind of ultrasound detector is best suited for sensing acoustic waves generated by therapeutic pulsed proton beams?

- ○ Standard clinical ultrasonic transducers, which offer a well proven solution of optimal sensitivity and bandwidth for imaging
- ○ Cardiac or small animal ultrasonic transducers are needed, to offer ultrahigh frequency operation for excellent spatial resolution to accurately resolve the Bragg peak position
- ○ Dedicated broadband transducers of high sensitivity and properly chosen central frequency are preferable due to the typically lower frequency range of proton-induced thermoacoustic emissions, compared to clinical ultrasound imaging

References

[1] Particle Therapy Co-operative Group https://ptcog.ch/index.php

[2] Wilson R R 1946 Radiological use of fast protons *Radiology* **47** 487–91

[3] Parodi K and Polf J C 2018 *In vivo* range verification in particle therapy *Med. Phys.* **45** e1036–50

[4] Montanari C C and Dimitriou P 2017 The IAEA stopping power database, following the trends in stopping power of ions in matter *Nucl. Instrum. Methods Phys. Res., Sect.* B **408** 50–5

[5] Ziegler J F, Ziegler M D and Biersack J P 2010 SRIM—the stopping and range of ions in matter (2010) *Nucl. Instrum. Methods Phys. Res. Sect.* B **268** 1818–23

[6] Wang L V and Hu S 2012 Photoacoustic tomography: *in vivo* imaging from organelles to organs *Science* **335** 1458–62

[7] Toulemonde M, Surdutovich E and Solov'yov A V 2009 Temperature and pressure spikes in ion-beam cancer therapy *Phys. Rev. E Stat. Nonlin. Soft Matter. Phys.* **80** 031913

[8] Pedroni E, Scheib S, Böhringer T, Coray A, Grossmann M and Lin S *et al* 2005 Experimental characterization and physical modelling of the dose distribution of scanned proton pencil beams *Phys. Med. Biol.* **50** 541–61.

[9] Wang L V and Wu H-I 2009 *Biomedical Optics: Principles and Imaging* (Hoboken, NJ: Wiley)

[10] Albul V I 2005 Acoustic field generated by a beam of protons stopping in a water medium *Acoust. Phys.* **51** 33

[11] Jones K C, Witztum A, Sehgal C M and Avery S 2014 Proton beam characterization by proton-induced acoustic emission: simulation studies *Phys. Med. Biol.* **59** 6549–63

[12] Agostinelli S, Allison J, Amako K, Apostolakis J, Araujo H and Arce P *et al* 2003 Geant4—a simulation toolkit *Nucl. Instrum. Methods Phys. Res., Sect.* A **506** 250–303

[13] Treeby B E and Cox B T 2010 k-Wave: MATLAB toolbox for the simulation and reconstruction of photoacoustic wave fields *J. Biomed. Opt.* **15** 021314

[14] Sulak L, Armstrong T, Baranger H, Bregman M, Levi M and Mael D *et al* 1979 Experimental studies of the acoustic signature of proton beams traversing fluid media *Nucl. Instrum. Methods* **161** 203–17

[15] Hayakawa Y, Tada J, Inada T, Wagai T and Yosioka K 1989 Acoustic pulse generation in water by pulsed proton beam irradiation and its possible application to radiation therapy *Jpn. J. Appl. Phys.* **28** 217

[16] Hayakawa Y, Tada J, Arai N, Hosono K, Sato M and Wagai T *et al* 1995 Acoustic pulse generated in a patient during treatment by pulsed proton radiation beam *Radiat. Oncol. Investig.* **3** 42–5

[17] Terunuma T, Sakae T, Hayakawa Y, Nohtomi A, Takada Y and Yasuoka K *et al* 2007 Waveform simulation based on 3D dose distribution for acoustic wave generated by proton beam irradiation *Med. Phys.* **34** 3642–8

[18] Xiang L, Han B, Carpenter C, Pratx G, Kuang Y and Xing L 2012 X-ray acoustic computed tomography with pulsed x-ray beam from a medical linear accelerator *Med. Phys.* **40** 010701

[19] Hickling S, Xiang L, Jones K C, Parodi K, Assmann W and Avery S *et al* 2018 Ionizing radiation-induced acoustics for radiotherapy and diagnostic radiology applications *Med. Phys.* **45** e707–21

[20] Stantz K, Alsanea F and Moskvin V 2013 Best in physics (therapy) – use of radiation-induced ultrasound to image proton dosimetry *Med. Phys.* **40** 546–6

[21] Jones K C, Vander Stappen F, Bawiec C R, Janssens G, Lewin P A and Prieels D *et al* 2015 Experimental observation of acoustic emissions generated by a pulsed proton beam from a hospital-based clinical cyclotron *Med. Phys.* **42** 7090–7

[22] Assmann W, Kellnberger S, Reinhardt S, Lehrack S, Edlich A and Thirolf P G *et al* 2015 Ionoacoustic characterization of the proton Bragg peak with submillimeter accuracy *Med. Phys.* **42** 567–74

[23] Kellnberger S, Assmann W, Lehrack S, Reinhardt S, Thirolf P and Queirós D *et al* 2016 Ionoacoustic tomography of the proton Bragg peak in combination with ultrasound and optoacoustic imaging *Sci. Rep.* **6** 29305

[24] Patch S K, Kireeff Covo M, Jackson A, Qadadha Y M, Campbell K S and Albright R A *et al* 2016 Thermoacoustic range verification using a clinical ultrasound array provides perfectly co-registered overlay of the Bragg peak onto an ultrasound image *Phys. Med. Biol.* **61** 5621–38

[25] Lehrack S, Assmann W, Bertrand D, Henrotin S, Herault J and Heymans V *et al* 2017 Submillimeter ionoacoustic range determination for protons in water at a clinical synchrocyclotron *Phys. Med. Biol.* **62** L20–30

[26] Jones K C, Nie W, Chu J C H, Turian J V, Kassaee A and Sehgal C M *et al* 2018 Acoustic-based proton range verification in heterogeneous tissue: simulation studies *Phys. Med. Biol.* **63** 025018

[27] Yu Y, Li Z, Zhang D, Xing L and Peng H 2019 Simulation studies of time reversal-based protoacoustic reconstruction for range and dose verification in proton therapy *Med. Phys.* **46** 3649–62

[28] Patch S K, Santiago-Gonzalez D and Mustapha B 2019 Thermoacoustic range verification in the presence of acoustic heterogeneity and soundspeed errors – robustness relative to ultrasound image of underlying anatomy *Med. Phys.* **46** 318–27

[29] Fontanarosa D, van der Meer S, Bamber J, Harris E, O'Shea T and Verhaegen F 2015 Review of ultrasound image guidance in external beam radiotherapy: I. Treatment planning and inter-fraction motion management *Phys. Med. Biol.* **60** R77–114

[30] O'Shea T, Bamber J, Fontanarosa D, van der Meer S, Verhaegen F and Harris E 2016 Review of ultrasound image guidance in external beam radiotherapy part II: intra-fraction motion management and novel applications *Phys. Med. Biol.* **61** R90–137

[31] Das C J, Razik A, Netaji A and Verma S 2020 Prostate MRI-TRUS fusion biopsy: a review of the state of the art procedure *Abdom Radiol.* **45** 2176–83

[32] Oraevsky A A, Clingman B, Zalev J, Stavros A T, Yang W T and Parikh J R 2018 Clinical optoacoustic imaging combined with ultrasound for coregistered functional and anatomical mapping of breast tumors *Photoacoustics* **12** 30–45

[33] Habermehl D, Henkner K, Ecker S, Jakel O, Debus J and Combs S E 2013 Evaluation of different fiducial markers for image-guided radiotherapy and particle therapy *J. Radiat. Res.* **54** i61–8

[34] Scherman Rydhög J, Perrin R, Jølck R I, Gagnon-Moisan F, Larsen K R and Clementsen P *et al* 2017 Liquid fiducial marker applicability in proton therapy of locally advanced lung cancer *Radiother. Oncol.* **122** 393–9

[35] Scherman Rydhög J, Irming Jølck R, Andresen T L and Munck Af Rosenschöld P 2015 Quantification and comparison of visibility and image artifacts of a new liquid fiducial marker in a lung phantom for image-guided radiation therapy *Med. Phys.* **42** 2818–26

[36] Bertholet J, Knopf A, Eiben B, McClelland J, Grimwood A and Harris E *et al* 2019 Real-time intrafraction motion monitoring in external beam radiotherapy *Phys. Med. Biol.* **64** 15TR01

[37] Prall M, Kaderka R, Saito N, Graeff C, Bert C and Durante M *et al* 2014 Ion beam tracking using ultrasound motion detection *Med. Phys.* **41** 041708

[38] van der Meer S, Bloemen-van Gurp E, Hermans J, Voncken R, Heuvelmans D and Gubbels C *et al* 2013 Critical assessment of intramodality 3D ultrasound imaging for prostate IGRT compared to fiducial markers *Med. Phys.* **40** 071707

[39] Ballhausen H, Li M and Belka C 2019 The ProMotion LMU dataset, prostate intra-fraction motion recorded by transperineal ultrasound *Sci Data* **6** 269

[40] Symonds P and Jones G D D 2019 FLASH radiotherapy: the next technological advance in radiation therapy? *Clin. Oncol. (R Coll. Radiol.)* **31** 405–6

[41] Diffenderfer E S, Verginadis I I, Kim M M, Shoniyozov K, Velalopoulou A and Goia D *et al* 2020 Design, implementation, and *in vivo* validation of a novel proton FLASH radiation therapy system *Int. J. Radiat. Oncol. Biol. Phys.* **106** 440–8

IOP Publishing

Emma Harris, Davide Fontanarosa, Saskia Camps and Frank Verhaegen

Chapter 12

Future directions for ultrasound imaging in radiotherapy

Emma Harris and Frank Verhaegen

This chapter takes a forward-looking perspective to explore the future role of ultrasound in radiotherapy and the technological advances that will be required to support its wider use. The future role of ultrasound in adaptive radiotherapy and proton therapy is considered and the potential for automation including robotics and artificial intelligence which will overcome some of the barriers to implementation posed by the lack of staff experience and training in ultrasound is discussed. We also review new ultrasound probe technology which may pave the way for systems that are more easily integrated within the radiotherapy workflow. Finally, we highlight the functional and biological imaging nature of ultrasound imaging techniques such as elastography, contrast enhanced ultrasound imaging and ultrasound molecular imaging and how these techniques may be used to help clinicians tailor treatment for individuals by monitoring the response of tissues to radiation therapy.

12.1 Introduction

Ultrasound-guided radiotherapy systems introduced into the clinic have been developed using ultrasound imaging hardware and software that was widely available in the diagnostic setting. This is largely understandable: this technology was well established, safe and, because it was readily available, cost effective. Arguably, however, it may not produce optimal results when used in the radiotherapy setting. Throughout this book we have highlighted the extra demands that radiotherapy places on the equipment. These include (1) the lack of staff training and experience with ultrasound, (2) greater time pressures, (3) the requirement to acquire computed tomography (CT) or magnetic resonance (MR) images with the probe in place, (4) the requirement to acquire images remotely, and the requirement

doi:10.1088/978-0-7503-2552-3ch12

to not compromise the quality of the treatment, which means that (5) the probe should not attenuate the radiotherapy beam and (6) there should be zero, or little and reproducible, probe pressure. Also, the need to measure tissue motion and deformation with 6 degrees of freedom (3 translational and 3 rotational) demands (7) volumetric imaging and, for tissues which are subject to respiratory motion, (8) high volume acquisition rates. These differences present new challenges for the designers of ultrasound equipment that can be used for radiotherapy guidance, and as such require innovative technological solutions presenting exciting physics and engineering research opportunities, which are discussed in this chapter.

Automation and robotics may be able to address (1), (2) and (4), these were described in chapters 5, 9 and 10, and their future implementation is discussed in section 12.2. Section 12.3 reviews new ultrasound probe technologies that may be used to address challenges (5) to (8). This chapter then goes on to explore how ultrasound-guided radiotherapy (USgRT) may in the future be applied beyond established current clinical use to adaptive radiotherapy in section 12.4 and proton therapy in section 12.5. Finally, ultrasound is not only an anatomical imaging modality but has functional and molecular imaging capabilities. The prediction and assessment of tumour response, is now established as an essential component for optimal care in radiation therapy and whilst MR, positron emission tomography (PET) and CT have been explored for this purpose, the functional and molecular imaging capabilities of ultrasound have been largely overlooked. Section 12.6 discusses how ultrasound may be used to determine tumour response using techniques such as ultrasound elastography, contrast enhanced ultrasound and ultrasound tissue characterisation.

12.2 The future of automation

To gain greater clinical acceptance and to eliminate the human element in ultrasound imaging (from holding and moving the probe to interpreting the images), it is necessary to automate all aspects of the USgRT workflow. For image acquisition this would entail the following steps: selection of probe location and orientation for optimal viewpoint and avoidance of interference with the radiation beams [1], selection of image acquisition settings for optimal contrast for the intended application (anatomical or physiological imaging); automatic calibration of the ultrasound probe [2]; positioning of the probe with a robotic system [3, 4]; automatic real-time image acquisition, triggered for intrafraction imaging by the radiation system; automatic assessment of image quality [5].

For the image processing, automating as many steps as possible would also be beneficial. This could entail the following steps: for systems that acquire inherent 2D images a reconstitution into a 3D (or 4D) image is needed; transfer to other parts of the informatics system such as the planning system and record and verifiy system; registering to other imaging modalities such as CT or MR; processing the images to automatically extract relevant information such as organ contours [6, 7], tissue texture and possibly radiomics features.

In many fields of radiotherapy and radiology, the use of artificial intelligence for image processing, which only in recent years became effective, is causing a revolution. The exponentially growing literature clearly shows the huge potential for these methods (machine learning, deep learning, neural networks etc) to automate and enhance many steps essential for radiotherapy. These methods may soon appear everywhere in radiotherapy practice and may improve speed and quality of many aspects of the workflow. A good example of this is the successful use of AI for image segmentation of 2D and 3D images (discussed in chapter 10) which paves the way for user independent USgRT.

12.3 New probe technology

3D ultrasound imaging was reviewed in detail in chapter 2 section 2.3; briefly, there are three techniques used to acquire volumetric ultrasound images: freehand scanning, mechanical scanning and electronic scanning. Commercial USgRT systems employ freehand scanning and mechanical scanning, but there has been very little exploration of the use of the electronic scanning technique for USgRT with just a few studies reported in the literature (see chapters 9 and 10). The benefits of electronic scanning which can be achieved using 2D matrix arrays include fast (> 10 Hz) volumetric imaging, elevational focussing and a smaller, lighter probe than the one which uses mechanical scanning. Two-dimensional matrix arrays are relatively expensive, access to B-mode data is challenging and has only been accomplished by some research groups with the help of the scanner manufacturers [8, 9]. Wider access to real-time raw (uncompressed) B-mode data is essential if these probes are to be explored by research groups for application to USgRT. Access to radiofrequency (RF) data, or even unbeamformed data, from these systems is unlikely with manufacturers handling the problem of massive channel counts by beamforming on the probe. Some diagnostic ultrasound research groups are now exploring experimental 2D matrix arrays with dedicated ultrasound research platforms (see for example [10–14]). These dedicated systems allow access to unbeamformed RF data, and manipulation and optimisation of ultrasound sequences which can be tailored for specific tasks, such as tissue tracking for motion monitoring. To date there has been no research activity on the benefits of using RF data for tissue tracking in the context of radiation therapy. Tissue tracking can be easily hampered due to image decorrelation as tissue rotates and deforms [15]; RF data, which contains both amplitude and phase data, may be useful to overcome this problem. New row-column addressable (RCA) devices also offer 3D ultrasound imaging without the drawback of large channel counts [16, 17]. In comparison with a fully addressed 2D matrix array in which all elements are used to form an image (this is achieved in commercial systems), the contrast and spatial resolution is poorer, because a stronger focus is achieved in the elevation direction by the 2D matrix array. However, when a limited number of channels are available (e.g., 128), the spatial and contrast of resolution of RCA is superior to the 2D matrix array [16].

The requirement for low probe pressure scanning is a challenge that cannot be addressed if the current 'torch-light' form factor of the ultrasound transducer is maintained. Flexible or conformable arrays are an exciting development under investigation for applications such as home monitoring or disease of obstetrics in remote environments. One idea is to use a belt on which are a widely dispersed array of small patches containing ultrasound arrays [18, 19]. The belt can lie over the abdomen of the patient, or be worn like a belt. One can envisage that such a device could be used to form a low pressure image of the abdomen, which would be useful for obtaining an extended field of view image of abdominal targets and adjacent organs at risk. The issue of acoustic obstructions such as gas, would be overcome because many multiple views would be available from which to selectively build up an image of the volume tissue. These ideas have recently been realised using an extended conformable (28 cm × 28 cm) array of 36 RCAs [20]. One challenge listed above was the requirement that the probe may obstruct the radiation beam if it needs to be in place during therapy. Using the idea of a conformable belt, it is possible that a small number of patches could be arranged in such a way that alternative views of abdominal targets could be achieved, i.e., from in between the ribs or from the back for the patient. The belt is also low profile and would therefore be less likely to obstruct the beam.

12.4 Adaptive radiotherapy

Ultrasound imaging plays an important role in ultrasound-guided surgery, ultrasound-guided biopsy and image guided radiotherapy. All these applications require millimetre accuracy and precision, but radiotherapy requires fully quantitative 3D–4D images, which makes the latter application more demanding. Radiotherapy uses images that are quantitative in spatial coordinates and in distances between structures. This is essential for accurate irradiation.

Despite these new developments, the current radiotherapy standard is cone beam CT (CBCT) based in-room imaging. This technology is now ubiquitous in most linac rooms, after its introduction about two decades ago, and it is heavily used for verifying patient setup. Its advantages are: the technology is reasonably cost effective allowing it to be used in every linac room; the procedure is quick and easy; staff is already familiar with CT images and these can easily be registered with CBCT images including copying contours; the images allow dose calculations, although with less accuracy than CT images. Its disadvantages are: image quality can be poor in some patients or organs, requiring implanted markers, real-time intrafraction motion tracking is not obvious and the (ideally) daily imaging delivers extra radiation dose to normal tissues.

Besides the advantages of ultrasound guidance already mentioned throughout this book, some recognised disadvantages need urgently to be addressed for optimal use in adaptive applications, among which: older/current systems show interoperator variability, they need extensive staff training, the images are not easily readable by many physicians, and image registration may depend on scanning mode; imaging contrast strongly depends on the patient, and can be so poor as to be unusable for a significant fraction of patients: these may then require fiducials and CBCT, and these patients would need to be preselected; acoustic coupling with the patient must always be ensured also in complex dynamic situations (patient breathing/coughing/moving etc); ultrasound imaging is prone to artifacts; ultrasound images cannot be used directly for dose calculations; automation (quality assurance, contouring, tracking, registration etc) is needed to be fully useful; some regions are hard to scan, for example bone or lung; scanning protocols can be hard to optimise/standardise (even with an automated system).

Other imaging modalities are currently considered excellent candidates for adaptive applications, among which the most important is MR. There is general consensus that this modality is capable of high soft tissue imaging contrast, which does not depend strongly on the patient, allows for real-time easy to interpret imaging, and allows for functional scanning. But the disadvantages should not be ignored, among which are: high cost; it is not an add-on technology; MR images cannot be used directly for dose calculation; dosimetry (and QA) is complex and with higher uncertainty than for regular linacs; and it is not suitable for all patients, because, for example, it can cause claustrophobia (in particular for pediatric applications) and some implants/implanted devices are not compatible with the treatment. In general, MR-guided radiotherapy is often considered as the most promising image guidance modality for adaptive radiotherapy, and while this may be true to some extent in the high-income nations, this will patently not be the case for the rest of the world.

Possibly all the technologies listed here may one day be used complementary [21, 22]: e.g. CBCT and MR for head and neck and lung, MR and ultrasound for abdomen, pelvis and breast, MR and CBCT for brain. Perhaps the biggest role for ultrasound is in real-time motion tracking of natural landmarks to quantify intra-fraction motion, and to assess structural tissue changes caused by response of tumour or normal tissue to radiation. Both are currently not performed routinely in radiotherapy, but may become important for adaptive radiotherapy or when margin reduction is desired. Other forms of imaging may be too slow to achieve the same goal. Ideally, automatic contour propagation in the presence of motion should be accompanied by automatic dose recalculation and real-time display of dose differences compared to the planned dose. Also, new forms of radiotherapy such as ultrahigh dose rate Flash radiotherapy may require new strategies for motion management.

12.5 Integration into proton therapy

The current applications of image-guided radiotherapy in particle beam therapy are limited, but with the growing popularity of this form of therapy the need for image guidance in this field will also increase. Currently, US imaging plays only a marginal role in proton therapy, with very few studies published so far [23, 24]. Several teams are investigating the combination of MR image guidance and proton therapy, but this will require a very long development time and it is not obvious how to integrate MR technology with existing proton gantries. So also for this form of radiotherapy CBCT is currently the workhorse, albeit in less widespread use than for photon radiotherapy. Skin surface tracking is also gaining popularity for particle therapy monitoring [25].

Verification of proton range is paramount, therefore various methods have been proposed such as PET imaging of positron annihilation, prompt gamma imaging and, most recently, proto-acoustic signal measurement with specialised US transducers, to localise proton energy deposition locations [26–29]. None of these methods have achieved clinical acceptance, besides a few prototypes and feasibility studies. All of these methods offer significant development and clinical challenges. US range verification could be combined with anatomical US imaging, possibly in combination with microbubbles US contrast media [30], but much work remains to be done. This is discussed in another chapter in this book (see chapter 11).

Extending the use of proton therapy from the field of cancer into e.g. cardiology [31] or nephrology for radio-ablation of certain aberrational anatomical structures may also offer new opportunities for real-time US image guidance for precise targeting. Ultrasound image guidance may also be beneficial for proton radiotherapy of pediatric patients, due to their long life expectancy (less imaging dose), the lower probability of radiation-induced second cancers with proton therapy and their favourable anatomy for ultrasound imaging.

With the rapid growth of proton/light ion therapy, there may be opportunities to integrate US imaging with particle beamlines to enable real-time organ monitoring. Challenges such as interfacing real-time ultrasound technology with scanning particle beams will have to be met.

12.6 Ultrasound for the measurement of tumour response to radiotherapy

In addition to standard B-mode imaging which is employed in USgRT, there are several alternative ultrasound imaging techniques that can be used to image tumours. Doppler and contrast ultrasound can be used to image the tumour vasculature. The rapid formation of new blood vessels, or angiogenesis, is a hallmark of cancer [32] and associated with tumour aggressiveness, or metastasis [33]. Vascular imaging improves the sensitivity and specificity of cancer detection, and CT, MRI and ultrasound imaging metrics of the vasculature are becoming established as useful imaging biomarkers of cancer and prognosis [34–36]. Novel microbubble ultrasound contrast agents which are targeted to molecules overexpressed by tumours open up the possibility of ultrasound as a molecular imaging technique offering greater specificity for the detection of cancer [37]. Ultrasound elastography enables interrogation of tissue stiffness and can provide either a relative measure of stiffness of the tumour compared to surrounding tissue, or quantitative measure such as shear wave speed which is related to Young's modulus. Tumours are often stiffer than normal tissues, and this increased stiffness can be exploited by ultrasound in order to detect them. Ultrasound elastography has most notably been applied to breast cancer, where it has been investigated as an adjunct to B-mode imaging to improve specificity with varied success [38]. Ultrasound tissue characterisation (UTC) typically refers to the spectral analysis of the backscattered ultrasound RF signal [39, 40], but may also include the statistical characterisation of the envelope detected B-mode signal, which includes textural analysis of the images. UTC can provide characterisation of tissue micro- and macrostructure, and has been shown to be useful for the detection and classification of cancer. For a recent review of these techniques please refer to Oelze and Mamou [41]. Changes in the tumour microenvironment, including the vasculature, are elicited in response to radiation therapy [42], and there is clear potential for functional and molecular ultrasound techniques to play an important role in the assessment of response. The introduction of USgRT potentially paves the way for greater use of ultrasound in the context of radiation treatment. Indeed, three-dimensional imaging and established workflows for multimodality image registration offer advantages for longitudinal studies of cancer. Below is a brief description of these techniques and a review of their use for therapy response, for a more detailed discussion please refer to O'Shea *et al* [43].

12.6.1 Doppler and contrast enhanced ultrasound

Doppler and contrast ultrasound can be used to interrogate the blood supply, providing information on the tumours blood volume and blood velocity. Contrast enhanced ultrasound uses microbubbles to provide information about smaller blood vessels, including capillaries. Insonification of microbubbles at or near their resonant frequency causes the microbubbles to expand and contract, leading to the emission of high amplitude echoes. In this way, the signal from smaller volumes of blood (containing microbubbles), and hence from smaller vessels (~ 40 μm) can be detected. More recently, methods such as acoustic angiography [44] and super resolution ultrasound imaging [45] have been introduced, that further increase the sensitivity and resolution of contrast ultrasound. Dynamic-contrast enhanced ultrasound can be used to investigate the kinematics of blood flow through the tumour vasculature by plotting the ultrasound image against time to form a time-intensity curve (TIC). Metrics derived from contrast enhanced ultrasound images and the TIC can be used as imaging biomarkers of disease and disease progression [46] and numerous studies have shown them be useful for monitoring tumour response to cancer therapies including: antiangiogenic therapy (e.g. [47–50]); radio-frequency ablation (e.g. [51, 52]); and chemotherapy (e.g. [53–55]). There is some clinical evidence to suggest that contrast ultrasound may be applied to monitoring tumour response to radiotherapy. For example, promising results for liver lesions [56–59], and cervical cancer [60, 61] have been published. Interestingly, there appears to be a growing number of preclinical studies of contrast ultrasound for tumour response to radiation, recent examples include Kwon *et al* [62, 63] and Kasoji *et al* [62, 63]. In addition, the use of ultrasound molecular imaging, has also been investigated for the measurement of response to ion therapy *in vivo*. This work showed that ultrasound signals from microbubbles targeted to αvβ3-integrin and ICAM-1, both markers of angiogenesis, were enhanced post therapy [64].

12.6.2 Ultrasound elastography

Ultrasound strain elastography uses external compression of tissue (stress) and measures the resulting strain (or deformation); because the applied stress to the tissues is unknown the method cannot be quantitative (i.e., the elastic or Young's modulus cannot be determined through the stress/strain relationship). The measured strain is therefore only a qualitative measure of stiffness. By measuring the strain in both tumours and surrounding tissues, a relative measure of tumour stiffness, the strain ratio, can be determined. Acoustic radiation force (ARF) imaging uses an intense pulse of ultrasound to apply a force to the tissue inside the patient, rather than at the surface, and measures the resulting tissue displacement. Again, the stress is unknown and only a qualitative measure of stiffness can be achieved, with manufacturers typically choosing to display image pixels on a scale between 'hard' and 'soft'. Shear wave elastography typically employs ARF, but instead of measuring tissue displacement, the speed of the resulting shear wave emitted in a plane perpendicular to the propagation of the pulse is measured. The shear wave speed is directly related to Young's modulus, and therefore systems can provide quantitative measures (shear wave speed or Young's modulus) of tissue stiffness. Ultrasound elastography (strain and shear wave), has been shown to have significant promise for measuring tumour response to neoadjuvant chemotherapy for breast cancer [65–67], with a statistically significant decrease in tumour stiffness in response to therapy. Shear wave and strain elastography have been shown to detect a reduction in tumour stiffness in response to chemoradiation of rectal [68] and cervical [60, 69] cancer, respectively. These studies showed that the reduction was detectable within two weeks of the start of chemoradiation. The studies in cervical cancer also showed a statistically significant difference in the strain ratio (ratio of strain in the tumour to normal cervix) of the patients that had complete response compared to those that only had complete response or relapsed. Clinical studies in other sites have yet to be performed, however, shear wave elastography is becoming commonly used in the assessment of liver disease and for localisation prostate cancer, and therefore there is a clear opportunity to investigate the role of elastography in the response of tumours in these sites.

12.6.3 Ultrasound tissue characterisation

As acoustic energy propagates through tissue it is attenuated via scatter and absorption processes. Scattering by components of tissue which have diameters smaller, or on the order of the wavelength, of the sound are frequency dependent (discussed in detail in chapter 2). As a consequence, the frequency content of ultrasound which is backscattered from tissues is characteristic of those tissues. Spectral analysis of the backscattered signal can be used to interrogate the frequency content of the RF signal. After correction for the spectral content of the incident ultrasound wave and frequency dependent attenuation, metrics which are related to the scatterer size, concentration and the difference in acoustic impedance between the scatterers and surrounding tissue can be determined. Spectral analysis has been used to monitor the effect of neoadjuvant chemotherapy of breast cancer [70–72] and has also been applied to the measurement of response of choroidal melanoma to proton radiotherapy [73, 74] and the response of lymph nodes (involved in head and neck cancer) to chemoradiation [75].

In addition to spectral characteristics, the texture of B-mode images has also been shown to change in response to therapy, in studies which use statistical and model-based descriptions of the distribution of the grey-levels in the tumour. One study proposes the use of fractal dimension and the lacunity of the grey-levels to characterise tumour heterogeneity as a predictor of response to therapy [76] although this was not tested in a therapy setting. These techniques have also been investigated for the measurement of response of normal tissues to radiation such as the parotid gland which opens up another potential avenue for the application of ultrasound: the assessment of radiation toxicity [77].

References

[1] Camps S, Verhaegen F, Vanneste B G L, de With P H N and Fontanarosa D 2018 Automated patient-specific transperineal ultrasound probe setups for prostate cancer patients undergoing radiotherapy *Med. Phys.* **45** 3185–95

[2] Schlosser J, Kirmizibayrak C, Shamdasani V, Metz S and Hristov D 2013 Automatic 3D ultrasound calibration for image guided therapy using intramodality image registration *Phys. Med. Biol.* **58** 7481–96

[3] Schlosser J, Gong R H, Bruder R, Schweikard A, Jang S and Henrie J *et al* 2016 Robotic intrafractional US guidance for liver SABR: System design, beam avoidance, and clinical imaging *Med. Phys.* **43** 5951

[4] Schlosser J, Salisbury K and Hristov D 2010 Telerobotic system concept for real-time soft-tissue imaging during radiotherapy beam delivery *Med. Phys.* **37** 6357–67

[5] Camps S M, Houben T, Carneiro G, Edwards C, Antico M and Dunnhofer M *et al* 2020 Automatic quality assessment of transperineal ultrasound images of the male pelvic region, using deep learning *Ultrasound Med. Biol.* **46** 445–54

[6] Ermacora D, Pesente S, Pascoli F, Raducci S, Mauro R and Rumeileh I A *et al* 2015 Automated computed tomography-ultrasound cross-modality 3-D contouring algorithm for prostate *Ultrasound Med. Biol.* **41** 2646–62

[7] Mason S A, O'Shea T P, White I M, Lalondrelle S, Downey K and Baker M *et al* 2017 Towards ultrasound-guided adaptive radiotherapy for cervical cancer: Evaluation of Elekta's semiautomated uterine segmentation method on 3D ultrasound images *Med. Phys.* **44** 3630–8

[8] Ipsen S, Bruder R, O'Brien R, Keall P J, Schweikard A and Poulsen P R 2016 Online 4D ultrasound guidance for real-time motion compensation by MLC tracking *Med. Phys.* **43** 5695

[9] Lediju M A, Byram B C, Harris E J, Evans P M and Bamber J C 2010 3D Liver tracking using a matrix array: implications for ultrasonic guidance of IMRT *2010 IEEE Int. Ultrasonics Symp.* (Piscataway, NJ: IEEE) pp 1628–31

[10] Harnut S and Christensen-Jeffries K 2018 3-d super-resolution ultrasound imaging using a 2-D sparse array with high volumetric imaging rate *2018 IEEE Int. Ultrasonics Symp. (IUS)* (Piscataway, NJ: IEEE) pp 1–9

[11] Petrusca L, Varray F, Souchon R, Bernard A, Chapelon J-Y and Liebgott H *et al* 2017 A new high channels density ultrasound platform for advanced 4D cardiac imaging *2017 IEEE Int. Ultrasonics Symp. (IUS)* (Piscataway, NJ: IEEE)
[12] Roux E, Varray F, Petrusca L, Cachard C, Tortoli P and Liebgott H 2018 Experimental 3-D ultrasound imaging with 2-D sparse arrays using focused and diverging waves *Sci. Rep.* **8** 9108
[13] Roux E, Badescu E, Petrusca L, Varray F, Ramalli A and Cachard C *et al* 2017 Validation of optimal 2D sparse arrays in focused mode: phantom experiments *2017 IEEE Int. Ultrasonics Symp. (IUS)* (Piscataway, NJ: IEEE)
[14] Papadacci C, Bunting E A and Konofagou E E 2017 3D Quasi-static ultrasound elastography with plane wave *in vivo IEEE Trans. Med. Imaging* **36** 357–65
[15] Harris E J, Miller N R, Bamber J C, Symonds-Tayler J R N and Evans P M 2010 Speckle tracking in a phantom and feature-based tracking in liver in the presence of respiratory motion using 4D ultrasound *Phys. Med. Biol.* **55** 3363–80
[16] Rasmussen M F and Jensen J A 2013 3-D ultrasound imaging performance of a row-column addressed 2-D array transducer: a measurement study *2013 IEEE Int. Ultrasonics Symp. (IUS)* (Piscataway, NJ: IEEE) pp 1460–3
[17] Seo C H and Yen J T 2009 A 256 x 256 2-D array transducer with row-column addressing for 3-D rectilinear imaging *IEEE Trans. Ultrason. Ferroelectr. Freq. Control* **56** 837–47
[18] Daft C M W 2010 Conformable transducers for large-volume, operator-independent imaging *2010 IEEE Int. Ultrasonics Symp.* (Piscataway, NJ: IEEE) pp 798–808
[19] Sada M and Tanabe M 2020 Preliminary study of self-shape estimation of ultrasonic flexible probe using direct waves among elements for medical ultrasound imaging *Jpn. J. Appl. Phys.* **59** SKKE25
[20] Lu J and Jiang X 2019 Conformable row-column ultrasound arrays for abdominal imaging *2019 IEEE Int. Ultrasonics Symp. (IUS)* (Piscataway, NJ: IEEE) p 1753–6
[21] Giger A, Stadelmann M, Preiswerk F, Jud C, De Luca V and Celicanin Z *et al* 2018 Ultrasound-driven 4D MRI *Phys. Med. Biol.* **63** 145015
[22] Lee W, Chan H, Chan P, Fiorillo T, Fiveland E and Foo T *et al* 2017 A magnetic resonance compatible E4D ultrasound probe for motion management of radiation therapy *2017 IEEE Int. Ultrasonics Symp. (IUS) (Washington, DC)* pp 1–4
[23] Schwaab J, Prall M, Sarti C, Kaderka R, Bert C and Kurz C *et al* Ultrasound tracking for intra-fractional motion compensation in radiation therapy *Phys Med.* **30** 578–82
[24] Schwaab J, Kurz C, Sarti C, Bongers A, Schoenahl F and Bert C *et al* 2015 First steps toward ultrasound-based motion compensation for imaging and therapy: calibration with an optical system and 4D PET imaging *Front. Oncol.* **30** 25
[25] Desplanques M, Tagaste B, Fontana G, Pella A, Riboldi M and Fattori G *et al* 2013 A comparative study between the imaging system and the optical tracking system in proton therapy at CNAO *J. Radiat. Res.* **54** i129–35
[26] Assmann W, Kellnberger S, Reinhardt S, Lehrack S, Edlich A and Thirolf P G *et al* 2015 Ionoacoustic characterization of the proton Bragg peak with submillimeter accuracy *Med. Phys.* **42** 567–74
[27] Kellnberger S, Assmann W, Lehrack S, Reinhardt S, Thirolf P and Queirós D *et al* 2016 Ionoacoustic tomography of the proton Bragg peak in combination with ultrasound and optoacoustic imaging *Sci. Rep.* **6** 29305
[28] Alsanea F, Moskvin V and Stantz K M 2015 Feasibility of RACT for 3D dose measurement and range verification in a water phantom *Med. Phys.* **42** 937–46

[29] Hickling S, Xiang L, Jones K C, Parodi K, Assmann W and Avery S *et al* 2018 Ionizing radiation-induced acoustics for radiotherapy and diagnostic radiology applications *Med. Phys.* **45** e707–21
[30] Carlier B, Heymans S V, Nooijens S, Toumia Y, Ingram M and Paradossi G *et al* Proton range verification with ultrasound imaging using injectable radiation sensitive nanodroplets: a feasibility study *Phys. Med. Biol.* **65** 065013
[31] Bert C, Engenhart-Cabillic R and Durante M 2012 Particle therapy for noncancer diseases *Med. Phys.* **39** 1716–27
[32] Hanahan D and Weinberg R A 2011 Hallmarks of cancer: the next generation *Cell.* **144** 646–74
[33] Folkman J 1995 Seminars in medicine of the Beth Israel Hospital, Boston. Clinical applications of research on angiogenesis *N. Engl. J. Med.* **333** 1757–63
[34] Miles K A 1999 Tumour angiogenesis and its relation to contrast enhancement on computed tomography: a review *Eur. J. Radiol.* **30** 198–205
[35] Lohrke J, Frenzel T, Endrikat J, Alves F C, Grist T M and Law M *et al* 2016 25 Years of contrast-enhanced MRI: developments, current challenges and future perspectives *Adv. Ther.* **33** 1–28
[36] Eisenbrey J R and Forsberg F 2010 Contrast-enhanced ultrasound for molecular imaging of angiogenesis *Eur. J. Nucl. Med. Mol. Imaging* **37** S138–46
[37] Thumar M D and Liu M D 2019 Applications in molecular ultrasound imaging: present and future *Adv. Ultrasound Diag. Ther.* **3** 62–75
[38] Liu B, Zheng Y, Huang G, Lin M, Shan Q and Lu Y *et al* 2016 Breast lesions: quantitative diagnosis using ultrasound shear wave elastography-a systematic review and meta-analysis *Ultrasound Med. Biol.* **42** 835–47
[39] Lizzi F L, Greenebaum M, Feleppa E J, Elbaum M and Coleman D J 1983 Theoretical framework for spectrum analysis in ultrasonic tissue characterization *J. Acoust. Soc. Am.* **73** 1366–73
[40] Oelze M L, Zachary J F and O'Brien W D 2002 Characterization of tissue microstructure using ultrasonic backscatter: theory and technique for optimization using a Gaussian form factor *J. Acoust. Soc. Am.* **112** 1202–11
[41] Oelze M L and Mamou J 2016 Review of quantitative ultrasound: envelope statistics and backscatter coefficient imaging and contributions to diagnostic ultrasound *IEEE Trans. Ultrason. Ferroelectr. Freq. Control* **63** 336–51
[42] Good J S and Harrington K J 2013 The hallmarks of cancer and the radiation oncologist: updating the 5Rs of radiobiology *Clin. Oncol. (R Coll. Radiol.)* **25** 569–77
[43] O'Shea T, Bamber J, Fontanarosa D, van der Meer S, Verhaegen F and Harris E 2016 Review of ultrasound image guidance in external beam radiotherapy part II: intra-fraction motion management and novel applications *Phys. Med. Biol.* **61** R90–137
[44] Shelton S E, Lindsey B D, Gessner R, Lee Y, Aylward S and Lee H *et al* 2016 Acoustic angiography: a new high frequency contrast ultrasound technique for biomedical imaging *Sensing and Analysis Technologies for Biomedical and Cognitive Applications 2016* ed L Dai, Y Zheng, H Chu and A D Meyer-Bäse (Bellingham, WA: SPIE) 987109
[45] Christensen-Jeffries K, Couture O, Dayton P A, Eldar Y C, Hynynen K and Kiessling F *et al* 2020 Super-resolution ultrasound imaging *Ultrasound Med. Biol.* **46** 865–91
[46] Lee H, Kim H, Han H, Lee M, Lee S and Yoo H *et al* 2017 Microbubbles used for contrast enhanced ultrasound and theragnosis: a review of principles to applications *Biomed. Eng. Lett.* **7** 59–69

[47] Lamuraglia M, Bridal S L, Santin M, Izzi G, Rixe O and Paradiso A *et al* 2010 Clinical relevance of contrast-enhanced ultrasound in monitoring anti-angiogenic therapy of cancer: current status and perspectives *Crit. Rev. Oncol. Hematol.* **73** 202–12

[48] Leen E, Averkiou M, Arditi M, Burns P, Bokor D and Gauthier T *et al* 2012 Dynamic contrast enhanced ultrasound assessment of the vascular effects of novel therapeutics in early stage trials *Eur. Radiol.* **22** 1442–50

[49] Lassau N, Chami L, Chebil M, Benatsou B, Bidault S and Girard E *et al* 2011 Dynamic contrast-enhanced ultrasonography (DCE-US) and anti-angiogenic treatments *Discov. Med.* **11** 18–24

[50] Lassau N and Pitre-Champagnat S 2016 Dynamic contrast-enhanced US for monitoring of anti-angiogenic treatments *2016 IEEE Int. Ultrasonics Symp. (IUS)* (Piscataway, NJ: IEEE) pp 1–7

[51] Du J, Li H-L, Zhai B, Chang S and Li F-H 2015 Radiofrequency ablation for hepatocellular carcinoma: utility of conventional ultrasound and contrast-enhanced ultrasound in guiding and assessing early therapeutic response and short-term follow-up results *Ultrasound Med. Biol.* **41** 2400–11

[52] Calio B P, Lyshchik A, Li J, Stanczak M, Shaw C M and Adamo R *et al* 2018 Long term surveillance of renal cell carcinoma recurrence following ablation using 2D and 3D contrast-enhanced ultrasound *Urology* **121** 189–96

[53] Cao X, Xue J and Zhao B 2012 Potential application value of contrast-enhanced ultrasound in neoadjuvant chemotherapy of breast cancer *Ultrasound Med. Biol.* **38** 2065–71

[54] Schirin-Sokhan R 2012 Response evaluation of chemotherapy in metastatic colorectal cancer by contrast enhanced ultrasound *WJG* **18** 541

[55] Ang J 2012 Contrast-enhanced ultrasonography assessment of gastric cancer response to neoadjuvant chemotherapy *WJG* **18** 7026

[56] Krix M, Plathow C, Essig M, Herfarth K, Debus J and Kauczor H U *et al* 2005 Monitoring of liver metastases after stereotactic radiotherapy using low-MI contrast-enhanced ultrasound--initial results *Eur. Radiol.* **15** 677–84

[57] Li H, Liu J, Chen M, Li H and Long L 2018 Therapeutic evaluation of radiotherapy with contrast-enhanced ultrasound in non-resectable hepatocellular carcinoma patients with portal vein tumor thrombosis *Med. Sci. Monit.* **24** 8183–9

[58] Detsky J S, Milot L, Ko Y-J, Munoz-Schuffenegger P, Chu W and Czarnota G *et al* 2018 Perfusion imaging of colorectal liver metastases treated with bevacizumab and stereotactic body radiotherapy *Phys. Imag. Radiat. Oncol.* **5** 9–12

[59] Shiozawa K, Watanabe M, Ikehara T, Kobayashi K, Ochi Y and Suzuki Y *et al* 2016 Evaluation of contrast-enhanced ultrasonography for hepatocellular carcinoma prior to and following stereotactic body radiation therapy using the CyberKnife® system: a preliminary report *Oncol. Lett.* **11** 208–12

[60] Xu Y, Zhu L, Ru T, Wang H, He J and Zhou Z *et al* 2017 Three-dimensional power Doppler ultrasound in the early assessment of response to concurrent chemo-radiotherapy for advanced cervical cancer *Acta Radiol.* **58** 1147–54

[61] Huang Y F, Cheng Y M, Wu Y P, Chen H H W, Hsu K F and Wu Y H *et al* 2013 Three-dimensional power Doppler ultrasound in cervical carcinoma: monitoring treatment response to radiotherapy *Ultrasound Obstet. Gynecol.* **42** 84–92

[62] Kwon J, Rajamahendiran R M, Virani N A, Kunjachan S, Snay E and Harlacher M *et al* 2020 Use of 3-D contrast-enhanced ultrasound to evaluate tumor microvasculature after nanoparticle-mediated modulation *Ultrasound Med. Biol.* **46** 369–76

[63] Kasoji S K, Rivera J N, Gessner R C, Chang S X and Dayton P A 2018 Early assessment of tumor response to radiation therapy using high-resolution quantitative microvascular ultrasound imaging *Theranostics* **8** 156–68
[64] Palmowski M, Peschke P, Huppert J, Hauff P, Reinhardt M and Maurer M *et al* 2009 Molecular ultrasound imaging of early vascular response in prostate tumors irradiated with carbon ions *Neoplasia* **11** 856–63
[65] Evans A, Armstrong S, Whelehan P, Thomson K, Rauchhaus P and Purdie C *et al* 2013 Can shear-wave elastography predict response to neoadjuvant chemotherapy in women with invasive breast cancer? *Br. J. Cancer* **109** 2798–802
[66] Jing H, Cheng W, Li Z-Y, Ying L, Wang Q-C and Wu T *et al* 2016 Early evaluation of relative changes in tumor stiffness by shear wave elastography predicts the response to neoadjuvant chemotherapy in patients with breast cancer *J. Ultrasound. Med.* **35** 1619–27
[67] Sadeghi-Naini A, Falou O, Tadayyon H, Al-Mahrouki A, Tran W and Papanicolau N *et al* 2013 Conventional frequency ultrasonic biomarkers of cancer treatment response *in vivo Transl. Oncol.* **6** 234–43
[68] Rafaelsen S R, Vagn-Hansen C, Sørensen T, Lindebjerg J, Pløen J and Jakobsen A 2013 Ultrasound elastography in patients with rectal cancer treated with chemoradiation *Eur. J. Radiol.* **82** 913–7
[69] Mabuchi S, Sasano T, Kuroda H, Takahashi R, Nakagawa S and Kimura T 2015 Real-time tissue sonoelastography for early response monitoring in cervical cancer patients treated with definitive chemoradiotherapy: preliminary results *J. Med. Ultrason.* **42** 379–85
[70] Khairalseed M, Javed K, Jashkaran G, Kim J-W, Parker K J and Hoyt K 2019 Monitoring early breast cancer response to neoadjuvant therapy using h-scan ultrasound imaging: preliminary preclinical results *J. Ultrasound Med.* **38** 1259–68
[71] Sannachi L, Tadayyon H, Sadeghi-Naini A, Tran W, Gandhi S and Wright F *et al* 2015 Non-invasive evaluation of breast cancer response to chemotherapy using quantitative ultrasonic backscatter parameters *Med. Image Anal.* **20** 224–36
[72] Dobruch-Sobczak K, Piotrzkowska-Wróblewska H, Klimonda Z, Roszkowska-Purska K and Litniewski J 2019 Ultrasound echogenicity reveals the response of breast cancer to chemotherapy *Clin. Imag.* **55** 41–6
[73] Boudinet M, Berges O, Le Huerou J-Y, Lumbroso-Le Rouic L, Desjardins L and Laugier P 2007 Quantitative echography in the follow-up of patients treated with proton-beam irradiation for primary choroidal melanomas *Ultrasound Med. Biol.* **33** 1046–56
[74] Maschi C, Thariat J, Herault J and Caujolle J P 2016 Tumour response in uveal melanomas treated with proton beam therapy *Clin. Oncol. (R Coll. Radiol.)* **28** 198–203
[75] Tran W T, Suraweera H, Quaioit K, Cardenas D, Leong K X and Karam I *et al* 2019 Predictive quantitative ultrasound radiomic markers associated with treatment response in head and neck cancer *Future Sci. OA* **6** *FSO433*
[76] Al-Kadi O S, Van De Ville D and Depeursinge A 2016 Multidimensional texture analysis for improved prediction of ultrasound liver tumor response to chemotherapy treatment *Medical Image Computing and Computer-Assisted Intervention—MICCAI 2016* ed S Ourselin, L Joskowicz, M R Sabuncu, G Unal and W Wells (Cham: Springer) pp 619–26
[77] Ying M, Wu V W C and Kwong D L W 2007 Comparison of sonographic appearance of normal and postradiotherapy parotid glands: a preliminary study *Ultrasound Med. Biol.* **33** 1244–50

Appendix A

Answers to quiz questions

Chapter 2

Q1: The speed of sound is:

○ greater in tissues with high compressibility
✔ lower in tissues with low compressibility
○ greater in tissues with low stiffness

Q2: Ultrasound is attenuated most by:

✔ the ribs
○ the liver
○ the breast

Q3: The depth of penetration of ultrasound:

○ increases with increasing pulse length
○ increases with increasing depth of focus
✔ increases with decreasing ultrasound transmit frequency

Q4: The spatial resolution of ultrasound depends on:

○ the wavelength of ultrasound and the strength of the elevational focus
✔ the wavelength of ultrasound, the pulse length, the strength of the lateral and elevational foci
○ the wavelength of ultrasound, the pulse length, the depth of the lateral and elevational foci

Chapter 3

Q1: Optical tracking devices require that the following condition must be met:

✔ The line of sight between the optical marker on the probe and the camera must not be obstructed
○ The ultrasound probe must be acquiring images.
○ There must be no operators in the treatment room

doi:10.1088/978-0-7503-2552-3ch13

Q2: Spatial calibration describes the geometric alignment of different coordinate systems. Which two approaches are generally used to calibrate ultrasound image coordinates to room coordinates?

- ○ Optical tracking and mechanical tracking
- ✔ Defined phantom (DP) and hand-eye (HE)
- ○ Six degrees of freedom (6 DOF) and three degrees of freedom (3 DOF)

Q3: Calibration accuracy is affected by cumulative uncertainties from a range of sources, including phantom alignment and tracking accuracy. Some sources are ultrasound-specific and affect the registration accuracy of:

- ○ Intermodality ultrasound guidance systems only
- ○ Intramodality ultrasound guidance systems only
- ✔ Both inter- and intramodality ultrasound guidance systems

Q4: What is a possible effect of the application of ultrasound probe pressure on the skin of the patient?

- ○ Anatomical structure displacement
- ○ Anatomical structure deformation
- ✔ Anatomical structure displacement and deformation

Chapter 4

Q1: Ultrasound probe set-up and image quality assessment are predominantly manual tasks. Why are these tasks particularly challenging in a radiotherapy environment?

- ○ Ultrasound scanners cannot acquire images during radiotherapy delivery
- ✔ Radiotherapy staff typically has limited experience with ultrasonography
- ○ The ultrasound probe must never be held by the operator

Q2: The clinical requirements of ultrasound in radiotherapy are similar to those of diagnostic ultrasound. One important difference in ultrasound image guidance is the need to maintain a consistently small probe pressure. Why?

- ○ To ensure the patient remains relaxed at all times
- ✔ To ensure the patient geometry at each treatment session is consistent
- ○ To avoid annoying the radiotherapy oncologist

Q3: Which of these is not a common ultrasound imaging artifact?

- ○ Shadowing
- ○ Reverberation
- ✔ Cavitation

Q4: Why is automated quality assessment important?

- ✔ Automated quality assessment can reduce interobserver variation and improve image guidance accuracy
- ○ Automated quality assessment improves ultrasound acquisition frame rates
- ○ Manually assessing image quality is physically impossible

Q5: Peak detection, minimum detection and averaging are all methods of what?
- ✔ Combining regions of overlap from multiple ultrasound images
- ○ Measuring lateral resolution in spatially compounded images
- ○ Calculating sub-aperture translations for spatial compounding

Chapter 5

Q1: Why is it not possible to create a radiotherapy treatment plan based on ultrasound images?
- ○ The field of view of a typical ultrasound image is too limited
- ✔ The ultrasound images do not provide physical density information, which makes it impossible to calculate radiation dose
- ○ Soft-tissue interfaces are poorly visible on ultrasound images

Q2: Why should beams passing the ultrasound probe be avoided?
- ○ The beams would destroy the ultrasound probe
- ✔ Attenuation and scattering may impact the delivered dose
- ○ The US image quality would degrade

Q3: How can the impact of ultrasound probe blocking beams be mitigated?
- ○ The ultrasound probe must be removed before each beam delivery
- ○ Only ultrasound probe positions from lateral viewports are used
- ✔ Inverse planning can be used to identify preferable ultrasound probe positions

Q4: Why is it important to consider a safety margin around the ultrasound probe?
- ✔ The ultrasound probe and the beams may move during treatment
- ○ To avoid a collision between the ultrasound probe and the patient
- ○ To prevent the beam source from colliding with the ultrasound probe

Chapter 6

Q1: Why is it important to, prior to each treatment fraction, set up the patient the same way as during the simulation stage?
- ✔ This was the setup based on which the treatment plan was designed
- ○ This setup was the most comfortable for the patient
- ○ This setup is the easiest to reproduce

Q2: Which of the following statements is correct?
- ○ Intermodality systems compare anatomical information from ultrasound images acquired at simulation stage with ultrasound images acquired at treatment stage
- ○ Intramodality systems compare anatomical information from CT scans (simulation stage) with ultrasound images (treatment stage)
- ✔ None of the above

Q3: Which of the following challenges can be associated with ultrasound-guided patient setup? (select all correct answers)
- ✔ Probe pressure effects
- ○ Patient discomfort
- ✔ Simultaneous acquisition of CT and ultrasound

Q4: Interfraction motion of a radiation therapy treatment site can be the result of….

○ Rectal and bladder filling
○ Changes in tumour volume size
✔ All of the above

Chapter 7

Q1: What is the advantage of using ultrasound for intrafraction motion monitoring?

○ Every radiotherapy department has an ultrasound image guidance system
✔ Ultrasound is the only imaging modality that can provide volumetric soft tissue imaging in real time
○ The ionising radiation dose associated with all other imaging modalities makes it impossible to rely on them for intrafraction motion monitoring

Q2: Regularisation is a technique used in both direct and indirect monitoring. Which of these is not a regularisation method used in intrafraction monitoring?

✔ Temperature regularisation
○ Spatial regularisation
○ Temporal regularisation

Q3: Intrafraction motion compensation requires accurate target localisation with low latency. What is the suggested maximum latency for a real-time motion compensation system?

○ 3 s
○ 10 μs
✔ 500 ms

Q4: Various clinical applications of intrafraction monitoring have been studied both *in vivo* and *in vitro*. What is the most common ultrasound intrafraction monitoring application?

○ MLC tracking
○ Breast SBRT
✔ Prostate radiotherapy

Chapter 8

Q1: In an adaptive radiotherapy workflow ultrasound will not provide:

✔ Accurate electron density information
○ Visualisation of soft tissue boundaries
○ Real-time volumetric images for dynamic replanning

Q2: Why is the acquisition of a CT scan prior to each treatment fraction not part of a standard clinical routine?

✔ CT equipment is commonly not available in the radiotherapy room
○ The patient can experience serious discomfort during the scan acquisition
○ It does not provide any clinically relevant information

Q3: In a comparison of uterine visibility on CBCT and ultrasound and ultrasound-CBCT fusion. Mason *et al.* (2019) did not find:

✔ Observers were much more confident when delineating the uterus on CBCT alone

○ Observer concordance in uterine delineation was equal for CBCT and ultrasound

○ Observer concordance in uterine delineation was greatest for ultrasound-CBCT fusion

Chapter 9

Q1: What is NOT an advantage of using robotic ultrasound guidance in radiotherapy?

○ Increase reproducibility of image acquisition and motion compensation

✔ Avoidance of treatment beam angles intersecting with the robot

○ Reduce impact of operator dependency

Q2: What are possible applications of robotic ultrasound probe manipulation?

○ Adapting contact pressure dynamically and positioning remotely during treatment

○ Keeping a constant probe position to cause variable target deformation

✔ Applying much higher probe pressure for better image quality

Q3: What is described by the term 'hand-eye calibration' in the context of robotic ultrasound guidance?

✔ Geometric alignment of the robot with the treatment room and the ultrasound probe

○ Adjustments of the robot joints and force measurements

○ Detection of malfunctioning acoustic elements in the ultrasound probe

Q4: What was the focus of most second-generation robotic platforms?

✔ Use of compliant, force-sensitive systems

○ Reduction of robot complexity

○ Reliance on two-dimensional ultrasound

Q5: What is NOT one of the major sources of error for robotic ultrasound guidance?

○ Misalignment due to erroneous calibration matrices (robot – isocentre / robot – ultrasound)

✔ Positioning inaccuracy of the robot (manufacturer level)

○ Force measurement inaccuracies at low force levels

Chapter 10

Q1: Which of the following statements about machine learning is true?

○ Unsupervised learning approaches are the most commonly used for medical imaging tasks

✔ For supervised learning approaches, the number of training images used can have a large impact on algorithm performance

○ None of the statements above is true

Q2: What type of CNN layer is used to transform the image features learned by the algorithm in a segmentation task to the original image resolution?

○ Convolutional layer

○ Pooling layer

✔ Up convolutional or transposed convolutional layer

Q3: Which of the approaches can be applicable to weakly supervised deep learning? (select all correct answers)

✔ A small subset of the available training data is labelled

○ A label is available for every voxel in an US image

✔ The available data labels are different from the expected output labels

Q4: Complete the following sentence with one (or more) of the statements below: 'The deep learning algorithms tested for USgRT applications…'

○ always showed a better performance compared to traditional (non-machine learning) image processing techniques

✔ showed promising results, but there is room for improvement and for further exploration of weakly-supervised and unsupervised methods

✔ were mostly based on supervised learning methods

Chapter 11

Q1: How are thermoacoustic emissions produced during pulsed proton therapy delivery?

✔ Upon tissue irradiation, a localised (in space and time) energy deposition, especially pronounced at the Bragg peak, can lead to thermal expansion and related acoustic emissions, with properties depending on the initial beam characteristics (especially energy deposition pattern and time profile)

○ Upon tissue irradiation acoustic waves result from photoacoustic emissions induced by the prompt gamma produced along the beam penetration depth, until the energy drops below threshold for nuclear interaction

○ Thermoacoustic emissions can only be produced by continuous beams of ionising irradiation

Q2: What defines the mean frequency of the ionoacoustic signal originating from the Bragg peak?

○ The ionoacoustic signal frequency depends only on the temporal ion pulse shape

○ The mean signal frequency is independent of the generation mechanism and only determined by the ultrasound detector properties

✔ The ionoacoustic signal mean frequency is mainly defined by the Bragg peak space distribution and partly by the temporal ion pulse shape

Q3: Which kind of ultrasound detector is best suited for sensing acoustic waves generated by therapeutic pulsed proton beams?

○ Standard clinical ultrasonic transducers, which offer a well proven solution of optimal sensitivity and bandwidth for imaging

○ Cardiac or small animal ultrasonic transducers are needed, to offer ultrahigh frequency operation for excellent spatial resolution to accurately resolve the Bragg peak position
✔ Dedicated broadband transducers of high sensitivity and properly chosen central frequency are preferable due to the typically lower frequency range of proton-induced thermoacoustic emissions, compared to clinical ultrasound imaging

www.ingramcontent.com/pod-product-compliance
Ingram Content Group UK Ltd.
Pitfield, Milton Keynes, MK11 3LW, UK
UKHW051855100926
8556IPUK00005B/633

9 780750 3255